INTRODUCTION TO
E M S   Systems

This book is dedicated to my students,
past, present, and future, for it
is in these students that the future
of EMS will be realized.

INTRODUCTION TO
E M S Systems

Bruce J. Walz, PhD, NREMT-P

Associate Professor and Chair
Department of Emergency Health Services
University of Maryland, Baltimore County
Baltimore Maryland

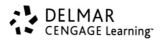
DELMAR
CENGAGE Learning

Australia Canada Mexico Singapore Spain United Kingdom United States

DELMAR
CENGAGE Learning

Introduction to EMS Systems
Bruce J. Walz

Health Care Publishing Director: William
Brottmille

Acquisitions Editor: Marie Linvill

Developmental Editor: Darcy M. Scelsi

Editorial Assistant: Jill Korznat

Executive Marketing Manager: Dawn
F. Gerrain

Channel Manager: Tara Carter

Production Editor: James Zayicek

For product information and technology assistance, contact us at
Cengage Learning Customer & Sales Support, 1-800-354-9706
For permission to use material from this text or product,
submit all requests online at **cengage.com/permissions**
Further permissions questions can be emailed to
permissionrequest@cengage.com

Library of Congress Control Number: 2001028225

ISBN-13: 978-0-7668-1984-9

ISBN-10: 0-7668-1984-1

Delmar
Executive Woods
5 Maxwell Drive
Clifton Park, NY 12065
USA

Cengage Learning is a leading provider of customized learning solutions with
office locations around the globe, including Singapore, the United Kingdom,
Australia, Mexico, Brazil, and Japan. Locate your local office at:
international.cengage.com/region

Cengage Learning products are represented in Canada by
Nelson Education, Ltd.

For your lifelong learning solutions, visit **delmar.cengage.com**
Visit our corporate website at **www.cengage.com**

Printed in the United States of America
2 3 4 5 6   14 13 12 11 10
ED152

Contents

Chapter 6: Medical Oversight   **99**

Chapter 7: Educational Systems   **113**

Preface

One of the courses I enjoy teaching each semester is an introductory course on Emergency Medical Services (EMS) and emergency health services. This course serves not only as the introductory course for emergency health services, but is also an elective for other health-related majors. To present the many aspects of EMS in enough detail for the students to understand, and also make the presentation interesting, is a daunting task. It has been made even more difficult by the lack of a suitable textbook. The only books that presented an overview of EMS systems were written for EMS system medical directors. To remedy this situation, I decided to write my own introductory textbook specifically designed for college students enrolled in an introductory EMS systems class. This book is the result of that effort.

ABOUT THIS BOOK

This book is an introductory textbook designed for use in a survey course on EMS systems at the college level. It is also useful as a general reference on EMS systems for students, field providers, administrators, medical directors, instructors, government officials, and anyone with an interest in learning more about EMS.

The framework for this book is the 14 attributes of an EMS system presented in the *Emergency Medical Services Agenda for the Future (EMS Agenda)*. The *EMS Agenda* is a national consensus document that presents a vision for the continued development of EMS in the United States. I chose the *EMS Agenda* attributes because they reflect a contemporary approach to the delivery of EMS. Most earlier books on EMS systems follow the 15 components of an EMS system outlined in the *EMS Systems Act of 1973*. While these components played a major role in the historical development of EMS in the United States, they are no longer indicative of modern EMS. In addition to following the 14 attributes, I have also taken a historical perspective in my presentation. Modern EMS is now over 30 years old. Each year, more and more of the pioneers of EMS pass on, leaving only their legacy behind. I feel it is important that today's students and providers of EMS have a firm understanding of how modern EMS came to be and the rationale for the many aspects of EMS we take for granted.

It is impossible to write a book that addresses all of the many variations in EMS systems nationwide. In addition to state variations, there are regional, county, local, and even service level variations in how EMS systems are designed and function. Although I have tried whenever possible to provide a generic explanation or example, the reader is cautioned that local practice and protocol might be different. Just because something is done differently does not make it wrong or less effective. Or, the fact that a system the reader may be familiar with does not do something as presented in this book does not make that system less effective or correct. It is my intention for the reader to develop a broader perspective of EMS systems. Likewise, this book is not intended to be comprehensive in nature. It is an overview of EMS systems. A bibliography is provided for readers interested in learning more about a particular topic.

HOW TO USE THIS BOOK

This book is designed to be used within a semester long, college level introductory course on EMS. It is assumed that the reader will have familiarity with, or access to a copy of, the *EMS Agenda* (available at www.nhtsa.gov).

Each chapter begins with a case study. The case study is designed to present a "real life" example of each system attribute. For readers new to EMS or with little experience, the extensive case study in Chapter 1 is designed to provide an overview of an EMS system and highlight each of the 14 attributes. Reference may be made to the case study throughout each chapter to illustrate important concepts.

Because this book is intended for use in an educational setting, objectives are presented for each chapter. These may be used by the course instructor to define or supplement the learning outcomes for the course. The objectives also provide a means for readers to assess their comprehension of the chapter. Students might find it helpful to "answer" each of the objectives after reading the chapter to determine their knowledge and comprehension of the material. Additionally, key terms are presented to identify important words or concepts found throughout the chapter. The key terms appear in bold at first usage in the text. After reading the chapter material, study questions are provided to allow students to assess their understanding of the chapter and to reinforce key ideas.

Appendices are provided to present in-depth information on particular chapter material. Of special note is Appendix A which contains the complete text of the EMS Systems Act of 1973. This federal legislation was the impetus for the development of most state EMS systems and provided the framework for the development of modern EMS.

ABOUT THE AUTHOR

Bruce J. Walz, PhD, NREMT-P, is an associate professor and chair of the Department of Emergency Health Services at the University of Maryland, Baltimore County (UMBC). The department provides undergraduate and graduate education in emergency health services management as well as undergraduate paramedic education. As a professor, he teaches management and clinical courses as well as serving on graduate thesis committees. He has been in the University System of Maryland since 1979, having served with the Maryland Fire and Rescue Institute until 1987 when he joined the faculty of UMBC. He has been department chair since 1994.

Bruce Walz has been involved in many aspects of EMS education and development. Most notably, he served as a group leader for the development of the 1998 National Standard Paramedic Curriculum and the 1999 National Standard Intermediate Curriculum. He is a charter member of the National Association of EMS Educators and served as president in 1998. He is currently on the Board of Directors. Additionally, he serves as a site visitor for the Committee on Accreditation of Educational Programs for the EMS Professions (CoAEMSP) and is on the editorial board of *Prehospital Emergency Care*. He wrote the chapter on education in the National Association of EMS Physician's medical director's handbook *Prehospital Systems and Medical Oversight*. He has presented at numerous international, national, and regional EMS conferences.

In addition to his professional experience, Bruce Walz has been active in the volunteer fire service since 1970. He has served in many administrative and line positions including president and chief officer. In 1975 he was certified as one of the first 50 Cardiac Rescue Technicians in the State of Maryland. In 1990, he became a nationally registered EMT–Paramedic and is currently licensed in Maryland. He is approved as a Maryland paramedic instructor. He is nationally certified as a Fire Officer IV and Fire Instructor IV.

Bruce Walz received a doctorate from the University of Maryland, College Park, a master's degree from Hood College Graduate School, and a bachelor's degree from Western Maryland College.

ACKNOWLEDGEMENTS

Writing this section is perhaps harder than writing the individual chapters. But I cannot begin any attempt to acknowledge the many people who made this book possible without first acknowledging my parents who set me on the path to professional and personal success.

It would be impossible to list all the individuals in my emergency services career who gave me the knowledge and experience to write this book. But I would like to mention my fellow firefighters and paramedics at the Winfield Community Volunteer Fire Department and the Mount Airy Volunteer Fire Company. There are no finer individuals with whom to serve. And I would like to acknowledge all of my peers and students in Carroll County, Maryland.

Perhaps the group that has suffered the most from my writing this book is the faculty and staff of the Department of Emergency Health Services at UMBC. They have had to endure my "working at home" days and lack of attention to departmental matters as I wrote this book while still serving as chair and maintaining a teaching load. Without their understanding, assistance, and guidance this project would never have been possible. I especially want to thank William Hathaway, Instructor Emeritus, for the foundation work he did related to our introductory course and the personal historical perspective he provided. I also want to thank Dwight Polk for his continued encouragement and experience in the publishing arena. Thanks also go to Stephen Dean for his assistance with the human resources and transportation chapters. But most of all, I want to thank LeVora Perry, my administrative assistant. She not only helped with the typing and preparation of chapters, but she also "ran interference" and handled departmental matters to provide me with the time necessary to complete this book.

I would like to thank Daniel Storer for agreeing to write the foreword. Dr. Storer is one of the true gentlemen of EMS.

And finally, I want to thank Lynn Borders Caldwell for starting me on the road to publication. And from Delmar, Darcy Scelsi and Doris Smith for their never-ending "encouragement" to finish the book on time.

CONTRIBUTORS

William Hathaway, MS
Instructor Emeritus
Department of Emergency Health Services
University of Maryland, Baltimore County

Brian Maguire, MSA, EMT-P
Associate Graduate Program Director
Department of Emergency Health Services
University of Maryland, Baltimore County

Jeffrey Mitchell, PhD, CTS
Clinical Associate Professor
Department of Emergency Health Services
University of Maryland, Baltimore County and
President, International Critical Incident Stress Foundation

Roger Stone, MD, MS, FACEP, FAAEM
Adjunct Assistant Professor
Department of Emergency Health Services
University of Maryland, Baltimore County
Clinical Assistant Professor, Emergency Medicine
University of Maryland School of Medicine
EMS Medical Director, Montgomery & Caroline Counties in Maryland and
Associate EMS Medical Director, Carroll County in Maryland

Kevin Seaman, MD, FACEP
Medical Director and
Clinical Assistant Professor
Department of Emergency Health Services
University of Maryland, Baltimore County and
Medical Director, Howard County, Maryland
MIEMSS Region III Medical Director

Matthew J. Levy, BS, NREMT-P
Department of Emergency Health Services
University of Maryland, Baltimore County

Jennifer Lee Jenkins, MS
George Washington University
School of Medicine and Health Sciences

Mic Gunderson
President
Institute for Prehospital Medicine/Mobile Healthcare Forum and
Lecturer, Department of Emergency Health Services
University of Maryland, Baltimore County

REVIEWERS

I would like to thank all of those who contributed their expertise in reviewing the manuscript.

Regina M. Twisdale, AS, MICP
Camden County College
Gibbsboro, New Jersey

Michael E. Carroll, EMT-P
United Ambulance Service
Lewiston, Maine

John Steven Molnar, NREMT-P
Meridia Health System
Euclid, Ohio

Bobby Baker, BS, NREMT-P
Ivy Tech State College
Evansville, Indiana

Thomas J. Rahilly, PhD, EMT-CC
Nassau County EMS Academy
Plainview, New York

Rebecca Hill, LPN
DeKalb Technical College
Clarkston, Georgia

William Raynovich, EdD, (abd), MPH, BS
University of New Mexico
Albuquerque, New Mexico

Donna Ferracone, RN, MA, BA
Grafton Hills College
Redlands, California

Dave Sarazin, Med, NREMT-P
Lake Superior College
Duluth, Minnesota

Terry DeVito, RN, Med. EMT-P, CEN
Capital Community Technical College
Enfield, Connecticut

Gloria Bizjak
Maryland Fire and Rescue Institute
University of Maryland
Berwyn Heights, Maryland

Kevin L. Hendrickson, CCEMT-P, NREMT-P, NAEMD
Ivy Tech State College
Evansville, Indiana

Keith Holtermann, RN, REMT-P, MBA, DrPH(c)
The George Washington University
Washington, DC

Foreword

It is an honor and a pleasure to contribute to this textbook. This book is an excellent example of a growing testimony that EMS providers are professional and not just technicians. The intended use for this text is as an introductory textbook for use in a survey course on EMS systems at the college level. However, this text will serve as an excellent introduction for anyone interested in a better understanding of EMS systems. The "case study " approach used in this text helps the reader understand the application of the principles expressed and helps the reader become involved as the information unfolds. This text will be useful to EMS administrators, EMS medical directors, EMS educators, and anyone searching for a reference to explain EMS and how its systems are structured. The text is clearly stated and organized in an easy to use manner. Currently there are no other texts written specifically for this purpose.

In addition to being unique in its intended use, the text's content follows the recommendations of the *EMS Agenda for the Future*. The *EMS Agenda for the Future* is a consensus document published in 1996 to reflect the current vision for the future of EMS in this country. The *Agenda* addresses 14 attributes of EMS, including EMS education. This book follows the vision of the 1996 *EMS Agenda for the Future*.

The author, Bruce J. Walz, PhD, NREMT-P, is an Associate Professor and Chair of the Department of Emergency health Services at the University of Maryland , Baltimore County (UMBC). Dr. Walz has long been a recognized EMS education leader, dedicated to excellence in education and the promotion of EMS providers as professionals. He is a charter member of the National Association of EMS Educators and served as the organization's president in 1998. During a visit to UMBC, I observed a class of Emergency Health Services students learning how to evaluate articles from the medical literature for significance. Research is emphasized both in Dr. Walz's EMS educational program and his textbook. Research is important to every academic program. This textbook and the achievements of the author, are examples of how EMS education is being elevated to new educational and professional heights.

I recommend this textbook to anyone searching for a better understanding EMS and its systems, whether they are new to EMS or seasoned EMS administrators, educators, and providers.

Daniel L. Storer, MD
Adjunct Professor, Department of Emergency Medicine.
University of Cincinnati College of Medicine

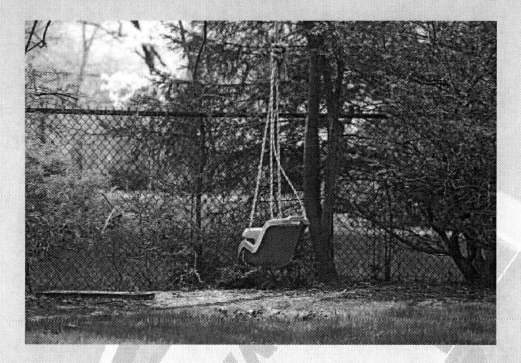

Case Study

A mother takes her five-year-old daughter outside to play on the family swing set. The little girl is the youngest of four children and the swing has been in the backyard for sometime. The mother absentmindedly pushes the little girl who keeps asking to "go higher, go higher." Suddenly, a rope breaks, stressed by many years of use and exposure to the weather. The little girl is propelled forward and flies through the air. She lands in a tumble on the hard ground and remains motionless. The panic-stricken mother cries out, "My baby, my baby!" The next-door neighbor, who is working in his garden, looks up and sees the crumpled little body lying on the lawn. He immediately runs over to help. The sobbing mother kneels by her daughter and turns her onto her back. The little girl has abrasions on her face and arms, her right leg is angulated outward, and she is listless. The neighbor arrives and remarks that she seems to be breathing. He then tells the mother that he is going to call 911 and rushes back to his house.

At the local fire station, approximately a mile from the scene of the accident, the crew is finishing their morning checkouts. Three miles away at the intersection of two major cross streets, a paramedic unit of the local ambulance company is staged according to a systems status management plan.

The local 911 center receives the neighbor's call for help. The center has an enhanced 911 computer system that displays the caller's address and phone number. The call taker confirms that the incident is at the residence

(continues)

CHAPTER 1

Introduction to Emergency Medical Systems

Outline

next door, asks the neighbor to remain on the line, and transfers the call to the ambulance company dispatcher and the fire board. Simultaneously, the local engine company and the staged ambulance begin their response to the little girl's home. The 911 dispatcher asks the caller to remain on the phone and to return to the incident scene, if possible. The neighbor responds that he is on a portable phone. As he runs back to the scene, the dispatcher begins to interrogate him to determine the child's condition. After accomplishing this, she gives him prearrival first aid instructions, which the neighbor relays to the frantic mother.

The engine crew, consisting of four personnel, two of whom are trained as emergency medical technicians–basic (EMT-B) and the other two as first responders, arrive on the scene. The EMT-Bs stabilize the little girl's head and neck, check for an open airway, and assess her pulse. Oxygen is applied and the child's right leg is stabilized. One of the firefighters comforts the mother and obtains information about what happened as well as pertinent information about the little girl.

The ambulance arrives and the paramedic assesses the child. She determines that the girl has a closed head injury as well as a fractured right femur. She contacts her dispatch center and requests a helicopter for evacuation to a pediatric trauma center located 57 miles away. While waiting for the helicopter, the paramedic intubates the child and establishes an interosseous infusion in the uninjured leg. The child is fully immobilized on a pediatric spine board and loaded into the ambulance. The engine company responds to the local high school athletic field to establish a landing zone for the helicopter. The ambulance arrives and awaits the helicopter, which has a 15 minute estimated time of arrival. The paramedic is patched through by radio to the pediatric trauma center and updates the attending physician on the child's status; she remains stable.

The helicopter, staffed by a team of two critical care flight paramedics, arrives and the little girl and her mother are placed on board. The ambulance paramedic transfers her findings to the flight crew. The helicopter lifts off and is on its way to the trauma center. A flight paramedic relays information to the medical staff via medical communications radio. Upon landing, a physician and nurse anesthetist meet the helicopter on the landing pad. The team rapidly moves the patient to the resuscitation area. A social worker greets the overwhelmed mother and escorts her to a quiet area.

The little girl is quickly surrounded by a team of health care providers, all working in controlled chaos under the direction of a pediatric traumatologist. The child is assessed, blood is drawn for analysis, and the little patient

(continues)

is sent for a CAT scan. The traumatologist receives the lab results, CAT scan report, and x-rays. He determines that the child has a small epidural hematoma, a transverse fracture of the right humerus, and two fractured right ribs. The senior resident advises that the little girl is starting to come around and resist the endotracheal tube. The attending advises the resident to sedate her so as not to increase intracranial pressure. She is moved to the ICU and an orthopedic specialist is called to manage her fractured femur. The traumatologist visits with the mother and father, who has recently arrived, and informs them that their daughter should be all right. She will be kept sedated for a few days. The bleeding in her head has stopped and surgery is not indicated. The leg will be cast and the ribs will not need any special treatment. After visiting with the parents, the traumatologist returns to his office and dictates a report of the incident which will be reviewed by the hospital quality management team with a copy forwarded to the staff epidemiologist.

After transferring the little girl to the helicopter, the ambulance returns to service. The paramedic completes her report and makes a note that this would be a good case to present during bimonthly case reviews. She also makes a mental note to call the pediatric trauma center to find out how the girl is doing.

Two days after the incident a graduate student from a nearby university interviews the child's parents. The student informs the parents that he is doing research on pediatric trauma and asks if they would mind answering a few questions. The parents agree and the student adds another case to his research database.

The little girl progresses well and is taken off sedation three days postincident. Her mental functions are good and there is no indication of permanent damage. A social worker continues to assist and support the family. She arranges for the parents to receive instruction in how to manage their daughter's recovery and interaction with her siblings.

One week postincident the child returns home with her leg cast. She is surrounded by her siblings and relatives. Life in the family returns to near normalcy. The mother returns with the little girl to the trauma center on a regular basis for follow-up care and evaluation. The cast is eventually removed and the little girl is sent for physical therapy. Six months later the social worker contacts the parents for a follow-up evaluation. The case of the little girl is finally closed and she again leads a normal life.

Objectives

Upon completion of this chapter, the reader should be able to:

*   State the three main parts of a system.
*   List the 15 components of an EMS system as defined by the EMSS Act of 1973.
*   List additional components necessary for a well-functioning EMS system.
*   List the 14 attributes of an EMS system as presented in the EMS Agenda for the Future.
*   List the seven critical patient groups.
*   Identify the role of an EMS lead agency.

Key Terms

Critical patient areas	EMS Agenda for the Future
Emergency Medical Services Systems Act of 1973	EMS system
	Lead agency

THE EMERGENCY MEDICAL SERVICES SYSTEM

This scenario describes a typical incident handled by a well-coordinated emergency medical services (EMS) system. The little girl was able to return to a normal life because a diverse group of components came together in an orderly fashion to assist her. This coordinated effort is known as an **EMS system**.

In order to understand an EMS system, you must first understand what makes up the system. In the classic sense, a system has three major components—input, process, and output. Input is what enters the system and is affected by it. The input is processed or changed in some way by the system with the resulting product being the output. The transformation process is sometimes referred to as a "black box," a term derived from the many complicated electronic components of early missile systems. Field soldiers may not have understood what each component of a weapons system did within the box; just that it worked in some particular way to produce a particular outcome.

There are many different types of systems. Some can be open, meaning that they interact with the environment, others are closed. Systems can also be described as man-made or natural, concrete such as the circulatory system, or abstract as in the social system. Systems can also be simple or complex. Complex systems are made up of a series of subsystems.

This case study illustrates the concept of a system. The input was the injured child. The process was the response, her treatment, and rehabilitation. The output was a healthy child able to live a normal and productive life. This system, known as an EMS system, is not a simple one; it is very complex and consists of a number of components and subsystems.

Components of an EMS System

The components of an EMS system were originally specified in the **Emergency Medical Services Systems (EMSS) Act of 1973** (see Chapter 3), which was passed as Public Law 93-154 by the United States Congress. This law defined an EMS system and provided funding for systems that met these requirements. The components, as specified in this legislation, are outlined in Figure 1-1.

The law defines an EMS system as follows:

> The term "emergency medical services system," which provides for the arrangement of personnel, facilities, and equipment for the effective and coordinated delivery in an appropriate geographical area of health care services under emergency conditions (occurring either as the result of the patient's condition or of a natural disaster or similar situations) and which is administered by a public or nonprofit private entity which has the authority and the resources to provide effective administration of the system.

Communications

Manpower

Training of Personnel

Use of Public Safety Agencies

Transportation

Mutual Aid Agreements

Facilities

Accessibility of Care

Critical Care Units

Transfer of Patients

Standard Medical Record Keeping

Independent Review and Evaluation

Consumer Information and Education

Consumer Participation

Disaster Linkage

Figure 1-1 Components of an EMS System

The fifteen components were delineated as a means to assist local planners and administrators in the establishment of EMS systems and as benchmarks for the evaluation of existing programs.

Communications One of the first components of the EMS system to be activated was the 911 system. Through this component, all of the other components are notified and made available to the patient. In addition, the various prehospital responders are able to communicate with one another and with medical control. Communication is a major component of any EMS system.

Manpower Trained personnel respond to the call for help. These included firefighters, EMT-Basics, EMT-Intermediates, paramedics, nurses, physicians, and other allied health personnel. An EMS system cannot function effectively without adequate personnel.

Training of Personnel Regardless of the title of the personnel responding, they will be of little or no use if they are not trained. Thus all personnel who interact with the little girl have received some degree of training with many being certified or licensed at a particular provider level.

Use of Public Safety Agencies The close cooperation of the fire department and ambulance company exemplifies the use of public safety agencies in the provision of emergency care. Cooperation with police agencies is also part of public safety involvement.

Transportation Realizing the nature of the little girl's injuries, the paramedic arranged for medical evacuation via helicopter. Transportation of patients to the proper source of care is central to the functioning of an EMS system. As in this case, multiple agencies—private ambulance, fire department, and helicopter service—worked together as a seamless team to transport the child.

Mutual Aid Agreements The seamless interaction of the fire department, private ambulance company, and helicopter service was accomplished through mutual aid agreements. Such agreements allow agencies to share resources across and within jurisdictional boundaries.

Facilities The paramedic's transport decision illustrates the need for prioritization and categorization of treatment facilities. She realized that the patient needed to be transported to a specialty center and not to the local emergency department. Thus facilities and their categorization are another important aspect of the EMS system.

Accessibility of Care Upon arrival at the trauma center, the staff, without regard for her parent's ability to pay for the service, immediately cared for the injured child. The universal provision of emergency care, regardless of ability to pay, is part of the accessibility of care system component.

Critical Care Units After being resuscitated and stabilized in the trauma center's admitting area, the little girl was transferred to a critical care unit, also part of this complex system.

Transfer of Patients Once recovered, the child was transferred to a rehabilitation unit and finally home to her family with referral to a local rehabilitation service. The ability to move patients through the system from one service to another is an example of the transfer of patients component.

Standard Medical Record Keeping Both the paramedic and the traumatologist completed reports on the incident. These are only two examples of the types of standard medical record keeping that occurred as a result of this incident.

Independent Review and Evaluation The standard medical records will be reviewed by various personnel and researchers as a basis for an independent review and evaluation of the system. Additionally, the work of system researchers, such as the graduate student who interviewed the family, will provide a research basis for system review and evaluation.

Consumer Information and Education This complex system would not have functioned if the neighbor had not known to call 911 for help. Through a series of advertisements in the local newspaper, citizens were introduced to the local 911 system and taught how to activate it in an emergency. This consumer information and education activity helped to ensure that a vital component of the EMS system, namely the public, was ready to function as part of the system.

Consumer Participation A member of the regional EMS advisory council, providing consumer participation in the local EMS system, suggested the idea for the local 911 promotion, which allowed the EMS system to effectively respond to a call for help.

Disaster Linkage This example involved only one injured victim, but some incidents involve multiple injuries or even mass casualties. The EMS system is prepared to respond to all types of emergencies.

Revision of the 15 Components

Since 1973, the 15 components have remained a vital part of any EMS system. However, other necessary components have been identified that must be considered in the functioning of contemporary EMS systems. These components include medical direction, system financing, regulation and policy, and trauma systems.

Medical Direction EMS involves the practice of medicine, but there is no mention in the 15 components of physician involvement in the development or delivery of EMS. Thus many EMS systems were developed without direct physician involvement or oversight. As emergency medicine developed as a specialty, the role of the emergency medicine physician in the EMS system became ambiguous. Mechanisms for ensuring quality, which must have physician involvement, were slow to develop.

System Finance Federal funds were available for the initial development of EMS systems. However, the need to plan for and integrate long-term funding resources for

EMS systems was not delineated. Consequently, as federal funds for EMS dried up, many systems were left without a dedicated means of support. Likewise, changes to insurance and Medicare reimbursement schedules were not made to allow for system reimbursement for EMS services.

Regulation and Policy The EMSS Act of 1973 contained specific requirements for the development of an EMS system using federal funds. The act encouraged the development of an EMS lead agency and the necessary authority for the EMS system to function. However, with the demise of federal funding, many states did not have regulations or legislation in place to effectively administer an EMS system. As EMS systems developed and became more complex, laws and regulations to control and regulate the system became more of a necessity. This was especially true as new players, such as commercial providers and public trusts, entered the field of EMS.

Trauma Systems Although trauma resulting from auto crashes was one of the major forces behind the development of EMS, the initial 15 components did not specifically address the concept of a regional or statewide trauma system. Facilities and critical care units addressed part of the trauma system, but there was no total, coordinated approach. Problems in trauma care came to the forefront with the passage of the Trauma Care Systems Planning and Development Act of 1990.

EMS AGENDA FOR THE FUTURE

The traditional 15 components have served EMS well for 30 years. However, as the nature of health care delivery changed, especially in areas related to technology and cost containment, the components of an EMS system needed to be redefined. This redefinition is presented in the **EMS Agenda for the Future**. Supported by the National Highway Traffic Safety Administration and the Health Resources and Services Administration, Maternal and Child Health Bureau, the Agenda puts forth a vision for out-of-facility EMS:

> EMS of the future will be community-based health management that is fully integrated with the overall health care system. It will have the ability to identify and modify illness and injury risks, provide acute illness and injury care and follow-up, and contribute to treatment of chronic conditions and community health monitoring. EMS will be integrated with other health care providers and public health and public safety agencies. It will improve community health and result in more appropriate use of acute health care resources. EMS will remain the public's emergency medical safety net.

The 14 Attributes of an EMS System

Similar to the 15 components, the emergency medical services attributes presented in the Agenda define a modern EMS system. The 14 attributes are listed in Figure 1-2. Each chapter will discuss these attributes with more depth.

Integration of Health Services
EMS Research
Legislation and Regulation
System Finance
Human Resources
Medical Direction
Education Systems
Public Education
Prevention
Public Access
Communication Systems
Clinical Care
Information Systems
Evaluation

Figure 1-2 Attributes of an EMS System

Integration of Health Services Historically, EMS has been viewed as a public safety function. However, the focus of EMS has changed to that of a provider of urgent out-of-facility medical care. EMS is becoming recognized as a legitimate component of the overall health care system.

EMS Research Early EMS practice was based on conjecture and "best guesses." Research is needed in EMS to provide a scientific basis for how EMS are delivered and practiced. Research provides a basis for continued improvement of the system.

Legislation and Regulation To be effective and receive the necessary resources to function, EMS must be recognized as an official and regulated activity of government. This can only occur if the proper legislation and resulting regulations are in place.

System Finance Many EMS systems were established through the EMSS Act of 1973 and supported by federal funding. When federal funding was phased out, systems had to rely on other funding sources to survive. Additionally, insurance and Medicare funding have not met the needs of EMS systems. A secure funding source is necessary for the continued development of EMS systems.

Human Resources This attribute is a modernization of the original components of manpower, training, and public safety involvement.

Medical Direction EMS now involves the practice of medicine, but early EMS systems were developed without a requirement for physician input or oversight. The addition of this attribute recognizes the role of the physician in patient care and in the medical oversight of EMS operations.

Education Systems This attribute expands on the original training component. Education is recognized as an ongoing need of EMS providers as well as a necessity for the professional growth of EMS.

Public Education The original components of consumer education and involvement addressed the need to not only make the public aware of EMS, but also to have input from citizens regarding system development and operation. This attribute focuses on the need to educate the public about health concerns.

Prevention The original concept of EMS was as a reactive service to support injured and sick people. Now, the trend is changing to become proactive and to provide opportunity to reduce injury, illness, and death through prevention.

Public Access The idea of universal access to all in need of EMS has been a foundation of EMS system development. This attribute is a carryover of the component of public access.

Communication Systems Communication remains the foundation of all EMS systems. With new technology, communication has the potential to play an even bigger part in the access, delivery, and coordination of EMS.

Clinical Care This attribute focuses on the medical care provided by EMS. It recognizes the need for effective, efficient, and efficacious care by trained professionals during all aspects of emergency care. This attribute differs from the components of facilities and critical care units which focused on hospital-based care.

Information Systems In 1973 when the first EMS systems were being formed, the importance and necessity for information and its management could not have been foreseen. Now, all aspects of life are intimately connected with data and information management. This attribute addresses the importance of data collection, management, and analysis in EMS.

Evaluation No system or service can continue to function without some means of measuring its effectiveness. One of the original components was review and evaluation. This component focused on the overall evaluation of an EMS system. The attribute evaluation not only addresses system outcome measures, but all aspects of EMS system operation, both structural and clinical.

Although defining a modern EMS system, it should be noted that a number of the attributes are similar to the original 15 components. This is because an EMS system needs certain, basic components to function as a system. Two examples of this are human resources, which replaces the component manpower, and communication systems, which provides a broader view of the basic role of communications.

The attributes also recognize the changes in health care management that have occurred over the past years. The first attribute, integration of health services, is designed to ensure that EMS is part of the total health care delivery system. It also acknowledges the possible linkages to other community health resources. The next section of this chapter addresses EMS subsystems. These are combined into the attribute of clinical care.

CRITICAL PATIENT AREAS

The EMSS Act not only outlined the 15 components of a comprehensive regional EMS system, but also identified seven **critical patient areas**. Each of these special patient populations has specific needs that are best met through an established subsystem of the total community EMS system. The seven critical patient groups are:

1. Major accidental trauma
2. Burn injuries
3. Spinal cord injuries
4. Acute coronary care/heart attacks
5. Poisonings
6. High-risk infants and mothers
7. Behavioral and psychiatric emergencies

These patient groups provide unique challenges for system planners and administrators. Each group has special needs and can be viewed as a separate system within the larger scheme of the local EMS system. For instance, much attention in EMS system development has been focused on the trauma patient. Central to the survival of a trauma victim is the need for rapid evacuation to a medical facility capable of providing intensive resuscitative and surgical care. To meet this need, many EMS systems have established specialized trauma centers and helicopter transport components as well as communication systems to ensure that the trauma victim receives the right care, at the right time, and in the right facility. However, such systems cannot be divorced from the total community EMS system. Just as a helicopter can be used to transport a trauma victim from the scene of an accident, it can also be used as part of a community wide coronary care system to provide interfacility transport of cardiac patients to specialty centers. The hallmark of a well-coordinated EMS system is the total integration of all components as well as the flexibility to provide for the special needs of diverse patient populations.

EMS LEAD AGENCY

No EMS system, no matter how sophisticated or complex, can function efficiently without a central point of focus. System planning, implementation, administration, and evaluation must all be coordinated through a central organization. The need for such centralized coordination was recognized in the EMSS Act which required each jurisdiction forming an EMS system to designate a **lead agency** within its public

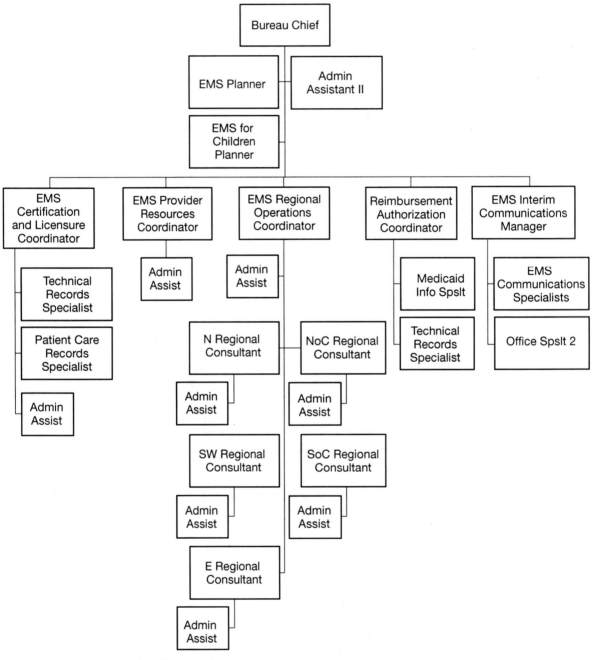

Figure 1-3 Structure of an EMS Agency

health authority. The lead agency would be the focal point for EMS system planning and implementation as well as the official agency for receipt of federal funds and assistance. An example of the organizational structure of a lead agency is shown in Figure 1-3.

Although initially required in the EMSS Act of 1973, with the end of direct federal funding of EMS systems in the 1980s, many state EMS agencies were reduced in size and function. Although all states have a designated state EMS director, they may not have a formal state EMS agency. The range of staffing for state EMS offices runs from four to almost 100 and the functions and authority of the offices varies greatly.

SUMMARY

EMS systems are a complex assemblage of components designed to serve the needs of diverse patient populations. Input into the system in the form of patients in need of emergency or emergent care are processed through a coordinated response and treatment process and emerge as either treated and recovering patients or stabilized for transfer to other parts of the much larger health care system.

Regardless of the nature of the system, a system will not work if it lacks coordination, integration, support, and constant feedback and review. By developing an understanding of EMS systems, the student of EMS will be better prepared to function optimally as a viable component of an EMS system. It is important for the student of EMS to have a working knowledge of the components of a modern EMS system.

STUDY QUESTIONS

1. Draw a diagram of a system and label the three main components.
2. List the 15 original components defined by the EMSS Act of 1973.
3. Compare the 15 components to the 14 attributes of an EMS system.
4. List seven patient groups that need special attention in an EMS system.
5. Identify the EMS lead agency in your state.

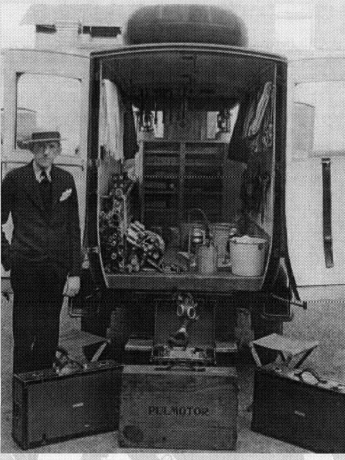

Courtesy of the Julian Stanley Wise Foundation

Case Study

The scene is the storage room of a local rescue squad.

"Hey Mike, look at these old pictures I found," remarks Charlie, a younger member of the squad.

"Look at that old ambulance and the funny uniforms the guys are wearing. How did they ever do EMS like that?" responds Mike.

"Did they even have or call it EMS back then?" asks Charlie.

Mike responds, "I don't know, I guess so, I mean there was always EMS, right?"

CHAPTER 2

History of Emergency Medical Systems

Objectives

Upon completion of this chapter, the reader should be able to:

- Identify significant events and people that have shaped the development of EMS.
- Summarize the history of EMS in the United States.

Key Terms

911 emergency number system

"Accidental Death and Disability: The Neglected Disease of Modern Society"

Alms houses

Basic and Advanced Red Cross First Aid

"The Blueprint"

Cardiopulmonary resuscitation (CPR)

Chain of survival

Defibrillate

Dispensary

Division of Emergency Medical Services

Emergency Medical Services for Children

Emergency Medical Services Systems Act of 1973

Emergency rooms

EMS Council

Evacuation

First responder

Heroic medicine

Hospital Survey and Construction Act

Medevac

Medicaid

Medicare

National Highway Safety Act of 1966

National Highway Traffic Safety Administration

One for Life Program

Rescue Squad

Restorative

Resuscitator runs

Socialized medicine

System status management

The golden hour

Trauma center

Trepanning

White Paper

HISTORY OF EMERGENCY MEDICAL SYSTEMS

A student once commented that "the problem with history is there is so much of it." Volumes have been written concerning both our history and health care in the United States, so writing a single chapter requires a good deal of condensing. This chapter attempts to put the development of EMS systems within the context of our growth as a nation, noting the significant events and developments that have led to our current EMS system.

The basic tenet of EMS is that the patient will be treated by the right people, in the right place, at the right time. In order to accomplish this, three key elements must be in place. First, we must have personnel with the medical knowledge, technology, and facilities necessary to effectively intervene. Second, we must have the communications and transportation equipment and technology in place to ensure that the patient can be treated in a timely manner. Third, we need society's support—conceptually, politically, and financially—in order to mold the first two elements into a system.

PREINDUSTRIAL ERA (1600–1850)

The importance of this era to EMS development is almost negligible, but it is useful to consider, if only to see where we started and to realize how far we have come. During the first 250 years of our history, the United States evolved from a scattering of settlements in the "new world" to a nation poised to fight a bloody civil war. From a few early colonists huddled along the East Coast, the United States had grown to a country of over 23 million, with states and territories spanning from the Atlantic to the

Pacific. During the colonial period and the early years of the republic, 95% of the population was involved in agriculture and, except for the large plantations of the South, these farms were relatively small family endeavors in remote and isolated areas. Several cities developed during this time as mercantile centers engaged in trade with Europe. The Industrial Revolution that had swept through England during this era, however, was only beginning to reach the United States. Transportation and communication were constrained to travel by foot, horse, or watercraft until well into the 1800s. The first practical steam-powered locomotive was not developed until 1825 and Samuel Morse's telegraph was not patented until 1837 (Brunner, 1999).

Early death due to illness and injury was a common occurrence that affected virtually every family. By far, the major cause of death was from infectious diseases. Malaria and respiratory illnesses such as influenza, pneumonia, and tuberculosis routinely afflicted much of the population. With little understanding of public health, the developing towns and cities often lacked a pure water supply and proper sewage treatment, which lead to dysentery, diarrhea, and typhoid. In addition to these endemic or community-based diseases, there were periodic epidemics such as yellow fever, smallpox, and cholera (Rothstein, 1987). Fatalities from the modern scourges of death—heart attack, cancer, and accidents—were minor by comparison.

For treatment and care, the individual was primarily dependent upon his family and a wide range of home remedies. If outside assistance was desired and available it might include physicians, but it might also include Indian doctors, botanical healers, and nostrum dealers whose patent medicines promised to cure a wide range of illnesses.

In England, clear distinctions existed among physicians, surgeons, and pharmacists; in the colonies these distinctions were often blurred, depending on need and training. If a physician was treating an illness he would focus on the outward signs and prescribe interventions. For centuries these interventions were based on the "humoral theory" which explained illness in terms of imbalances in the four humors: blood, phlegm, black bile, and yellow bile. Complementary theories focused on the tone of the blood vessels and nerves as well as on the balance of acids and bases (King, 1997).

In order to adjust these tones and balances, two treatment therapies developed. The first, **evacuation**, sought to rid the body of fluids that disrupted balance and tone. This was accomplished by various methods: drugs to increase urination, sweating, vomiting, and bowel movements; plasters to create blisters; and bleeding blood vessels by cutting, cupping, or leeches. Drugs such as opium were used to calm hyperactivity and an appropriate diet was prescribed. The adage "feed a cold and starve a fever" is clearly traceable to this therapy. There is strong evidence to suggest that George Washington's death was considerably hastened by an overzealous application of bleeding which was then termed **heroic medicine** (Starr, 1982). If the patient survived his illness and treatment, the second therapy, **restorative**, was begun. This regimen consisted of an array of tonics, drugs, and food, as well as cold water and even electrical stimulation. All were applied with the intent of building up and further strengthening the body (King, 1997).

Surgical procedures were equally primitive. Armed with only a basic, and frequently incorrect, notion of how the human body functioned, surgeons had no effective means of controlling pain, visualizing internal injuries, replenishing blood loss, or dealing with infections, which they neither understood nor had the medicines to effectively treat.

A well-trained surgeon would be called upon to lance boils, remove superficial tumors, externally manipulate intestines to reduce hernias, pull teeth, and treat burns. A surgeon could splint fractures and remove bullets, arrows, and splinters, although infection frequently followed. Severe injuries to the head and torso were virtually untreatable although some surgeons would remove a portion of the skull, in a process called **trepanning**, to reduce pressure on the brain (Boyd, Edlich, & Micik 1983).

Severe injuries to the extremities were usually addressed by amputations which were gruesome, but often successful if the dressings were properly tended. With only opium or alcohol available as an anesthetic, the patient was held steady by strong assistants and speed was essential. A skilled surgeon could remove a leg in less than two minutes, but it was not without risk. A well-known British surgeon of the time, who prided himself on his speed, is reported to have amputated his patient's leg and his scrotum as well, inadvertently slashed his assistant, who subsequently died of infection; and caused the death by heart attack of an observer who thought he had also been slashed (Boyd et al., 1983).

Pharmacists fulfilled a major role in health care during this period, providing the drugs prescribed by physicians and surgeons as well as prescribing medicines of their own. By the 1800s, more than two hundred remedies were a regular part of a pharmacist's inventory, providing the means to balance and strengthen the body's systems. Although most of the remedies were of marginal benefit, several are still in use or were found to contain effective ingredients. A favored drug, cinchona, or Peruvian bark, was prescribed as early as the seventeenth century as a cure for fevers, including malaria. In fact, the drug contained quinine which is still used to treat malaria, although it would have been ineffective against other fevers. Ipecac, a drug that was used to induce vomiting and to remove "foul humors" is still used to remove poisons from the stomach. Opium was used in several forms and was effective as a sedative and antidiarrheal agent.

A seriously ill or injured patient during this time period did not have a general hospital to go to for care. Most care was provided in the home with supportive care provided by family members. As towns and cities developed, however, there was a growing need for facilities to care for those who did not have families to rely on. These facilities, called **alms houses** provided care to a broad class of the needy including orphans, the poor, the mentally ill, as well as the sick and injured who did not have family support or could not afford to purchase care. As time went on, this diverse population of the needy was segmented and sent to more specialized facilities. Many of these alms houses would later become general hospitals, as in Maryland where the Baltimore County Alms House became the Baltimore City Hospital (Starr,

1982). Another facility that developed during this time was the city **dispensary**. Several were founded in the late 1700s in major commercial centers such as Philadelphia (1786), New York (1791), Boston (1796), and Baltimore (1800) (Starr, 1982). Dispensaries were similar to alms houses in that they administered to the poor, but unlike alms houses they focused on medical care. Because dispensaries brought together a large group of patients requiring medical care, they became excellent training facilities for medical schools. Over time many of these dispensaries were incorporated as outpatient departments in medical school teaching hospitals.

The medical training of physicians during this era was haphazard and, in fact, formal training was not even required in order to open a practice. A few physicians studied at the universities of Europe, but the majority received their training through apprenticeships or were self-taught. As time went on, medical schools were established at American colleges and universities, and by 1850 there were 42 medical colleges. The majority of these programs were in rural western areas and were generally poor quality with a small, nonsalaried faculty presenting lectures. To obtain a degree, a student was expected to first attend and then repeat lectures, which might include dissection labs, during two four-month sessions over two years (Starr, 1982). Many programs required students to bring their own cadavers, which led to a justifiable distrust of medical institutions by the public, particularly by those people who had just lost a family member. Several of our present medical schools, which had their beginnings in this time period, have interesting histories of townspeople storming the grounds in search of deceased loved ones.

With the proliferation of training programs and the growing numbers of persons presenting themselves as physicians, several state medical societies were temporarily successful in having state licensure laws established in the 1830s, but the concept was unpopular and all such laws were subsequently repealed in this era (Starr, 1982).

One could easily write off the entire era, from an EMS perspective, except for three events: the early efforts to provide resuscitation to victims of sudden death, which led to the establishment of humane societies in the United States; the discovery and use of general anesthesia in surgical operations; and the development and the use of ambulances in the health care field.

Resuscitation

Although there are early records in texts and works of art from different cultures depicting what appear to be attempts at resuscitating victims, for most of our Western history, death was believed to be irreversible except through divine intervention. Galen, an ancient Greek physician (120–210 A.D.) whose writings were regarded as inviolate for centuries, believed that the "furnace of life" was turned on at birth and turned off at death and could not be restarted (Eisenberg, 1957). It wasn't until the Renaissance (fourteenth–sixteenth centuries) that people began to question Galen's teachings of human anatomy and the Enlightenment period (eighteenth century) before physicians and scientists of the day began to actively intervene in cases of sudden death. Still acting on an incomplete understanding of the physiology of the body, a variety of methods were tried to restore breathing, including warming, tickling, suspending the body upside down, compressing the chest in a variety of ways, applying electricity, and blowing air and smoke into the lungs and rectum.

Interestingly, in 1732, a Scottish physician named William Tassach used mouth-to-mouth ventilation to revive a miner overcome by smoke and fumes. The fact that his experience was recorded and the information circulated, has led to the recognition of him as the first physician to use mouth-to-mouth ventilation. Unfortunately, the technique enjoyed only a short period of support; it was later rejected in favor of the bellows and rediscovered some 240 years later (Eisenberg, 1957). Based on several reported successes at resuscitation, in 1767 a group in Amsterdam, responding to the large number of deaths due to drowning, established the Amsterdam Rescue Society. Following their success, similar societies were established in Italy, France, Russia, and England. American physicians who had trained in Europe formed similar rescue societies in Philadelphia (1780), New York (1784), and Boston (1786) (Eisenberg, 1957). Although we would certainly disagree with some of the medical techniques advocated, the idea of preplanning an emergency response, education, and keeping sound statistics is remarkably similar to the EMS systems of today. There was also a strong current of volunteerism in these efforts, in that rescuers normally refused compensation for their efforts.

Anesthesia

The use of general anesthetics in surgery began with Dr. Crawford Long in 1842 who removed a tumor from a patient who was inhaling ether (Brunner, 1999). After a demonstration by Dr. William Morton at the Massachusetts General Hospital in 1846, the use of general anesthesia was quickly adopted and was in general use by both sides during the American Civil War. The advantage was obvious for both the patient and surgeon, and was the first step toward the development of modern surgical procedures.

Transportation

Baron Dominique–Jean Larrey, chief physician in Napoleon's army, is credited with developing the first prehospital transport system in 1792 (Eisenberg, 1957). Using a fast two-wheeled horse-drawn cart, casualties were triaged and treated in the field and then evacuated to aid stations if required. In the United States the concept was known, but it was only after several large Civil War engagements that an organized system of evacuation of the wounded was developed (Figure 2-1).

As the preindustrial era ended, none of the elements necessary to establish an effective EMS system existed or could even be conceived. Medical knowledge and facilities were just beginning to move away from their ancient forms and institutions. Trans-

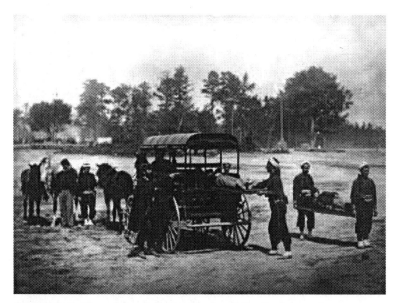

Figure 2-1 The civil war brought about the first use of
ambulances in the United States.
(Courtesy of the Library of Congress, Selected Civil War Photographs,
photo no. LC-B8171-7636.)

portation and communication were slow and based on the same means that had been used for centuries. Health care remained primarily a concern for the individual and his family and focused primarily on alleviating the ravages of infectious diseases.

INDUSTRIAL ERA (1850–1970)

During this 120-year period, our population grew from 23 million to 203 million as a result of natural growth and as succeeding waves of immigrants arrived to seek new lives. Industrialization and innovation brought new products and inventions that fundamentally changed our lives and expectations.

Railroads, automobiles, then aircraft linked even distant locations to within hours and neighboring locations to within minutes. Communication went from the useful, but cumbersome telegraph to telephones, radio, and television, making information and the knowledge of events almost instantaneous.

Large cities developed as our culture moved from an agricultural base to an industrial base. Accompanying this change, municipal, state and federal governments assumed greater responsibility for the health and welfare of the citizenry.

During this era, Americans were called on to fight a succession of major wars and to endure cyclical economic hardships from recessions to depressions. Though painful, each contained lessons that brought about changes in the role of government and health care. Due to a rising standard of living, and improved health care and public health programs, mortality rates dropped significantly. In 1850 life expectancy was 38 years, by 1900 it was 48 years, and by 1970 it had nearly doubled to 71 years.

During this period medical interventions gained credibility and reliance upon physicians and hospitals became routine. Medical science was revolutionized through the development of new technologies and understandings. Following the invention of the stethoscope in 1816, a succession of new tools were developed to assist physicians in evaluating their patients and understanding and treating their illnesses and injuries.

With the use of anesthesia, surgical procedures proliferated. No longer constrained by time because of their patient's pain, physicians tried and perfected new procedures. Antiseptic techniques, which were finally accepted near the end of the nineteenth century, coupled with the discovery of blood types, which allowed the safe transfusion of blood, helped to make many surgical operations routinely successful. The gruesome amputations in the field hospitals of the Civil War were in stark contrast to the modern operating rooms of the 1960s where kidneys, livers, and hearts were changing owners in operations that made front page news.

This era also witnessed the successful organization of American medicine through the creation of the American Medical Association (AMA) which was established in 1846. Though it struggled initially, the AMA became powerful by the turn of the century and was able to establish standards for physicians, medical schools, and hospitals. Hospitals, which had at the beginning of the era functioned chiefly as institutions of last resort for the poor, became integral to the practice of medicine and the training of physicians and nurses. In addition to the overall improvements in medicine, several developments during this time period had a direct bearing on the development of EMS systems.

Causes of Death

One of the more significant events that occurred during this era was the change in the leading causes of death. In 1900 most deaths were caused by pneumonia, influenza, tuberculosis, and diarrhea (Brunner, 1999). As a result of public health measures and medical care that could prevent as well as treat many infectious diseases, by 1970 the leading causes of death were heart disease, cancer, and cerebrovascular disease. In addition, accidents became the leading cause of death for individuals between the ages of 1 and 37 (Brunner, 1999).

First Aid Training

As industrial development continued, and society became more mobile, there was an increasing need for a standardized approach to the delivery of immediate life saving care to the sick and injured. This standardization came in the form of **Basic and**

Advanced Red Cross First Aid. These courses, offered by the American Red Cross, remained the standard for prehospital care well into the 1970s.

Although most people associate first aid care and emergencies with the American Red Cross (ARC), the original mission of the ARC was to provide assistance to victims of war (Pickett, 1923). The American Red Cross was incorporated in 1881 under the leadership of Clara Barton, a nurse who treated soldiers during the Civil War, and developed the concept of "treat them where they lie," did not begin offering first aid training until 1909.

The concept of first aid training, now called **first responder**, developed in the mining towns of Pennsylvania. Because of the hazards associated with coal mining, miners formed first aid clubs to teach each other first aid skills. The early teams received training from members of the St. John's Ambulance Association in England. As more and more teams were formed, first aid contests developed between the teams. Hearing about these first aid clubs, members of the American Red Cross Executive Committee observed a first aid club contest in 1908. In 1909, the ARC Central Committee organized the Red Cross First Aid Bureau. The bureau was managed by Colonel Charles Lynch who was detailed to the ARC from the U.S. Army Medical Corps. In 1910 Colonel Lynch authored the first ARC first aid textbook *Red Cross First Aid,* which remained the standard for ambulance personnel training until the widespread acceptance of emergency medical technician (EMT) training in the late 1970s. See Chapter 7 for additional information on training EMS personnel.

Resuscitator Calls

The 1930s and 1940s saw the development of portable oxygen-powered devices to help revive patients in respiratory arrest (not breathing). These large, heavy, mechanical devices were also used to administer supplemental oxygen to a breathing patient. Familiar brands of these devices were the E&J Resuscitator-Inhalator-Aspirator, MSA Pneolator, and Emerson Resuscitator (Ohio Trade and Industrial Education Service, 1959).

Firefighters during this time period did not have modern self-contained breathing apparatus and canister masks were just coming into use. As a result of this lack of respiratory protection, firefighters were routinely overcome by smoke and the products of combustion. To revive these firefighters, fire departments organized resuscitation squads and special vehicles to respond with an oxygen-powered resuscitator on what were called **resuscitator runs**. These early responses were, for many fire departments, the beginning of their involvement in the provision of EMS.

Motor Vehicle Injuries

America's love affair with the automobile resulted in increased road traffic and inevitably the number of auto accidents, or as they are now referred to auto crashes, began to climb. It was the concern over death and injury from auto crashes that brought the federal government into EMS. In the 1920s, the first uniform traffic codes were established nationwide. The Federal-Aid Highway Act of 1956 provided funding for the development of interstate highways and standards for road design and safety. The Kennedy administration was the first to express concern over the increasing number of citizens killed in traffic crashes. In 1965 a presidential commission published *Health, Medical Care and Transportation of the Injured,* which addressed the treatment and survival of auto crash victims. Perhaps the most significant federal response to highway deaths came in 1966 with passage of the Highway Safety Act of 1966. This act created the **National Highway Traffic Safety Administration** (NHTSA) with an EMS division within the Department of Transportation. The National Traffic and Motor Vehicle Safety Act of 1966 provided for the coordination and financing for states to develop highway safety programs.

Transportation

Horse-drawn ambulances similar to those used by the military in the Civil War began to appear as hospital-based units in the 1860s and became motorized units at the turn of the century. Most units remained hospital-based until World War II limited the manpower available to provide staffing and the responsibility then shifted to other groups (Page, 1978). In cities the responsibility was frequently assumed by existing fire department personnel, whereas in rural areas the service might be provided by volunteers associated with existing volunteer fire departments or newly formed independent units.

In 1928, Julian Stanley Wise founded the Roanoke (Virginia) Life Saving and First Aid Squad. This was the first volunteer **rescue squad** in the United States. Similar units developed in New Jersey. Some were spin-offs from fire departments; others were independently formed units.

Several private ambulance services also developed during this time, some providing only routine medical transport and others providing both emergency and routine transport. In many areas of the country the service was assumed by the local funeral home that could, with minor modifications, readily turn a hearse into an ambulance. In 1966, over 50% of the ambulances in the United States were run by funeral directors (Beebe & Funk, 2001). In many communities, the hearse was the only available vehicle capable of transporting a person lying down. Funeral directors were also readily available to respond to emergencies. Hearses could be easily converted to carry a stretcher and a magnetic red light was easily placed on the roof. Even though funeral directors provided a transport vehicle, many had little, if any, training in first aid.

The training of personnel was basic first aid at best and the emphasis was on speed, as in the phrase "scoop and swoop." Because the attendant did not provide much care there was no need for interior working space and the units were usually built along sleek lines that emphasized comfort and style rather than utility. For many attendants they were the grandest vehicles they had ever driven and it was with some resistance that they parted with them when prehospital care techniques made a different configuration imperative. By the end of the 1960s increasing numbers of ambulances were van-type chassis and their attendants had been trained to the Emergency Medical Technician–Ambulance (EMT-A) standards established by the NHTSA.

Military

During this period, the United States military participated in five major conflicts that influenced the development of modern EMS. First was the American Civil War. Battlefield casualties during the Civil War might not be collected for weeks after an engagement and many men died where they had fallen, days after their wounds were received. Through the efforts of the Sanitary Commission and individuals such as Clara Barton, attempts were made to provide relief to wounded soldiers on both sides of the conflict. Attempts by the Union Army to provide for wounded troops resulted in the first use of ambulances in the United States (Beebe & Funk, 2001).

Improvements in medical care and ground transport helped to reduce mortality in World War I and World War II, but many soldiers still died because of delays in proper treatment. World War I saw the introduction of new, more deadly weapons such as the machine gun, tank, and poison gas. World War I was also the first major conflict served by members of the International Red Cross working under the Treaty of Geneva (Pickett, 1923).

During World War II, professional soldiers serving as medics provided immediate care to wounded comrades. Pain control using morphine and fluid replacement with plasma were common practice. However, rapid evacuation of the wounded to surgical field hospitals still was not commonplace in the military.

The Korean Conflict of the 1950s saw the introduction of Mobile Army Surgical Hospitals (MASH) and the rapid evacuation of the wounded using helicopters to MASH and battle area based treatment hospitals. By the time of the Vietnam War, the use of helicopters for the evacuation of the wounded was well established. It is frequently pointed out that because of this system, an injured soldier in Vietnam was far more likely to survive his wounds than his American counterpart who had been in a serious automobile crash back home.

Cardiac Care

Efforts to revive victims of heart attacks and other sudden death occurrences continued in this era, culminating in 1960 in the development of modern **cadiopulmonary resuscitation (CPR)** using mouth-to-mouth ventilation and chest compression. The technique was the result of the combined efforts of doctors and researchers James Elan and Peter Safar, who were investigating the effectiveness of mouth-to-mouth resuscitation at Baltimore City Hospital, and James Jude, Guy Knickerbocker, and William Kouwenhoven, who developed the method of external cardiac massage at Johns Hopkins Hospital. The combined technique was first used successfully in a pre-hospital setting by Baltimore City firemen in 1960 (Eisenberg, 1957).

During this era the importance of ventricular fibrillation in heart attacks was discovered as well as the ability to **defibrillate** the heart using electrical shock. First employed in hospitals using an open-chest technique, electrical defibrillators were later refined to defibrillate without opening the chest and then redesigned to allow portability. In Belfast, Northern Ireland, Dr. Frank Pantridge, along with his resident Dr. John Geddes, developed the first mobile intensive care unit in 1966. Their modified ambulance carried a standard hospital defibrillator that could be moved into a residence and plugged into a wall circuit or operated in the ambulance by using two car batteries (Eisenberg, 1957). Pantridge's idea spread rapidly and several similar programs using physicians and specially equipped ambulances were initiated in the United States. Dr. Eugene Nagel, working with the Miami Fire Department, developed the first unit manned by firefighters trained in the use of defibrillators, the precursors of the paramedics of today.

Government Involvement

Another development that occurred during this era, which was to have important ramifications for the future of EMS, was the increased role of the federal government in funding health care and developing health care policy. Unlike many of the industrialized countries of Europe, the federal government had taken only a very limited role in health care in the United States. During the depression years of the 1930s, the Roosevelt administration had considered developing a national health program, but had dropped their plans when opposition to **socialized medicine** threatened to derail other federal social programs as well.

The first major federal funding for health care occurred in 1946 during the Truman administration with the enactment of the **Hospital Survey and Construction Act**, better known as the Hill-Burton Act. This legislation provided funds and loan guarantees for the construction and renovation of hospital facilities. Although the act did not directly address medical care, provisions within the legislation required participating hospitals to justify their needs through planning and to guarantee that a portion of their service would be provided without charge to the indigent in the community. The legislation was significant in that it marked the first major involvement of the federal government in health care funding.

The next major federal legislation concerning health care came during the Johnson administration (1965) with the enactment of **Medicare** and **Medicaid**. The legislation, which assisted in the funding of health care for the elderly and indigent, rapidly established the federal government as the single largest purchaser of health care and eliminated the detached and peripheral role that the federal government had taken toward health care in the past. Besides increasing the demand for health services for the elderly and the poor, the legislation opened the possibility for the future consideration of other federally supported health care programs.

EMS Development

The first efforts to develop a modern EMS system began to take shape during the 1960s. Concern over increasing deaths from auto crashes led to a presidential investigation. In 1966, the President's Commission on Highway Safety issued its final report, "Health, Medical Care and Transportation of the Injured," which focused on the problem of highway accidents and led to the **National Highway Safety Act of 1966**. This legislation in turn established 18 standards for improving highway safety. Standard 11 of the act specifically addressed emergency medical services. This legislation provided both technical support and funds to improve the prehospital care of accident victims. The legislation was significant because it was the first such federal legislation to specifically address EMS and many of the activities, including standards for ambulances and training, contributed to the future development of EMS systems.

In the same year, 1966, the National Academy of Sciences published **"Accidental Death and Disability: The Neglected Disease of Modern Society"** in which it enumerated the magnitude of the problem of trauma in terms of deaths, disability, and costs. The publication, frequently referred to as the **"White Paper"** made numerous recommendations regarding training, ambulances, communication, hospital care, record keeping, and research.

Attention to, and advancements in, coronary care also lead to numerous advances in the care of out-of-hospital victims of sudden cardiac death. Building on the work of Pantridge, and with the development of CPR and external defibrillation, pilot advanced life support programs were started in various parts of the country. Most significant was the work of Dr. Eugene Nagel with the Miami Fire Department in 1964. Dr. Nagel developed a "portable" field biotelemetry unit and in 1967 Miami Fire Department paramedics began functioning. But the field provision of advanced life support (ALS) was not limited to big city fire departments and hospitals. In 1968 Dr. Ralph Feichter trained 40 volunteers of the Haywood County Rescue Squad in North Carolina to deliver out of hospital coronary care (Page, 1978). This is the first recorded use of volunteers serving as paramedics.

The importance of advanced life support was also recognized by the American Medical Association at their 1967 Chicago Conference and again in 1969 at the Sixth Bethesda Conference of the American College of Cardiology which was titled "Early Care for the Acute Coronary Suspect."

In the late 1960s a pioneering surgeon, Dr. R Adams Cowley, coined the phrase **"the golden hour"** referring to the time a seriously injured patient had to receive definitive care if he were to survive. Emulating the military model, Dr. Cowley used Maryland State Police helicopters with a medically trained trooper to bring accident victims to his shock trauma unit at the University of Maryland Hospital. Although successful, the concept of the use of **trauma centers** and **Medevac** helicopters was not accepted until the late 1970s (Franklin & Doelp, 1980).

The history of training EMS personnel is covered in more detail in Chapter 7. However, it was during the 1960s that the first attempt to revise and standardize training for ambulance attendants occurred. In 1966, the federal Department of Transportation's EMS Division within NHTSA issued a request for proposal (RFP) to develop the basic EMS national standard training curriculum. In 1969, the EMS Committee of the National Academy of Science—National Research Council (NAS/NRC), published "Training of Ambulance Personnel and Others Responsible for Emergency Care of the Sick and Injured at the Scene and During Transport." This document was the first of a series of publications to address the need for specialized training of EMS personnel. It also identified the need to better equip ambulances.

MODERN ERA (1970–PRESENT)

By 1970 we had both the technology and the medical knowledge to develop EMS systems, but only the military on the battlefield had developed an effective response. Whether you lived or died as a result of your accident or heart attack depended very much on luck and where you were at the time.

Most hospitals operated **emergency rooms** as adjuncts to their main operations without full-time directors and staffed with whomever might be available, frequently the least trained of their medical staff. Even many large hospitals closed their operating rooms after 11:00 PM. Patients requiring emergency surgery had to wait until morning. If you were seriously injured and needed the care of a specialist, such as a neurosurgeon, and you were taken to a small community hospital, you might wait there for days or be transferred too late to be saved.

If you had a heart attack your family might watch in horror, not knowing how to summon help or what to do until help arrived. The responding ambulance attendants might know CPR, but you would be very lucky if they could defibrillate. Meanwhile families sat before their television sets watching a television drama called "Emergency" based on the exploits of Los Angeles County Fire Department paramedics. Conceived as entertainment television, "Emergency" introduced the entire country to the concept of EMS and made "paramedic" a household word.

1970s

Several groups and individuals were working for change. The "White Paper" and the Highway Safety Act legislation had a catalytic effect in identifying the problems and engaging professionals to develop solutions. Within the federal Department of Health, Education and Welfare, the **Division of Emergency Medical Services** (DEMS), which had initially been formed to prepare medical services in case of a nuclear attack, became a focal point for change. Working with the American Academy of Orthopaedic Surgeons and the American College of Surgeons, DEMS assisted in organizing several national conferences on EMS (Boyd et al., 1983). At the conclusion of the second national conference held in December 1971, a telegram was sent to President Richard M. Nixon urging him to take action to improve emergency medical services. In his subsequent State of the Union Message in January 1972, President Nixon announced that he was directing the Department of Health, Education and Welfare (DHEW) "to develop new ways of organizing emergency medical services and providing care to accident victims" (Boyd et al., 1983). As a result, in June 1972, DHEW initiated five EMS demonstration projects and two EMS communication programs in states and regions around the country. President Nixon firmly believed that EMS was a state and local responsibility and that the role of the federal government should be limited to technical support and guidance. The demonstration projects were intended to develop various approaches that could be copied, but it would be the responsibility of the states and local areas to adopt and fund their own projects (Boyd et al., 1983).

Congress had other ideas, however. As advocates for improving emergency care had pointed out, a medical breakthrough was not necessary. Improvements could be made immediately, across the nation, if start-up funding was made available. In early 1973 both the House and Senate adopted comprehensive legislation to fund nationwide EMS development. Also included in the bill at the last minute was an amendment to continue the operation of eight U.S. Public Health Service hospitals that the Nixon administration had sought to close. President Nixon objected to both the EMS provision, which he thought inappropriate and excessive, and the continued federal funding of the hospitals. As a result, he vetoed the bill in August 1973 (Boyd et al., 1983). Congress was still committed to the program, however, and after narrowly failing to override the president's veto, it adopted new legislation that did not include any provision for the Public Health Service hospitals. Persuaded that another veto would be overridden, President Nixon signed the **Emergency Medical Services Systems Act of 1973** (PL 93-154) into law on November 16, 1973 (see Chapter 3 for more information and a complete text of the EMS Systems Act of 1973) (Boyd et al., 1983). The law was designed to take a systems approach to EMS through the development of regional programs. It differed from the Highway Safety Act, which had primarily focused on prevention and the prehospital care of accident victims, in that it also addressed hospital care and rehabilitation of an expanded list of emergency medical conditions. Classified as a categorical project grant program, it offered matching funds on a competitive basis to regional EMS organizations that addressed the 15 components of an EMS system across seven emergency medical areas. The components and medical areas, which were illustrated in Chapter 1, are shown in Table 2-1.

Regions were essentially offered five years of funding proceeding from Planning (1 year) to Basic Life Support (2 years) and then Advanced Life Support (2 years). Separate grants were also offered for research. Regional development funds could be used across a broad spectrum of categories including training, equipment, supplies, and

Table 2-1   The Components and Emergency Medical Areas Outlined in the EMS Systems Act of 1973

Component	Emergency Medical Area
Communications	Major Accidental Trauma
Manpower	Burn Injuries
Training of personnel	Spinal Cord Injuries
Use of Public Safety Agencies	Acute Coronary Care/
Transportation	heart attacks
Mutual Aid Agreements	Poisonings
Facilities	High Risk Infants and Mothers
Accessibility of Care	Behavioral and Psychiatric
Critical Care Units	Emergencies
Transfer of Patients	
Standard Medical Record Keeping	
Independent Review and Evaluation	
Consumer Information and Education	
Consumer Participation	
Disaster Linkage	

travel. Regions were encouraged to use Highway Safety Act funds in appropriate categories to augment the EMS funding. Development and expenditures were closely monitored by DEMS, the federal lead agency headed by Dr. David Boyd, as well as the regional HEW offices. These agencies provided technical assistance and encouragement, as well as the grant funding for compliance in following the guidelines.

The original legislation was enacted for three years and was renewed with some modification for two additional three-year terms. However, the last renewal was curtailed by President Ronald Reagan's Omnibus Budget Reconciliation Act of 1981 which effectively ended the program. In all, approximately $300 million had been appropriated for the establishment and improvement of EMS delivery systems (NHTSA, 1996). In retrospect it is clear that the program brought about dramatic and fundamental change in EMS. Early planning by DEMS had envisioned a total funding level of approximately $500 million in order to fully establish a nationwide system (Boyd et al., 1983). We can only speculate as to what further progress could have been made if the program had not ended so abruptly.

Despite the difficulties, the program unquestionably spurred the development of EMS systems on a national basis. By 1981, some 303 EMS regions, covering the entire country, had been established and were taking some actions to improve EMS (Boyd et al., 1983). Every region had an **EMS council** made up of representatives of the major organizations for EMS delivery within their region. Through a series of national meetings sponsored by DEMS, local leaders were able to share their experiences and bring back ideas that had been successful in other regions. The federal program guidelines provided the goals and the monetary incentives to accomplish them. It was up to the regional councils to determine what steps to take to reach these goals. Failure to reach consensus on any specific component, as defined by the federal program guidelines, meant jeopardizing the entire funding so there was strong incentive to reach agreement. A region could not request funds to equip and train paramedics without also taking steps to categorize their hospitals.

The legislation had been passed in Congress with broad support from the medical community but opposition developed as some of the more difficult aspects of development had to be addressed. The designation of specialty referral centers, particularly trauma centers, became one of the major areas of contention. Designating one hospital in an area as the trauma center meant that other hospitals would be bypassed by the seriously injured patient on his way to definitive care. This struck at the heart of local medical pride and was seen as a financial threat to the bypassed hospitals. Opposition to the concept, as well as to the process of designation, grew, resulting in several lawsuits. In other regions the process of designation was delayed or so modified that the requirement had little effect in changing delivery patterns or improving care. An article in Time magazine several years after the program had ended pointed out that only two states had successfully established a statewide trauma system.

Another area of conflict developed between the EMS regions and their state governments. The federal program had deliberately bypassed state health departments in favor of regional organizations. Consequently many in state government felt that the federal program had interfered with state authority and prerogatives, and favored legislation that would give the states greater discretion.

The 1970s also were a time of great expansion for EMS training. In 1971, the first national curriculum for training of Emergency Medical Technician–Ambulance (EMT-A) was adopted. By 1977, a revision of the original EMT-A was needed and approved by NHTSA.

In 1970, the NAS/NRC EMS Committee appointed a task force to examine training of "advanced" EMTs through a proposed 480-hour program. Although advanced life support was being provided by specially trained firefighters and EMTs outside the hospital, the first legal recognition of ALS providers came with passage of the Wedworth–Townsend Paramedic Act by California. This law was the first legal recognition of paramedics and served as model legislation for other states. As more and more local paramedic programs developed, the NHTSA recognized a need for standard training similar to that of the EMT. A contract for the development of a national standard curriculum for the Emergency Medical Technician–Paramedic was developed in 1975. The final curriculum was presented to NHTSA for acceptance in 1976.

1980s

As stated earlier, EMS programs initiated and funded under the EMS Systems Act of 1973 effectively came to an end in 1981 with the enactment of the Omnibus Budget Reconciliation Act of 1981. Funding for the program was combined with other federal preventive health care programs, reduced in total, and then distributed to the states as block grants to be used as they deemed appropriate. Compliance to federal program guidelines was eliminated and the federal lead agency, DEMS, abolished. The legislation was not specifically targeted at EMS, but included a number of federal grant programs that had developed over the years. The action reflected the Reagan administration's concern both for reducing the federal budget and limiting the role of the federal government in what had traditionally been state and local functions.

The budget legislation was particularly serious for EMS because of the dependence that had developed between the federal program and the regional EMS agencies for both funding and leadership. While the regional structure made sense operationally, it lacked the traditional political structure to replace the lost federal funds. As a result, many of the regional offices collapsed as states and local governments decided that they were unable or unwilling to support the regional infrastructure. While much of the development toward an effective system had occurred because of the federal insistence on standards, their efforts had also provided a forum for an exchange of ideas with national EMS leaders and among managers of developing regional programs. Suddenly this national consensus building structure was gone, along with the funding.

A successful federal legislation began almost unnoticed in 1984 when the **Emergency Medical Services for Children** (EMS-C) program was established. The program, which is directed by the Maternal and Child Health Bureau within the Department of Health and Human Services, focuses on the special needs of children in EMS. Funding for the program has continued to grow and now represents the largest federal funding commitment to EMS since the end of the EMSS Act in 1981 (NHTSA, 1996). While its focus is children, many of the projects also benefit EMS in general.

While EMS funding was the first priority, national leadership and consensus building were also important and DOT's NHTSA emerged as the lead federal agency for EMS development. During the EMSS Act period, the agency had been placed in a subordinate role, but the agency has gradually increased both its perspective and its role in EMS development since that time. While direct matching funds for pre-hospital EMS projects have significantly decreased, the agency has sponsored a number of broader projects to encourage the adoption of standards and the strengthening of EMS systems.

The training of EMS providers continued to evolve during the 1980s. The basic training course for EMTs was expanded to 110 hours in 1983. In 1989, NHTSA put out a request for proposal to again revise the basic curriculum. Perhaps the most significant training development of the 1980s was the introduction of EMT-Intermediate (EMT-I). Not all states were able or willing to train all of their EMS personnel to the paramedic level. The EMT-I was seen as a means to provide ALS at a minimum level and with a training schedule more conducive to volunteers and rural providers. In 1980, the National Registry of Emergency Medical Technicians recognized EMT-I. The national acceptance of EMT-I took an approach in reverse to that of the basic and paramedic curriculum. Various local programs were developed that later were recognized by NHTSA. In 1982, NHTSA sponsored a study of EMT-I in conjunction with the National Council of State EMS Training Coordinators. A curriculum was developed in 1983 and approved by NHTSA in 1985.

1990s

In the immediate aftermath of the end of the federal EMS program, there was a general feeling of pessimism and failure, but too much progress had been made for a complete collapse of the system. Standards for training, equipment, and operations, though they were no longer enforced by the federal government, had been incorporated into the day-to-day operations. The concept of a systems approach to EMS was ingrained in the minds of EMS administrators and no one was advocating a return to the presystem status. Several strategies developed at the state and national level as administrators sought to make the best of the new conditions. The first concern was funding and two basic initiatives developed. The first was to develop a mechanism for the states to replace some of the federal funds and the second was to reintroduce federal legislation that would at least support portions of the system.

Many states and local governments began or continued to support EMS development through general tax funds, but several states also enacted special taxes to support EMS. Virginia gained nationwide recognition for its **One for Life Program** which added one dollar to its vehicle registration fee and earmarked the new revenue for EMS development. The program has been copied by several other states at varying levels of taxation. A variation that is used by several states involves adding an extra fine to moving vehicle violations and earmarking these revenues for EMS.

The results of efforts to reintroduce federal EMS legislation have been mixed. A few years after the cessation of the federal EMSS Act, a United States General Accounting Office (GAO) report indicated that while states had in part replaced the federal funding, there were three problematic areas that needed to be addressed: statewide trauma center planning, rural EMS, and completion of the 911 system. With support from several agencies and organizations, including the American Hospital Association which lobbied for funds to reimburse trauma hospitals for uncompensated care, the Trauma Care Systems Planning and Development Act was enacted in 1990. To develop the program, a new organization was created within the federal Department of Health and Human Services (the successor agency to HEW) called the Division of Trauma and EMS (DTEMS). Charged with addressing those areas identified by the GAO, the agency was hampered from the start by delays in funding. When funds were finally appropriated at the level of approximately $5 million per year, they were so paltry that only the state trauma planning portion could be addressed in any detail. Without funding to encourage participation and compliance, the planning effort did little more than create a paper exercise. The half-hearted effort ended with the loss of appropriations and the disbanding of DTEMS in 1995 (EMS Agenda for the Future).

The 1990s were a time of great change for EMS training and education. Changes in the nature of EMS, and the proliferation of state variations in provider training, lead to the convening of the National EMS Training Blueprint Task Force in 1992. The task force identified four levels of EMS provider and standardized the knowledge and skills necessary for each level in their final document "National EMS Education and Practice Blueprint." **The Blueprint** is discussed in more detail in Chapter 7.

Building on the recommendations of the Blueprint Task Force, NHTSA again called for the revision of the EMT curriculum. The resultant national curriculum for basic EMT changed the formal designation of the EMT from EMT-Ambulance (EMT-A) to EMT-Basic (EMT-B). The curriculum also made a fundamental change in the approach used to train EMT-Bs. As a result of the change to EMT-B, the paramedic curriculum was also revised and accepted in 1998.

Perhaps the most significant development of the 1990s was the creation of the EMS Agenda for the Future in 1995 and 1996. This national consensus document recognized the 14 attributes as essential to a well-functioning EMS system. It called for increased emphasis on education and research in EMS as well as integration of EMS into the national health care system. As a result of the "Agenda," the process of developing individual agendas for each of the 14 attributes was begun, with provider education the first area to be addressed. The close of the twentieth century saw EMS leaders, regulators, and educators working together to develop an EMS Education Agenda for the Future.

Twenty-First Century

As EMS moves into the next millennium, it continues to grapple with many of the same issues that have shaped its past. Changes in health care funding and insurance reimbursement remain a major area of concern. Economic changes have had a profound effect on the delivery of EMS by private, for-profit providers, with a number of major consolidators either going out of business or forced to sell off their assets. As a result, fire department based EMS have experienced a resurgence with renewed interest and support from fire service leaders.

Legislatively, there have been few initiatives by the federal government to reinvest in EMS. The most significant legislation is aimed at controlling the practices of health maintenance organizations (HMO) and defining what constitutes a medical emergency.

The role of NHTSA has changed over the past few years as a result of increased cooperation with the EMS-C program administered through the Maternal and Child Health

Bureau of the U.S. Department of Health and Human Services, Public Health Services, Health Resources and Services Administration. Maternal and Child Health and NHTSA signed a memorandum making each full partners in the role of a national lead agency for EMS. The EMS Education Agenda for the Future was accepted by NHTSA and the EMS community in 2000. This document, discussed in more detail in Chapter 7, defines and integrates the process of EMS education.

Other Developments

In addition to the developments cited above, there have been several other significant trends that have affected EMS since 1970. A question often posed today is "What group is best capable of providing prehospital ambulance service?" In the 1970s and early 1980s emergency ambulance service was almost entirely provided either by career municipal services, usually associated with fire departments, or by volunteer units that were also frequently fire department based. Typically, an urban fire department, or in some cases a separate municipal service, would be responsible for the city. The suburbs would be provided care by a combination of career and volunteer services and the remaining rural areas covered by volunteers. Funding for these units was usually provided by general tax support for the career services and by donations and local subsidies to the volunteers. Patients were seldom billed for care or transportation. Private ambulance services provided emergency care in some areas, but federal funding had not been intended for the private sector. Consequently, many of the private providers found they could not meet the new standards for training and equipment and either went out of business or settled for routine transports of subcritical patients. In other areas, private ambulance services were prohibited by local governments from providing emergency care.

Because of the increased costs of training and equipment, by 1985 increasing numbers of both municipal and volunteer organizations began charging patients for services to augment funds already provided. As the practice became more widespread, the role of the private ambulance service provider was reconsidered. Municipal services are inherently reliable but, like most government operations, also inherently inefficient. Because of changing social dynamics volunteer services often lacked the personnel necessary to make a timely response. Based on the concepts of **system status management** developed by Jack Stout, a pioneer in the economics of prehospital care, private ambulance services reentered the emergency care marketplace. Several of these private firms have expanded their operations by buying smaller companies and they represent a viable and competitive alternative to the traditional pattern of prehospital care (see Chapter 5).

Another area that has undergone significant change is the **911 emergency number system**. The 911 concept began in the United States during the Nixon administration primarily as a way of improving police services. Until the EMSS Act of 1973, development had progressed very slowly. However, with the incentive of new federal funds

Table 2-2   EMS Chronology

1797	Napoleon's chief physician implements a prehospital system designed to triage and transport the injured from the field to aid stations
1860s	Civilian ambulance services begin in Cincinnati and New York City
1915	First known air medical transport occurs during the retreat of the Serbian army from Albania
1920s	First volunteer rescue squads organize in Roanoke, Virginia, and along the New Jersey coast
1958	Dr. Peter Safar demonstrates the efficacy of mouth-to-mouth ventilation
1960	Cardiopulmonary resuscitation (CPR) is shown to be efficacious
1966	The National Academy of Sciences, National Research Council, publishes "Accidental Death and Disability: The Neglected Disease of Modern Society"
1966	Highway Safety Act of 1966 establishes the Emergency Medical Services Program in the Department of Transportation
1972	Department of Health, Education and Welfare allocates 16 million dollars to EMS demonstration programs in five states
1973	The Robert Wood Johnson Foundation appropriates 15 million dollars to fund 44 EMS projects in 32 states and Puerto Rico
1973	The Emergency Medical Services Systems (EMSS) Act provides additional federal guidelines and funding for the development of regional EMS systems; the law establishes 15 components of EMS systems
1981	The Omnibus Budget Reconciliation Act consolidates EMS funding into state preventive health and health services block grants, and eliminates funding under the EMSS Act
1984	The EMS for Children program, under the Public Health Act, provides funds for enhancing the EMS system to better serve pediatric patients

Table 2-2　*continued*

1985	National Research Council publishes "Injury in America: A Continuing Public Health Problem" describing deficiencies in the progress of addressing the problem of accidental death and disability
1988	The National Highway Traffic Safety Administration initiates the Statewide EMS Technical Assessment program based on ten key components of EMS systems
1990	The Trauma Care Systems and Development Act encourages development of inclusive trauma systems and provides funding to states for trauma system planning, implementation, and evaluation
1993	The Institute of Medicine publishes Emergency Medical Services for Children which points out deficiencies in our health care system's ability to address the emergency medical needs of pediatric patients
1995	Congress does not reauthorize funding under the Trauma Care Systems and Development Act

Source: National Highway Traffic Safety Administration and Maternal and Child Health Bureau. (1996). Emergency Medical Services Agenda for the Future (DOT HS 808 441). Washington, DC: US Government Printing Office.

from EMS, development increased rapidly and the concept gained national acceptance, even spawning a popular TV series, "Rescue 911."

The rationale for a single, easy-to-remember number to be used in emergencies is obvious, but having a mixed system that works in some areas, but not in others, is both confusing and dangerous. Even though federal funding through EMS development ended, states and local areas have continued to establish and improve their 911 systems. Many states and local governments have enacted legislation to create a special tax on telephone subscribers for 911 development and maintenance. A national survey in 1993 indicated that approximately 75% of the population was covered by 911 (Roush, 1994). As an adjunct to the development of 911, new programs have been developed to train dispatchers and call takers to better recognize medical emergencies and to provide emergency care instructions to callers until help arrives. The concept, which began in the 1980s, is now becoming the standard nationally (Roush, 1994).

CPR has also undergone changes during this period with increased emphasis on the **chain of survival** advocated by the American Heart Association. This concept—early access, early CPR, early defibrillation, and early advanced care—reinforces the importance of early intervention with CPR and defibrillation. Small, automatic defibrillators that require limited training are routinely used by early responding fire and police units and advocates envision a time when such devices will be as commonplace as fire extinguishers in offices, stores, and even homes.

The last development to be considered is not directly concerned with EMS, but represents a major shift in health care policy that could have a major effect on the emergency care system. For years the rising cost of health care has exceeded all other cost increases in our economy. Total cost for health care now accounts for one-seventh of our gross domestic product or approximately one trillion dollars a year. Unsuccessful attempts by the federal government to adequately control health care costs have lead to the growth of managed care organizations in the private sector. Though these organizations have had some success in reducing the rate of increase of health care costs, there is growing concern that emergency patients are not receiving proper care.

Table 2-2 presents an overview of the major events in the history of EMS.

SUMMARY

EMS systems are not a naturally occurring phenomenon. In our mixed market economy they are particularly susceptible to being pulled apart by special interests. As stated at the beginning of this chapter, the basic tenet of EMS is that patients will be treated by the right people, in the right place, and in the right time. Over the last 30 years we have made enormous progress toward this goal and as EMS professionals we must be the educated and vocal advocates to ensure that this trend continues to happen and to improve.

STUDY QUESTIONS

1. List at least two individuals who influenced the development of emergency care in the preindustrial era.
2. Discuss the importance of war in the development of EMS.
3. What is the "white paper" and what effect did it have on the development of modern EMS?
4. Discuss the role of traffic safety in the development of modern EMS.
5. What has the EMS Agenda for the Future contributed to modern EMS?

BIBLIOGRAPHY

Beebe, R. D., & Funk, D. (2001). *Fundamentals of emergency care.* Albany, N.Y.: Delmar Cengage Learning.

Boyd, D. R., Edlich, R. F., & Micik, S. (1983). *Systems approach to emergency medical care*. Norwalk, CT: Appleton-Century-Crofts.

Brunner, G. (Ed.). (1999). *The time almanac*. Boston: Information Please.

Eisenberg, M. S. (1957). *Life in the balance*. New York: Oxford University Press.

Franklin, J., & Doelp, A. (1980). *Sock trauma*. New York: St. Martin's Press.

King, D. (1997). *Sea of words* (2nd ed.). New York: Henry Holt & Co.

National Highway Traffic Safety Administration & Maternal and Child Health Bureau. (1996). *Emergency medical services agenda for the future* (DOT HS 808 441). Washington, DC: U. S. Government Printing Office.

Ohio Trade and Industrial Service. (1959). *Emergency rescue squad manual*. Columbus, OH: The Ohio State University.

Page, J. O. (1978). *Emergency medical services* (2nd ed.). Boston: National Fire Protection Association.

Pickett, S. E. (1923). *The American National Red Cross: its origin, purposes, and service*. New York: The Century Co.

Rothstein, W. G. (1987). *American medical schools and the practice of medicine*. New York: Oxford University Press.

Roush, W. R. (1994). *Principles of EMS systems* (2nd ed.). Dallas, TX: American College of Emergency Physicians.

Starr, P. (1982). *The social transformation of American medicine*. New York: Basic Books.

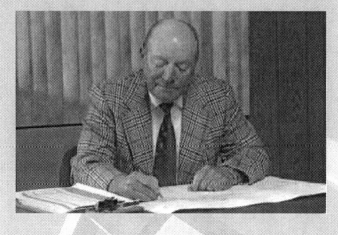

Case Study

The scene is a meeting of the Four County Regional EMS Council.

"We will now have a report from the Legislative Subcommittee. Bill?"

"Thank you, Madam Chair. I only have one piece of proposed legislation to report on. The state EMS office has drafted legislation setting a limit on how old an ambulance can be and still be licensed. At present, the licensing requirements do not include a limit on how old an ambulance can be."

"Bill, what is the proposed limit?" asks another council member.

"Five years based on the model year of the chassis."

"That could cause a problem for some of the smaller 'mom and pop' ambulance services that buy their ambulances used. They may not be able to afford newer models." states another member.

Bill responds, "You have mentioned the main concern that was voiced at the state meeting last week. There was also concern for some of the rural volunteer units that run older ambulances as back-up or second due units. The state rescue squad association is going to meet with the state EMS director to discuss this matter. They want to get this change dropped. If the state won't do that, then they will try to get it changed to require that vehicles over five years old go through the state vehicle inspection program."

"Ok, Bill" says the chair, "Let's move on to the standards committee. Robin?"

CHAPTER 3

Legislation and Regulation

Outline

Objectives

Upon completion of this chapter, the reader should be able to:

- Summarize Public Law 93-154.
- Differentiate between a law, regulation, and consensus standard.
- State the four sources of laws.
- Summarize federal legislation related to EMS.
- Describe how funding is related to legislation.
- Define 1200 money.
- Differentiate between categorical funding and block grants.
- State the purpose of federal regulations related to EMS.
- Define lead agency at both the federal and state level.

- State the role of NHTSA in federal EMS.
- Identify the major components of a state lead EMS agency.
- List the roles and responsibilities of a state lead EMS agency.
- List three areas common to state legislation.

Key Terms

1200 money	COBRA	Constitutional law
402 funds	Code of Federal	Lead agency
Administrative law	Regulations (CFR)	Public law
Block grants	Common law	Statutory law
Categorical funding	Consensus standards	

OVERVIEW OF LEGISLATION AND REGULATION

To fully appreciate the role of legislation and regulation in EMS, it is necessary to have a basic understanding of the governmental process. This basic understanding is necessary for EMS personnel so that they know the laws and regulations related to EMS, as well as how to be involved in the legislative process and influence the passage of such laws.

In simple terms, laws are created by a legislative body, enforced by an executive, and interpreted by the courts. This three-legged approach is central to our democratic form of government. Although most often evident at the federal level, this approach applies to state and local governments as well.

There are four sources of law: constitutional, statutory, common, and administrative. **Constitutional law** is derived from the United States Constitution. Examples of constitutional law include laws related to civil rights, privacy, and due process.

Laws passed by a legislative body become **statutory laws**. These are the laws found in a state's code of laws or on the local level as ordinances. When people think of breaking the law, they usually are referring to a statutory law.

Common law is law derived, in most areas of the United States, from English common law. It is also known as case law. Common law differs from statutory law in that it is not derived from the actions of a legislature, but from judicial precedent. It is applied by the courts based on the social needs of the community, thus it is less rigid and fixed than statutory law. An example of common law applied to EMS would be malpractice. What constitutes malpractice cannot be specifically defined; the standards must be established by judicial action.

The executive branch of government is charged primarily with enforcing laws. However, it may be given the authority to enact laws or regulations that are more specific or complex than those traditionally passed by a legislature. As an example, Congress has passed a law establishing the Occupational Safety and Health Administration (OSHA). It would be too time-consuming and involved for Congress to pass all the regulations needed to ensure occupational safety and health. Therefore, they pass enabling legislation that allows OSHA to make such laws and rules. These laws and regulations are known as **administrative law**. The promulgation of such laws follows an established rule making process. Just like other forms of law, failure to follow administrative law may result in fines, imprisonment, loss of professional status, or loss of the ability to conduct business.

Federal Regulation Process

Once a government agency has been given the authority to make a regulation, the agency must follow an established procedure involving publication of each step in the *Federal Register.* Agencies receive authority to make regulations by federal statute or executive order from the president. A government agency must publish a notice of proposed rulemaking in the *Federal Register.* This lets interested parties know that the agency is in the process of developing rules and regulations. Once the regulation is developed, the draft is published in the *Federal Register.* This step begins a public comment period of 30, 60, or 90 days. Information on how to make comments on the proposed rule as well as receive additional information are also published. At the close of the public comment period, the agency reviews the comments received and either approves the rule as proposed or makes changes as a result of public comments. The notice of final rulemaking ends the process with the publication of the final rule. The agency is required to provide responses to public comments received regardless of whether the comments are incorporated into the final rule.

In addition to formal laws, EMS systems and providers are also affected by standards established by nongovernmental agencies. Professional associations and groups often develop standards and requirements for their members. Trade groups (see Table 3-1) may establish standards for processes or products related to a particular occupation or service. These peer-developed standards are known as **consensus standards**. The process is similar to that used in the development of federal regulations. Usually, a committee of the association develops a draft standard. The draft is circulated among the membership for input and comment. The committee responds to received comments and develops a revised draft. After an established period of time for review, the revised proposed standard is presented to the full membership for ratification. Compliance with the standard is usually voluntary or may be required for continued membership in the group that set the standard. An example of a consensus standard in EMS is the list of minimum essential equipment for ambulances developed by the American College of Surgeons. Although consensus standards do not carry the force

Table 3-1 Trade and Professional Organizations Providing Consensus Standards for EMS

- Ambulance Manufacturers Division of the National Truck Equipment Association
- American College of Emergency Physicians (ACEP)
- Association of Air Medical Services (AAMS)
- ASTM Committee F-30
- Commission for the Accreditation of Air Medical Services (CAAMS)
- Committee on Accreditation of Emergency Medical Services Professions (CoAEMSP)
- National Association of EMS Physicians (NAEMSP)
- National Fire Protection Association (NFPA)

of law, they may be used in court proceedings to establish a standard of care. Therefore, EMS systems and providers should be aware of applicable standards.

It is not enough for EMS providers and administrators to know about laws, regulations, and standards and how they are made. They also need to be aware of proposed legislation and standards that may have a direct effect on them and/or their service. Political action may not be the most desirable activity for EMS personnel, but some degree of political savvy is necessary. Professional associations and trade groups often retain professional lobbyists to represent their interest to government. At the local level, a simple appearance at a town council meeting may be all that is needed to influence the political process.

THE FEDERAL ROLE

Federal involvement in EMS developed through efforts to reduce death and injury from automobile crashes. As early as the 1920s, the Department of Commerce convened the National Conference on Street and Highway Safety which led to the development of uniform traffic codes. However, traffic safety at this time was considered a state responsibility. The Federal-Aid Highway Act of 1956 called for the federal government to investigate means to improve highway safety.

It was not until the presidential election campaign of 1960 that John F. Kennedy observed that "traffic accidents constitute one of the greatest, perhaps the greatest of the nation's public health problems" (Kennedy, 1960). Upon becoming president, Kennedy directed further investigation of traffic safety and accident prevention. Federal investigation identified areas of deficiency as well as recognized that highway safety involved a systems approach. One component of the system so identified was the human element.

In 1965, the President's Commission on Highway Safety published "Health, Medical Care and Transportation of the Injured." This report made recommendations similar to the National Academy of Science/National Research Council report "Accidental Death and Disability—The Neglected Disease of Modern Society." Following the lead begun by the Kennedy administration, President Lyndon Johnson proposed a Traffic Safety Act in his State of the Union Message of 1966. Congress responded by passing the Highway Safety Act of 1966 and the National Traffic and Motor Vehicle Safety Act of 1966. Passage of these bills established a defined federal role in EMS involving coordination and financing for states to develop highway safety programs (see Chapter 2 for more information).

Legislation

The federal role in EMS is grounded in a series of legislative actions. Significant federal legislation related to EMS includes:

- The Highway Safety Act of 1966: Public Law 89-564 established the Emergency Medical Services Program in the Department of Transportation. This act identified highway safety as a public health concern worthy of federal attention.

- The Emergency Medical Services Systems Act of 1973: Public Law 93-154 (Appendix A) established a systems approach to the provision of EMS. The bill called for the establishment of comprehensive and integrated regional EMS systems. The 15 components of an EMS system were defined in the legislation as mandatory components of regional EMS systems. Funding for planning, establishment, expansion, research, and training for EMS systems was provided. This funding provided the start-up funding for many statewide and regional EMS systems across the country.

- The EMSS Act Amendments of 1976: Public Law 94-573 and The EMSS Act Amendments of 1979: Public Law 96-142 provided funding for EMS project grants in feasibility studies and planning, burn treatment, trauma, burn, and poison demonstration projects, and additional funding for training.

- Omnibus Budget Reconciliation Act of 1981: Public Law 97-35 marked the end of funding for EMS as established by the EMSS Act. Instead, funding was consolidated into preventive health and health services **block grants** (lump sums to be used for broad program areas) to the states. In addition to EMS, states had the option of funding programs in health incentives, urban rat control, hypertension, fluoridation, health education risk reduction, and home health care. Thus the level and extent of federal funds going to EMS was now controlled by the states. This shift in funding patterns had a major effect on EMS systems at the state level.

- Trauma Care Systems Training and Development Act of 1990: Public Law 101-590 was an attempt by the original sponsors of the EMSS Act to revitalize federal involvement in EMS. The act was directed toward the development of coordinated trauma systems and improved EMS communications. After moving through various congressional committees, the act was finally passed in 1989. Funding included in the bill was approved for fiscal year 1990–1991. The act established an office within the Health Resources Services Agency (HRSA) of the Department of Health and Human Services. This office was charged with developing model trauma systems and providing grants to state and local agencies to plan comprehensive trauma systems.

Funding

Federal funding for EMS began with the Highway Safety Act of 1966 which provided funding for development of EMS systems as a means to reduce highway fatalities. Section 402 of the act provided matching grants to the states for demonstration projects and studies. In 1972, the Health Services and Mental Health Administration of the Department of Health, Education, and Welfare was directed by the president to support development of five EMS demonstration projects. The projects were designed to develop comprehensive EMS systems. Contracts totaling $16 million were authorized. Passage of the EMSS Act in 1973 provided the most significant level of federal funding for EMS. The cost of the act was estimated to be $500 million. However, between 1974 and 1981, the federal government awarded grants under the act totaling $308,456 million (Boyd, Edlich, and Micik, 1983).

States, regions, and local jurisdictions were able to utilize federal funding for the development of comprehensive EMS systems. The act limited funding to five years and required that at least 25% of each annual appropriation be given to rural areas. To ensure proper development of EMS systems, the act required recipients to utilize the 15 components of an EMS system as outlined in the act. In addition, local matching funding was required. Matching funding means that for each federal dollar provided, the state or region had to provide a dollar of their own funds. This approach ensured that the local recipients were involved and committed to the funded project. In 1974, it was estimated that $1.5 to $1.75 million would be needed to maintain a comprehensive EMS system after federal funding ended (United States General Accounting Office, 1986).

Funding through the EMSS Act and amended versions is often referred to as **1200 money**. This is derived from the various sections of the act:

- Section 1202/1 and 1202/2: Feasibility studies and planning
- Section 1203: Establishment and initial operation
- Section 1204: Expansion and improvement
- Section 1205: Research
- Section 1221: Burn demonstration

- Section 1221: Trauma, burn, and poison demonstration
- Section 776 and 789: Training

Federal funding for EMS continued under the EMSS Act until 1981. Change in the political philosophy concerning the role of government, coupled with a desire to reduce the federal budget deficit, resulted in passage of the Omnibus Budget Reconciliation Act of 1981. This act changed the way the federal government provided funding to states. Primarily the federal government controlled funding under the EMSS Act. Thus states had less direct involvement in the development of EMS systems. The type of funding provided by the EMSS Act is known as **categorical funding**, funding provided to support specific programs or initiatives. The OBRA Act of 1981 changed funding to block grants, which provide lump sums of money to states to address broad programmatic or target areas. The state is given more authority to set priorities and commit funds than under categorical funding.

The OBRA Act of 1981 moved funding for EMS through the "1200 monies" into the Preventive Health and Health Services block grant program of the Department of Health and Human Services (DHHS). The block grant program reduced the federal role in EMS, turning responsibility for funding local EMS over to the states. States were now free to determine the level and use of funds provided for EMS. As a result of this change, initial funding for EMS under the block grants decreased in many states. This reduction was due in part to a lower level of funding by the federal government under the block grants. To overcome this short fall, states used a number of strategies to maintain funding levels. These included using funds remaining from categorical funding programs, transferring funds among block grants, or increasing the use of state funds. Because EMS programs had enjoyed a high level of federal support and control, some states were reluctant to assume this role initially.

As state support for EMS stabilized in the 1980s, significant changes occurred in many state EMS programs. Competition for funding resulted in state EMS lead agencies evolving from planning and development agencies with strong central control into offices supporting a regulatory and technical assistance role. This role change often came about as the result of staff and budget downsizing. In some states, however, alternative funding sources were developed, often tied to vehicle or license registration fees, to maintain funding of a comprehensive statewide EMS system.

Although direct federal funding for EMS was reduced, federal funds were still flowing to the states through highway safety funding administered by NHTSA. This funding source still continues today. Known as **402 funds** these block grants cover six primary areas: EMS, occupant restraints, speed enforcement, drug and alcohol enforcement, traffic records, and highway construction. Given that the states have control over how the block grant money is used, it is easy to see that EMS may not be considered a high priority.

Concerned over the effect of the DHHS block grants created by the Omnibus Budget Reconciliation Act of 1981, two of the original sponsors of the EMSS Act introduced the Trauma Care Systems Training and Development Act of 1990. This legislation authorized grants to states to develop trauma care systems, improve rural trauma systems, and establish a national Advisory Council on Trauma Care Systems. Funding to support 911 service was added in fiscal year 1993. Grants were also to be made available to trauma centers for uncompensated care resulting from drug-related violence and for residency programs in emergency medicine. Although $5 million was appropriated for the act, this amount was insufficient to meet grant demands and funding for uncompensated care was never supported. The provisions of the act were terminated in 1995 and the Division of Trauma and Emergency Medical Systems within the Bureau of Health Resources Development of HRSA was closed. Since this time, there has been no further federal legislative interest in EMS.

COBRA Statute

In addition to passing legislation to provide for the general welfare of the population and the associated funding to support such legislation, the federal government also passes legislation to address specific problems or citizen concerns. An example of such legislative action is what has come to be called **COBRA**. COBRA, also known as the Emergency Medical Treatment and Active Labor Act (EMTALA) or antidumping laws, provides for the necessary stabilization of emergency medical conditions and active labor regardless of the patient's ability to pay. The law derives its name from Section 9121 of the Consolidated Omnibus Budget Reconciliation Act of 1985 which contained the EMTALA legislation. It is a common political practice for senators and representatives to add unrelated amendments to legislative bills in hopes of getting the legislation approved.

COBRA applies to hospitals that have an emergency department. The law requires that the hospital provide initial stabilizing care to all patients regardless of their ability to pay. The law also establishes guidelines for the transfer of patients from one facility to another. The onus for the law came out of the practice by some hospitals of either refusing to treat uninsured patients, or "dumping" them to another facility. Of primary concern to EMS systems are the requirements for an authorized patient transfer. Services providing interfacility and critical care transports come under the scrutiny of the COBRA statute. To provide for the enforcement of COBRA, civil monetary penalties are specified in the statute for both the institution involved and the transferring physician. Depending on the size of the hospital, a fine of up to $50,000 per occurrence and loss of Medicare and Medicaid reimbursement can be imposed on both the hospital and the physician.

Federal Regulations

Federal regulations are laws promulgated by federal agencies. They are contained in the **Code of Federal Regulations (CFR)**. The authority to create regulations is contained in legislation passed by Congress and signed by the president or through a presidential executive order. Regulations address specific areas too detailed or dynamic to be codified in a **public law**. Because of the complexity of some federal regulations, the administrative head of a governmental agency will issue rulings. Rulings are similar to the interpretation of laws by the courts. They provide clarification and interpretation of complex or ambiguous provisions of laws or regulations.

It is beyond the scope of this text to list all of the federal regulations related to EMS. Some regulations apply directly to the delivery of EMS whereas others address the various components of an EMS system such as personnel. Representative federal regulations are presented below.

- 42 CFR 434.30—Contracts with Health Maintenance Organizations (HMOs) and Prepaid Health Plans (PHPs): Contract Requirements, Emergency Medical Services. This regulation defines the nature of contracts to provide emergency medical services with HMOs and PHPs that receive Medicare reimbursement. The regulation is administered by the Health Care Financing Administration (HCFA) of DHHS. The HCFA promulgates many regulations related to Medicare and Medicaid that apply indirectly to EMS because many EMS providers bill for service, especially interfacility transports.

- 42 CFR 489.24—Special Responsibility of Medicare Hospitals in Emergency Cases. This regulation defines the responsibilities of Medicare hospitals (a hospital that bills Medicare for patient services) under 42 USC 1395 dd—Emergency Medical Treatment and Active Labor Act (EMTALA). This regulation defines the requirements for Medicare hospitals under the law and sets fines and penalties for failure to comply with the requirements.

- 42 CFR 493—Laboratory Requirements. The Clinical Laboratory Improvement Amendments of 1988 (CLIA) were enacted to ensure that medical laboratory tests are properly performed. Enforced by HCFA, this regulation applies to the performance of medical laboratory tests in an ambulance, specifically blood glucose testing. The regulations require ambulance services to apply for a waiver to perform glucose testing if using devices approved for home use. If an ambulance service wishes to perform other medical tests, they must have their ambulances licensed as medical laboratories.

- 29 CFR 803—Medical Device Reporting (MDR). A Food and Drug Administration regulation, the MDR procedures require the reporting on any failure of biomedical equipment. If the cardiac monitor on an ambulance fails while in use, the incident must be properly reported to the FDA.

- 29 CFR 1910.1030—Bloodborne Pathogens. A regulation of the Occupational Safety and Health Administration (OSHA), Department of Labor, this section of the Code of Federal Regulations sets forth standards for the safe handling of blood and body fluids as well as requirements for personnel handling such materials.

Federal Lead Agency

At present, there is no single federal agency designated by law to serve as a **lead agency** for EMS in the United States. The National Highway Traffic Safety Administration's (NHTSA) EMS Office is the federal entity most closely filling this role. A lead agency is defined in the EMSS Act of 1973 as:

> The Secretary shall administer the program of grants and contracts authorized by this title through an identifiable administrative unit within the Department of Health, Education, and Welfare. Such unit shall also be responsible for collecting, analyzing, cataloging, and disseminating all data useful in the development and operation of emergency medical services systems, including data derived from reviews and evaluations of emergency medical services systems assisted under Section 1202, 1203, or 1204.

This section of the EMSS Act established the basic parameters of an EMS lead agency. Although functioning at a federal level, the basic tasks of the lead agency are also found within state level agencies. It is the role of the lead agency to gather and analyze data, provide technical assistance, EMS system component coordination, and administer grants. More prevalent at the state level, the lead agency may also be responsible for regulation.

The role of a federal lead EMS agency passed through various divisions and bureaus within DHEW and its successor, DHHS. The role changed as federal legislation related to EMS changed. With the end of categorical funding, a strong federal focus in EMS also ended. Today, the two federal agencies most involved in EMS within DHHS are the Health Care Finance Administration (HCFA) through its administration of the Medicare and Medicaid programs, and the Bureau of Maternal and Child Health within the Health Resources and Services Administration.

The federal agencies currently providing the most visible federal leadership in EMS are NHTSA and the Maternal and Child Health Bureau. Through its EMS Division, NHTSA provides technical assistance and program guidelines for EMS system development and review. It is NHTSA's philosophy that good EMS systems will ultimately improve survival from transportation-related incidents. The Maternal and Child Health Bureau has been instrumental in increasing awareness of the special EMS needs of children. Through a memorandum of understanding, these two federal agencies have agreed to combine efforts to promote EMS development nationwide. All of the recently revised national standard EMS training curriculums were developed with NHTSA and Maternal and Child Health funding and oversight.

THE STATE ROLE

The EMSS Act of 1973 also had a profound effect on EMS at the state level. Not only did the act provide funds to the states through the 1200 grants, but also required the establishment of state lead agencies. Prior to the act, many states had statewide organizations and associations that fostered the interest of rescue squads and ambulance units. However, there was no office at the state level devoted to the coordination and delivery of EMS. Likewise, states often lacked legislation specific to EMS and EMS services.

Charged with improving EMS nationwide, the Division of Emergency Medical Services attempted to establish an identifiable lead agency within the health service of each state. In large metropolitan areas, local lead agencies were also developed. The same was true of more rural areas that came together to form regional EMS systems. A primary incentive for many states and areas to cooperate was the requirement of a lead agency to receive and manage 1200 funds.

Lead agencies sought to bring together providers and consumers to develop a systems approach to EMS delivery. The agency provided coordination, technical expertise, and medical direction. They also administered the 1200 grants at the local level and provided fiscal oversight and management. Additionally, the lead agency was to work with professional groups, public and private agencies, and public safety to coordinate and develop the delivery of EMS.

The original intention of the EMSS Act was to support the development of regional lead agencies as opposed to working with state level health departments. It was thought that regional agencies would be more focused on EMS than specific state agencies. The regional approach also allowed areas with specific or common needs to work together. An example of such a region was Emergency Medical Services Development, Inc. (EMSDI), a nonprofit corporation composed of Baltimore, Maryland, and the five surrounding counties. This region later became Region III within the Maryland EMS system.

The regional and state agencies worked to establish legislation and regulation to accomplish their mission of EMS system coordination and control. In order to establish and develop an EMS system in a state, the lead agency needed the authority and regulatory ability to control system components. In many cases, the new roles given to personnel and system providers required legislative changes or entirely new laws. For the first time, prehospital providers and ambulance services found themselves regulated and licensed by the state.

As federal funding for EMS changed in the 1980s, states suddenly found themselves with functional lead agencies required by law, but with little or no funding support. States either had to make up the lost funds, or scale down the lead agency to fit available budget support. In those states with strong support for EMS, alternative funding sources were developed. Because EMS was tied to highway safety, a few states developed programs that earmarked a portion of vehicle registration or drivers license renewal fees to EMS. One such program was known as "Two for Life" referring to the two dollars passed on for EMS. Without federal 1200 dollars to administer, the roles and responsibilities of the state EMS lead agency changed. The lead agency was seen more as a source of technical assistance to developed and functioning local EMS systems than as a central point for control and funding.

Components of a State Lead Agency

State level EMS lead agencies in general have three major components: a state EMS director, a governing board, and a training and regulatory entity. The state EMS director (SEMSD) serves as the chief operating officer of the state EMS agency. The SEMSD may be appointed by the governor, secretary of health, or public safety director. The director reports either to a higher official or to the state EMS governing board. In most states, the SEMSD is not a physician. The SEMSD is responsible for seeing that EMS-related policy is developed and carried out as well as enforcing laws and regulations passed by the legislature. The National Association of State EMS Directors (NASEMSD) represents the interests of state directors at the national level and provides a forum for networking among the directors. In those states with strong statewide control of EMS, a state EMS medical director (SEMSMD) may assist the SEMSD. The SEMSMD is a physician responsible for coordinating statewide medical direction and quality assurance.

Following on a requirement of the EMSS Act, many states maintain a statewide EMS governing or advisory council. The council brings together representatives of the many attributes of an EMS system. If the council has policy-making authority, it is the body that passes regulations and issues policy statements that are carried out by the SEMSD and the lead agency. The council may work through the governor's office to propose legislation and request funding for EMS. If the role of the council is only advisory, it serves to provide guidance and initiative to the SEMSD. It may review the operation of the state lead agency and make recommendations, but it has no authority to make policy or allocate funds. It may make recommendations to the governor or other authority concerning system operations and legislation. In order to carry out its mission, the state EMS council may work through regional and local EMS councils.

The third common component of a state lead agency is a division or office responsible for regulation. This office is often combined with the training and certification function of the lead agency. The chief operating officer of this division is the state EMS training coordinator (SEMSTC). The SEMSTC is responsible for ensuring that the training and certification of EMS providers follow applicable regulations and laws. Licensing of vehicles, EMS services, and hospitals may also be included in the regulatory domain of this office. State training coordinators are represented by the National Council of State EMS Training Coordinators (NCSEMSTC).

The roles and responsibilities of the state lead agency vary by state. However, the following are common to most states:

- *Allocation of federal and state funding.* Although federal funding for EMS has been greatly reduced, current funding requires administration by the state lead agency. Likewise, state funds and grants for EMS usually flow through the lead agency. The lead agency is responsible for approving requests and fiscal oversight.

- *Certification or licensure of providers.* Approval of training for EMS personnel and authorization to function are handled at the state level. The lead agency sets standards and requirements for training programs and recognition of providers. The lead agency may also provide the certification testing for providers. Quality assurance and disciplinary matters are also addressed.

- *Regulation.* State EMS legislation often gives the lead agency regulatory authority. The agency may regulate ambulance services, flight services, personnel, vehicles, equipment, hospitals, and trauma centers. The regulatory process usually follows established state administrative policies and procedures, including enforcement.

- *Technical assistance.* The lead agency provides technical assistance in a number of areas including grant writing, system development, equipment selection, and vehicle design.

- *Medical direction.* Many states have a minimal statewide medical protocol. This protocol is developed either by a medical advisory committee or by the state medical director. The protocol usually outlines a minimum standard of care that can be augmented at the regional, county, or local level.

- *Legislative liaison.* The lead agency serves as a lobbyist for the EMS community. The lead agency monitors legislative actions, comments on proposed legislation, prepares legislation related to EMS, and informs the EMS community of new legislation that affects EMS operations.

- *Training.* The state agency may be responsible for the approval of EMS training-related activities including training sites, instructors, curriculum, and educational materials. In some states, training sites must be accredited either nationally or by the state.

- *Leadership.* The state agency serves as the focal point for EMS-related activity within the state. As such, the lead agency provides direction and policy related to EMS. This is often accomplished through development of a state EMS plan administered by the state lead agency.

State Legislation

Legislation related to EMS at the state level is as varied as the states themselves. Some states have very specific requirements including licensing of ambulances, personnel, and medical facilities. Others provide only minimal state level oversight. However, three areas of legislation common to all states include Good Samaritan laws, 911 service, and provider authorization.

Good Samaritan laws exist to provide legal relief to individuals who of their own accord stop and render aid at the scene of a medical or trauma emergency. In most cases, the person must do so without compensation and provide care consistent with his level of training. Good Samaritan laws provide coverage from acts that do not constitute gross negligence.

The federal government fostered the development of 911 as the universal access number for emergency assistance nationwide. At the state level, legislation requires local telephone service providers to provide 911 service. Regulation of 911 is accomplished through a statewide "Numbers Board."

With the development of new levels of emergency care providers, the states were forced to change their medical practice acts, especially in regard to advanced life support (ALS) providers. States passed laws and regulations governing the scope of practice, requirements, education, licensing, and relicensing of prehospital providers. Regulation of prehospital providers is one of the key roles of the state EMS lead agency.

SUMMARY

Legislation and regulation are an integral part of EMS. At the federal level, legislation passed by Congress has had a profound effect on the development of EMS nationally. Legislation has served to authorize funding for states to develop EMS systems. In addition to public laws, various agencies within the federal government have regulatory authority over EMS-related activities.

At the state level, EMS lead agencies provide leadership through legislative mandate to coordinate and assist EMS systems. The lead agency accomplishes its mission under the direction of a state director guided by an advisory council. The agency's mission is supported by regulatory authority.

Legislative and regulatory initiatives of the future will be directed toward the integration of EMS into the overall health care system, especially as it relates to the reimbursement of EMS services through federally supported health care programs. Future regulation will seek to improve the quality of the workplace environment and provide for the safety of EMS providers. Emerging regulation is just beginning to address issues related to workplace violence.

STUDY QUESTIONS

1. List the four types of laws and describe each.
2. Explain how consensus standards affect the delivery of EMS.
3. Select one federal legislative act involving EMS and describe its effect on EMS system development and funding.
4. Discuss the importance of the 1200 monies to the development of statewide EMS systems.
5. Define lead agency and cite an example of such an agency at the federal level.

6. List the major components of a state level EMS lead agency.

7. Describe the roles and responsibilities of a state level EMS lead agency.

BIBLIOGRAPHY

Boyd, D. R., Edlich, R. F., & Micik, S. H. (Eds). (1983). *Systems approach to emergency medical care.* Norwalk, CT: Appleton-Century-Crofts.

Kennedy, J. F. (1960). Quotation from campaign speech. In U.S. Department of Health, Education, and Welfare. (1968) *Report of the secretary's advisory committee on traffic safety.* Washington, DC: U.S. Government Printing Office.

United States General Accounting Office. (1986). *Report to Congressional requesters: Health care: States assume leadership role in providing emergency medical services.* (GAO/HRD-86-132). Washington, DC: U.S. Government Printing Office.

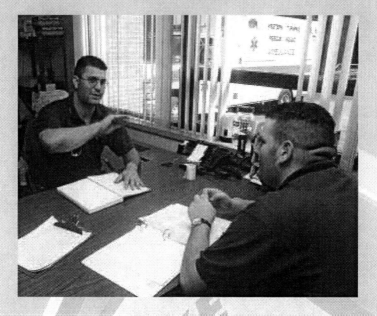

Case Study

The scene is the reception desk at Metro City Ambulance Corporation.

"Hello! How may I help you?" The receptionist asks.

"I'm here about the ambulance attendant job advertised in the Sunday paper," replies the visitor.

"You need to go to HR, down this hallway, second door on the left," advises the receptionist.

"What is HR?" asks the visitor.

"Oh, that's human resources, what they used to call personnel."

"Thank you," the visitor replies and walks down the hallway.

The scene is the office of Frank Church, director of human resources for Metro City Ambulance.

"Hello, my name is Frank Church. I'm the HR director," says Frank as he extends his hand.

"Pleased to meet you. My name is Sabrina Hollingston," says the visitor as she shakes his hand.

"Won't you be seated," the director says as he gestures toward a chair in front of his desk. "I understand you are interested in the EMT position we have open. Is that correct?"

(continues)

CHAPTER 4

Human Resources

Outline

Case Study (continued)

"Well, I'm not sure, I think so. I mean, I'm interested in the ambulance attendant position that was in the paper." Says Sabrina.

"Ms. Hollingston, do you have any experience with ambulance work? Are you familiar with EMS?" asks the director.

"I'm currently working as a medicine aid at Sunshine Eldercare. I've seen a lot of ambulance people coming to get patients and I thought I would enjoy that type of work," she replies.

"I see. Let me give you a little background. EMT stands for emergency medical technician. Actually, the full title is Emergency Medical Technician–Basic. EMTs are certified providers who have completed 120 hours of training to qualify them to provide patient care on an ambulance." Church explains.

"You mean like the paramedics on TV?" asks Sabrina.

"Not exactly." replies the director. "Paramedics are much higher trained providers than EMTs. EMTs handle basic level ambulance calls." he replies.

"Oh, I see." She replies.

"Now then, I can assume you will need to be trained. We, of course, provide our own training courses for our employees. Let's go through your application in case I have any questions."

Frank Church continues with his review of Sabrina's application.

Objectives

Upon completion of this chapter, the reader should be able to:

- Briefly state the historical development of current prehospital provider levels.
- Identify prehospital providers involved in the delivery of EMS.
- Identify hospital-based providers involved in the delivery of EMS.
- List examples of specialized EMS providers.
- State the role of allied health professionals in providing EMS.
- State the role of telecommunicators and emergency medical dispatchers in an EMS system.
- Identify sources of EMS providers.
- Identify two organized labor organizations serving EMS providers.
- State the role of CISM in resolving provider stress.

Key Terms

Career provider
Critical incident
Critical incident stress
 (CIS)
Critical incident
 stress debriefing
 (CISD)
Critical incident stress
 management
 (CISM)
Cumulative stress
Defusing
Demobilization

Emergency Medical
 Dispatch (EMD)
 dispatcher
Emergency Medical
 Technician–Basic
 (EMT-B)
Emergency Medical
 Technician–Intermediate
 (EMT-I)
Emergency Medical
 Technician–Paramedic
 (EMT-P)
First responder

Flight nurse
Flight paramedic
General stress
Intensivist
Post-traumatic stress
 disorder (PTSD)
Telecommunicator
Traumatic stress
Traumatologist
Volunteer
Wilderness medical
 training

HISTORICAL BACKGROUND

Prior to the development of modern EMS in the 1970s, transport vehicles were often staffed with only a driver, and little, if any, care was provided at the scene or during transport. The normal mode of operation was what has come to be known as "swoop and scoop." Services that maintained trained attendants most often utilized American Red Cross Standard and Advanced First Aid as the required training level. As noted in *Accidental Death and Disability: The Neglected Disease of Modern Society:*

> There are no generally accepted standards for the competence or training of ambulance attendants. Attendants range from unschooled apprentices lacking training even in elementary first aid to poorly paid employees, public-spirited volunteers, and specially trained full-time personnel of fire, police, or commercial ambulance companies. Certification and licensure of attendants is a rarity. (National Academy of Sciences, National Research Council, 1966)

Not only were ambulances inadequately staffed, but upon arrival at the hospital, the patient may not have fared any better. Many hospital emergency departments (ED) were little more than receiving areas for seriously injured patients or "charity" patients who lacked the means to visit a family doctor. Known frequently as "accident rooms," the role of the ED had been changing since World War II. A mobile society and the demise of the local family doctor who made house calls resulted in more Americans using the ED as their primary source of health care. Emergency rooms and their staffing are discussed in Chapter 13.

Early EMS system research and legislation identified the need to not only have well-trained and certified ambulance attendants, but also to categorize and accredit emergency departments. Building on the work of Cowley related to trauma systems and Boyd who developed the 15 components, the concept of a system's approach to trauma care developed (see Chapter 2). With the evolution of more sophisticated EDs and trauma centers, the need for specially trained physicians, nurses, and other allied health professionals emerged, leading eventually to current levels of EMS professionals.

PREHOSPITAL PROVIDERS

Today, the standard for ambulance attendants is Emergency Medical Technician–Basic (EMT-B). Advanced care is provided by the EMT-Paramedic. Other provider levels include EMT-Intermediate and first responder. Although defined by a national standard curriculum and practice blueprint (see Chapter 7), regional and state variations have resulted in over 40 different levels of prehospital providers. This chapter will focus on the nationally recognized EMT and first responder.

First Responder

In 1973, the U.S. Department of Transportation (USDOT) recognized the need to develop a basic EMS course for law enforcement officers. Police officers are often the first to arrive at the scene of automobile crashes. Prior to this time, law enforcement personnel were trained in American Red Cross first aid or had no training at all. The course developed by USDOT was called Crash Injury Management for Law Enforcement Officers or CIMFLEO. The course was made available to jurisdictions across the nation through federal grants to training agencies. The CIMFLEO course was 40 hours in length and covered basic airway management, CPR, bleeding control, and shock management. It also contained a module on basic automobile extrication using minimal hand tools.

As the training of law enforcement personnel progressed, the fire service realized a similar need for EMS training for firefighters. Although many fire departments provided EMS, not all department personnel were trained to provide even rudimentary first aid. This was especially true of engine company personnel. If an engine company arrived at the scene of an automobile crash before an ambulance, the crew could do little more than comfort the injured. Rather than require personnel to complete the more extensive EMT-A course that was designed for ambulance personnel, a need for a firefighter first responder course was recognized. This led to the revision of the CIMFLEO course into the Firefighter First Responder (FFFR) curriculum. Realizing that firefighters were not the only first responders, the course evolved into simply First Responder. Now a basic emergency care course was available to personnel such as highway workers, school personnel, camp counselors, the military, and industrial workers.

The **first responder** is described as an individual who is trained to provide initial life saving assessment and intervention utilizing minimal specialized equipment. First responders are trained to assist other EMS providers. In most states, certification as a first responder is for two years, renewable by completing a refresher course.

Emergency Medical Technician–Basic

The **Emergency Medical Technician–Basic**, or EMT-B, is the minimal level of training for ambulance personnel. Originally designated EMT-A for ambulance, EMT certification has evolved from a 72-hour course developed by USDOT into a 110-hour program of basic EMS instruction. The EMT-B is trained to assess the ill or injured patient and provide treatment based on assessment findings. Certification in most states requires completion of a course based on the USDOT EMT–Basic National Standard Curriculum and successful completion of a written and practical examination. Implementation of the *EMS Education Agenda for the Future: A Systems Approach* (see Chapter 7), will move EMT-B training from the auspices of a national standard curriculum to national EMS education standards based on a core content and scope of practice model (see Chapter 7). Some jurisdictions require EMT-Bs to participate in hospital-based clinical training programs. Certification is usually for two years with renewal requiring participation in continuing education activities. Although EMT-B is based on a national standard curriculum, not all EMT-Bs function at the same level. Due to variations across states, some EMT-Bs are able to perform more advanced skills such as endotracheal intubation to secure a patient's airway and field intravenous therapy to treat blood volume loss and establish a means for medication administration.

Emergency Medical Technician–Intermediate

The **Emergency Medical Technician–Intermediate** or EMT-I evolved to fill the gap between the basic EMT-B and the much more advanced EMT–Paramedic. In some areas of the country, especially rural areas, a provider with basic advanced life support skills was needed. Training and maintaining personnel at the paramedic level was not feasible or practical. In other EMS systems, it is more cost effective to have a cadre of EMT-Is supported by a limited number of paramedics. EMT-Is can respond to the majority of advanced life support (ALS) calls such as chest pain and trouble breathing as well as injuries associated with most car crashes. They may establish an airway by endotracheal intubation, defibrillate, interpret electrocardiograms, administer medications, start IVs, and perform chest decompression.

Intermediate training also currently follows a USDOT national standard curriculum, and like EMT-B, will change with the implementation of the *EMS Education Agenda for the Future*. The curriculum is modular, allowing states and jurisdictions to tailor training to local needs. The complete EMT-I course consists of 120 hours of classroom and laboratory instruction. Students must also complete clinical competencies in various hospital settings and through field experience. The total length of an EMT-I training course could reach 250 to 300 hours. Certification is for two years, renewable by participation in continuing education.

Emergency Medical Technician–Paramedic

The **Emergency Medical Technician–Paramedic** is the primary provider of advanced life support. In addition to having the knowledge of an EMT-B, the paramedic processes knowledge of pathophysiology and the disease process. The paramedic can perform a comprehensive physical assessment of the patient using a diagnostic approach. Having assessed the patient, the paramedic can provide treatment using advanced invasive procedures.

Preparation for becoming a paramedic involves between 1,000 and 1,200 hours of classroom and laboratory instruction along with extensive clinical and field experience. Prior to enrolling, the student should have knowledge of basic anatomy and physiology as well as preparation in mathematics, reading, and writing.

Specialized Prehospital Providers

In addition to the traditional first responders and EMTs, there are other prehospital providers trained to provide care to special patient populations. In most cases, these providers are paramedics who have received advanced or special training.

Flight Paramedics and Nurses Recognizing the need to transport severely injured victims promptly to a trauma center, and building on the experience of the military with helicopter medical evacuation, many hospitals and EMS services operate air medical units. Utilizing helicopters for on-scene response, air medical units are typically staffed by either a **flight paramedic** or **flight nurse**, or a combination of a flight paramedic and nurse. Pilots are also specially trained for air medical operations.

Training of flight paramedics and nurses is based on the USDOT *Air Medical Crew National Standard Curriculum* (ASHBEAMS, 1988). For the paramedic, the curriculum defines competencies as follows:

> The Flight Paramedic is a certified EMT-P who possesses all of the knowledge and skills required for EMT-P certification. The minimum entry requirements for a Flight Paramedic is the body of knowledge and skills identified by the required and optional objectives contained in the EMT–Paramedic DOT National Curriculum. Additional knowledge and training exceeding that of a Flight EMT-I is required of the Flight Paramedic, including:
>
> 1.   Endotracheal intubation/ventilation in the airborne environment
> 2.   Application of advanced principles of altitude physiology as it pertains to specific pathologies and patient management during transport.

Competency for the flight nurse is defined as follows:

> The Flight Nurse is a Registered Professional Nurse with a current license in the state of practice. The Flight Nurse possesses all of the knowledge and skills required of a Flight Paramedic, but is not required to be a certified Paramedic. The minimum entry requirement for a Flight Nurse is the body of

Tabe 4-1   Comparison of Provider Levels Based on National Standard Curriculum for Each Provider Level

	Provider		
First Responder	**EMT–Basic**	**EMT–Intermediate**	**EMT–Paramedic**
Training Hours			
40	110	≈250	≈1200
Clinical Field			
None	Optional clinical May include field ride-along on EMS unit	Clinical and Field	Clinical and Field
Prerequisites			
None	CPR	EMT-B	EMT-B Anatomy & physiology
Patient Assessment			
General assessment with vital signs	Complete assessment	History taking Clinical decision making ECG interpretation	Comprehensive and diagnostic based
Airway Management			
Manual maneuvers Pocket mask	Oral airways Oxygen	Oral intubation Combitube or PtL airway	Nasal intubation Surgical airway
Medical			
Initial stabilization AED use	Assessment-based support Assist with patient prescribed medicine administration AED use	Advanced assessment and definitive pharmacological intervention ECG monitoring and electrical therapy	Field diagnosis and advanced pharmacological intervention Increased knowledge base of pathophysiology 12-lead ECG monitoring and cardiac pacing

(continues)

Tabe 4-1   *(continued)*

Provider			
First Responder	**EMT–Basic**	**EMT– Intermediate**	**EMT–Paramedic**
Trauma			
Basic stabilization	Assessment and basic stabilization	Advanced assessment	Advanced assessment
Bleeding control	Bleeding and shock management	Fluid replacement	Increased knowledge base of patho- physiology
Basic shock management	Spinal immobi- lization	Chest decompression	Basic rescue techniques
Limited splinting	Traction splinting		
	Introduction to basic rescue		
Special Considerations			
Childbirth	Pediatrics	Intraosseous fluid replacement	Neonatology
	Geriatrics	Pharmacological interventions in behavioral emergencies	Abuse and assault
	Behavioral emergencies	Geriatrics	Patients with special special challenges
		Neonatal resuscitation	Acute intervention for chronic care patient
		Obstetric emergencies	
Operations			
Integration with EMS System	Introduction to EMS System	Wellness	Wellness
	Wellness	Prevention	Prevention and public education
	Vehicle operations	Research in EMS	Research in EMS
			Medical incident command
			Hazardous materials
			Crime scene awareness

knowledge and skills identified by the objectives in a National League for Nursing (NLN) accredited registered professional nursing program and a current license as a registered nurse (RN) in the state of practice. Additional education and training are as prescribed by the air-medical director.

In addition to the medical knowledge required by the curriculum, air medical crew members receive training in aircraft safety and orientation, communications, rules and regulations, survival, search and rescue, and air medical crew fitness. Crews engaged in interfacility transports may also be trained and certified in critical care transport. Flight crew members also adhere to standards established by professional organizations such as the American Society of Hospital-Based Emergency Air-Medical Services (ASHBEAMS), the National Flight Nurses Association (NFNA), and the National Flight Paramedic Association (NFPA).

Critical Care Transport Specialists The special needs of patients requiring transport between hospitals has led to the development of critical care transport specialists, who are usually paramedics or nurses who have received additional training in critical care topics. Federal legislation known as the "COBRA Law" requires that the level of care being provided a patient be maintained during transport to, and after arrival at, the receiving facility (see Chapters 3 and 13). To comply with the COBRA requirements transport services would utilize a nurse from either the sending or receiving facility to accompany the patient. Although a workable solution, there were many logistical and clinical problems inherent in this approach. Training paramedics and nurses specifically for this role and having them employed by the transport service eliminate many of the problems. Critical care transport is discussed further in Chapter 13.

Wilderness EMT Wilderness medical training was developed to meet the special challenges of extreme environments. The training focuses on extended patient management, extreme environments such as mountains, rural areas, and at sea, and availability of limited equipment. Courses are offered at the basic and advanced life support level and build on the USDOT National Standard Curriculum.

Specialized Response Providers Special response teams exist in a number of fire departments and law enforcement agencies. Medical care for personnel as well as victims is an integral part of their operations. Many teams either require their members to be cross-trained as EMTs or paramedics, or they utilize EMS personnel as part of the team. EMS personnel receive additional training in aspects of emergency care related to the mission of the team. Examples of such specialized personnel include SWAT team, hazardous material, and tactical rescue team EMTs and paramedics. Physicians may also be involved in high-risk mission teams.

HOSPITAL-BASED PROVIDERS

Once a patient arrives at the hospital, the provision of emergency medical care does not stop. It is continued by a team of highly trained medical professionals. In some systems that utilize a hospital-based EMS system (see Chapter 5), the paramedic may continue to provide care while the patient is in the emergency department. If the patient needs advanced care due to severe injury, he may be transferred or taken directly to a trauma center (see Chapter 13) staffed by another group of specialists.

Nurses

Nurses continue to play an important role in the EMS system beyond functioning in an emergency department. They serve in all aspects of EMS. Nurses may function as prehospital providers, ALS providers, critical care transport team members, educators, system coordinators, and flight, trauma, critical care, and pediatric nurses. Nurses were one of the first medical professionals to take an active role in the training of paramedics. Additionally, the broad-based, patient-centered nature of nursing education and practice makes nurses well suited to the many aspects of an EMS system. In the emergency department, nurses are often the first staff member that prehospital providers encounter. They not only provide a link between the field and the hospital, but they can also play a vital role in providing feedback and support to field personnel. In some systems, specially trained nurses are permitted to provide direct medical control to prehospital providers.

In 1970, the Emergency Nurses Association (ENA) was founded to advance emergency nursing practice. The ENA provides education as well as advocacy for the interest of all nurses involved in the delivery of emergency care. Through the *Journal of Emergency Nursing* and educational courses such as Trauma Nursing Core Course, Emergency Nursing Pediatric Care, and Advanced Trauma Nursing, the ENA provides a wide range of educational opportunities for nurses.

Physicians

Physicians play a critical role in the delivery of EMS. They not only provide specialized medical care, but also provide medical direction necessary for all other levels of providers to function. Historically, physicians have been considered the first EMS responders. Until after World War II, physicians would visit patients at home, an event commonly known as "house calls." Hospital-based ambulances routinely included an intern or resident as part of the crew. Physicians still respond on ambulances as primary crew members in many European and South American countries. In rural communities, it was not uncommon for the "town doc" to be summoned to major automobile crashes or farm and industrial accidents. Some rural physicians even ran their own small, community hospitals. Emergency department physicians are not the only physicians routinely involved in EMS. The first paramedic units were formed to provide out-of-hospital care for victims of sudden cardiac death. Building on the work of EMS pioneers such as Eugene Nagle, a cardiologist who was also an electrical engineer, cardiologists continue to be involved in EMS education, protocol development, and system design.

One of the first textbooks used for EMT training was *Emergency Care and Transportation of the Sick and Injured* (American Academy of Orthopaedic Surgeons, 1971) by the Committee on Injuries of the American Academy of Orthopaedic Surgeons (AAOS). The book had an orange cover and became known as the "orange book." The AAOS worked to develop an educational program and lesson guides for EMT training. Their efforts were instrumental in the development of a national standard curriculum. The AAOS continues to provide review and input into the development of EMS training curriculums.

A major portion of EMS activity is directed toward the trauma patient. Definitive care of serious trauma injuries usually requires surgical intervention. In a manner similar to the AAOS, the American College of Surgeons (ACS) continues its involvement in EMS. The College recognizes trauma as a surgical disease. Their Committee on Trauma works to establish standards for the care of the trauma patient. The ACS also developed Advanced Trauma Life Support (ATLS), a course designed to allow surgeons to assess and treat trauma patients in a systematic manner during the critical first hour after a traumatizing event.

Central to the care of trauma victims is the concept of the trauma center. As the trauma center concept expanded, the specialized nature of physicians working in the centers also evolved. Surgeons specializing in trauma victim resuscitation became known as **traumatologists**. The specialty of trauma surgery was developed. Nonsurgical physicians dealing with the continued care of critical patients became critical care **intensivists**.

In addition to the physician roles described above, members of almost all medical specialties provide consultation and support to EMS systems. The physician is the central core from which all other provider levels extend. Without physician authority and oversight, an EMS system would not be able to deliver the sophisticated care now commonly expected of such systems.

Allied Health Professionals

An EMS system could not function, and proper patient care be delivered, without the assistance and cooperation of numerous allied health professionals. Consider a patient transported to the ED with a simple fracture. An x-ray technician will be needed to take x-rays. An ED technician records vital signs. A surgical physician assistant applies the cast after the orthopedist has set the fracture. For a medical patient, other allied health professionals may include medical lab technicians, ECG technicians, and respiratory therapists. In addition to their hospital-based roles, some allied health professionals assist with the interhospital transfer of critical patients. Critical care transport teams may include a respiratory therapist to manage ventilator-dependent patients. Physician's assistants have been placed on special ambulances to provide limited primary care, especially to geriatric and underserved populations.

OTHER PROVIDERS

The delivery of prehospital emergency care involves not only personnel who provide direct patient care, but also personnel who provide valuable support functions critical to the system's operation.

Telecommunicators

More commonly known as dispatchers, **telecommunicators** provide a vital link between the public and the EMS service. In recent years, the role of the telecommunicator has expanded from just receiving calls for help to being an on-line resource and advocate for the caller in distress. Back in the "old days" a caller needed to just dial "O" for the telephone operator who would connect the caller to the fire department, police department, or hospital. If the caller could not give a good location or address, response was delayed. Now, a caller need only dial 911 to be connected to a telecommunicator who will not only take the call for help, but will also provide prearrival instructions and remain on the line until a unit arrives. Response to the correct address is ensured through an enhanced 911 system that displays the caller's phone location.

Telecommunicators receive specialized training and certification. A number of organizations and private companies provide telecommunicator training programs and materials. Basic telecommunicator courses are commonly conducted over four days and include topics such as roles and responsibilities, telephone and 911 operations, computer-aided dispatch (CAD) systems, and fundamentals of call handling. Complete training courses leading to certification are also available online.

Emergency Medical Dispatcher

Once a call for EMS assistance has been received by the call taker, it may be transferred to the **Emergency Medical Dispatch (EMD) dispatcher**. The call taker may also serve the dual function of EMD dispatcher. Through a systematic caller interrogation, the EMD dispatcher can determine the nature of the caller's distress. This information is matched to a series of protocol cards that provide the dispatcher with scripted prearrival instructions for the caller. This approach provides greater assistance and assurance to the caller. Under the old system the dispatcher would determine the caller's name and location and then hang up. The EMD dispatcher is also able to more accurately determine the proper EMS resources to send, thus improving system efficiency.

Firefighters

In many areas, the fire department also provides EMS service. However, there are still a significant number of fire departments that do not provide these services. Even though they have no formal EMS service, these fire departments are often called upon to provide assistance to EMS units. The fire department may routinely send a unit as a first responder. This may occur in departments with EMS service if no units are immediately available to respond or will be delayed. Training of firefighters in EMS runs the gamut from paramedic to no formal training. The typical training level for non-EMS fire personnel is first responder. As a minimum, many departments require proficiency in CPR. These minimal training levels allow personnel to provide basic, lifesaving support until an EMS unit arrives.

Changes in demand for fire department services, coupled with a renewed interest in EMS and budgetary restrictions, have resulted in various approaches to combine traditional firefighting activities with EMS delivery. One such approach is the paramedic engine company. A paramedic cross-trained as a firefighter is assigned to an engine company. On medical calls requiring advanced life support, the engine is dispatched along with a transport unit. The paramedic goes to the hospital in the ambulance and the engine can remain in service. If a fire call is received, the paramedic functions as part of the engine crew. This approach provides greater flexibility and more efficient utilization of specially trained personnel (see Chapter 5).

Police Officers

Not often thought of as EMS responders, police officers play a vital role in the delivery of EMS. The most obvious role is being that of a first responder. Because of the nature of police work, officers are often the first on the scene of incidents requiring EMS. Most police departments require officers to be trained to the first responder level and provide minimal first aid kits for patrol cars. In some areas of the country, the police play a much greater role in EMS. Select police officers are trained to the paramedic level and provide ALS upgrades to local ambulance services. Like paramedic engine companies, this approach also provides greater flexibility and utilization of public safety personnel.

SOURCES OF PROVIDERS

In general terms, prehospital providers can be placed into two groups—volunteer and career. This classification is based upon the nature of the organization for which they work and their status within that organization. However, this dichotomy is not absolute. It is possible for a provider to be a volunteer with one organization and work in a career position with another. There are also providers who are paid on call. This means that they receive compensation only when they respond to a call. For all other activities, they are essentially volunteers.

Volunteer Providers

The majority of EMS in the United States is provided by **volunteers**. These uncompensated providers deliver all levels of EMS from first responder to paramedic. Volunteers are most often found in rural and suburban areas. However, some significant urban areas are still served by volunteer providers, often with support from part-time paid personnel. In addition to providing emergency response, volunteers are often required to participate in fundraising activities to support their organization.

Although volunteer providers receive no monetary compensation, they receive many intangible rewards, the most important being a sense of having provided service to their community. To increase recruitment and retention of volunteers, other rewards such as insurance coverage, reduction or elimination of fees and taxes, worker's compensation, and length of service awards (retirement) are provided.

Training and education requirements for volunteers mirror those of career personnel. In combination departments, volunteers are often indistinguishable from career staff. State certification requirements for EMS providers are the same for volunteers and career employees. By not distinguishing between providers, the professionalism of all providers is maintained as well as respect among providers. One area where providers do differ, however, is in the format of training programs. Training for volunteers is often spread out over a longer time period and offered on weekends and evenings.

A constant area of concern for volunteer organizations is the retention of members. Increased training standards and workplace regulations require volunteer personnel to give more time just to be able to respond to emergency calls. It is not unusual for a new member to take a year's worth of training before being able to respond to an actual call. This presents a challenge to the organizational leadership to keep the member motivated. As a member's family and/or work situation changes, his ability to volunteer may also change, leading to conflicts at home, at work, and within the volunteer organization. To maintain sufficient volunteers, organizations must engage in recruitment efforts. Although a necessary activity, it is nonetheless another demand placed upon volunteers.

Career Providers

Career providers include all providers whose primary job is providing service. Employees of fire departments, hospitals, and commercial ambulance providers would be included in this category. Because career personnel do not have to be concerned with earning a living as well as volunteer organizational and fund raising issues, they can focus more directly on the job of providing EMS. In some areas, the provision of ALS is limited to career personnel due to training and skill proficiency requirements.

Career providers face not only the demands of providing prehospital care, but they are also subject to the stresses and demands found in any workplace environment. These may include unionization, pay disputes, discrimination, management issues, and workplace safety. Career providers often work in high volume systems, thus they have the opportunity to practice their skills more frequently than in traditional volunteer systems. However, working in an understaffed, high-demand system could lead to provider burnout. Because EMS is their livelihood, career providers cannot just slow down or quit. This often leads to conflicts and increased stress.

In suburban areas surrounding large urban centers, career personnel employed by the urban municipality were a source of trained volunteers. In many areas this trend continues, but increased demands by unions and labor regulations has had an impact on this source of volunteer providers. Likewise, family and financial demands often require career personnel to have second jobs, thus limiting their availability to volunteer.

ORGANIZED LABOR IN EMS

Organized labor has a very strong and influential presence in prehospital EMS. The fire service, the largest provider of prehospital care, is heavily organized. The International Association of Fire Fighters boasts over 225,000 members in the United States and Canada in 2,500 affiliate organizations (locals). The private sector is not as heavily unionized but workers in that sector are represented by several different labor organizations including the International Association of EMTs and Paramedics (IAEP), which is a division of the National Association of Government Employees, AFL-CIO; the Professional EMTs and Paramedics (PEP), which is a division of the International Brotherhood of Boilermakers; the Service Employees International Union (SEIU); and the Teamsters.

During the late 1990s the health care industry and, in particular, the private sector of the prehospital care industry, was targeted for unionization by labor organizations. Organizing efforts in the private sector have had mixed success in part due to the financial difficulties of the industry as a whole during this period.

The International Association of Firefighters (IAFF) has been a leader in advocating fire-based EMS in the country and has encouraged local governments to enter the emergency ambulance business. In the late 1990s operational responsibility for EMS was moved from a third service to the fire department in New York City. In the year 2000 the fire service was the primary provider of emergency ambulance service in the ten largest cities in the United States.

The IAFF also is a leader in the provision of EMS. IAFF Local I-39 in Kansas City, Missouri, was instrumental in creating the employee-owned ambulance service Emergency Providers, Incorporated. This company holds the contract with the Metropolitan Ambulance Services Trust to provide all emergency and nonemergency ambulance service in Kansas City, Missouri, and Kansas City, Kansas. Members of the local sit on the board of directors of the corporation whose profits fund the local's retirement program. Appendix B lists some organizations involved in EMS.

PROVIDER STRESS

Like any job or profession, the provision of prehospital emergency care has its sources of stress. They include, but are not limited to, schedule problems, time pressures, conflicts with supervisors and colleagues, having to miss important family occasions, low pay, sleep deprivation, a limited career ladder, as well as job conflict and job ambiguity. The stressors that are common in most professions as well as EMS are in a category called **general stress**. Everyone encounters general stress. It is not all bad. In fact, general stress has two versions, *eustress* and *distress*. Eustress is a positive, driving, and creative force that can help people make wonderful changes in their own lives while contributing to humankind. Distress covers the uncomfortable aspects of general stress such as heat, cold, crowding, contacts with human beings, and excessive workloads. Both the eustress and the distress versions of general stress are normal conditions of life. Stress is not harmful unless it becomes prolonged and/or severe. The biggest problem with general stress is that, if it is not monitored carefully, it can turn into a destructive form of stress known as **cumulative stress**.

Cumulative stress is the type of stress that develops when general stress is not properly resolved. Cumulative stress used to be called "burnout," but that term has become overused and misunderstood. The current term, cumulative stress, indicates a piling up of unresolved stress over time. The stress has, therefore, become excessive and prolonged. If someone does not do something about his or her cumulative stress, it will eventually have harmful effects on that person's health and performance as well as on his or her relationships and personality.

Unlike most other professions, the EMS field places additional burdens on its providers. Other common sources of stress for EMS providers include:

- Potential for exposure to infectious diseases
- Dealing with death and dying
- Incidents involving accidental injury or illnesses in infants and children
- Multicasualty incidents
- Severe injuries and mutilations
- Abuse and neglect of children
- Death of a coworker
- EMS system abuse

Situations such as the suicide of a colleague, line-of-duty death, serious injury to a fellow EMS worker, disasters, child deaths, accidentally killing or wounding someone, and events with a significant threat to the provider, are categorized as **critical incidents**. The type of stress that results from exposure to a critical incident is called **traumatic stress** or **critical incident stress (CIS)**. Critical incidents are pivotal experiences that can produce a disturbing stress reaction so powerful that it can cause people to become dysfunctional on the job and/or at home. Although critical incidents are very disturbing and painful experiences, CIS is a normal response of normal people to an abnormal event. The CIS response is not a sign of weakness or psychological imbalance. Most people do recover from the experience and are able to learn valuable lessons that can be used in future experiences.

If CIS is not resolved properly, however, it may turn from a normal response of normal people to an abnormal event into something much more serious and disruptive. It can turn into a psychological disorder called **post-traumatic stress disorder** (PTSD).

PTSD is characterized by three symptom categories that start or are made worse by exposure to the critical incident. The symptom categories are:

1. *Intrusion* (seeing, hearing, smelling, or feeling the event repeatedly or not being able to stop thinking about it)
2. *Avoidance* (any effort to avoid being exposed to stimulus or experience that reminds the person of the traumatizing experience)
3. *Arousal* (restlessness, sleeplessness, hyper alertness, difficulties paying attention or planning actions)

PTSD causes significant disturbance in a person's normal life. Many cannot work or are acutely disturbed by certain aspects of their work. Some have difficulties relating to their loved ones at home. Normal life pursuits are very difficult to achieve. People with PTSD can become disabled in many ways and they need professional treatment to recover from the condition. PTSD can be cured, but the cures can be a challenge. It is much easier to prevent it or mitigate it so that it is less disruptive to the lives of EMS personnel or others who might be exposed to the horrific events that can produce PTSD.

Critical Incident Stress Management

In the mid 1970s, Jeffrey T. Mitchell, Ph.D. of the University of Maryland, began work on a systematic program to prevent and mitigate traumatic stress reactions in emergency personnel. Today, the program is called **Critical incident stress management (CISM)**. Its use has spread to 27 countries and the system is fast becoming standard operating procedure in EMS services, fire departments, and law enforcement agencies. In fact, CISM is being utilized in businesses, industries, communities, and school systems in addition to emergency services organizations. CISM is a comprehensive, systematic, and multicomponent approach to deal with the traumatic stress caused by tragic critical incidents.

Although stress reactions are normal responses of normal people to abnormal events, they can produce painful emotional reactions that might interfere with work performance, health, and relationships. Under severe circumstances, healthy personalities may even be altered. The key to maintaining healthy personnel on the job is to mitigate acute stress responses and to reduce the amount and intensity of the stress symptoms caused by a critical incident. This is the primary function of a CISM program.

In a well-organized Critical Incident Stress Management program, a team of specially trained emergency personnel work together with mental health professionals and clergy personnel to provide a wide range of stress management services. The training of all of the CISM team members takes many hours. The nature and the depth of the training goes well beyond the limitations of this book so only brief descriptions of a limited number of CISM interventions will be provided in this chapter. People who are interested in obtaining additional details or actual CISM training should contact the International Critical Incident Stress Foundation or their local CISM resource.

Some CISM services are provided before tragedies occur. For example, CISM teams provide stress management training and education to prepare emergency personnel for what they might encounter in their work. They also assist organizations in writing policies and procedures that can lessen the stress associated with critical incidents.

CISM teams provide support during stressful situations. They work with the leadership of an organization to ensure that field crews are properly rested, get enough food and fluid, and are sheltered from the elements. Team members provide individual support as it may be required by the personnel. In large-scale incidents such as disasters, CISM teams provide brief group informational sessions when the work crews have finished their work. These sessions are called **demobilizations**.

Once a critical incident is concluded, CISM teams provide a variety of services to assist emergency personnel in recovering from their stressful experience. Groups that experienced events that are smaller or less intense than disasters might be provided a **defusing** within hours of the event. A few days later the same group might be given another procedure, which is just another step in CISM's comprehensive, systematic, and multipart approach to traumatic stress.

This second group procedure is more complex than the defusing and it is called a **Critical incident stress debriefing (CISD)**. It has been proven to be very effective in lowering the symptoms of stress associated with critical incidents. It has also accelerated the recovery of emergency personnel from traumatic events and has allowed the CISM team to identify those personnel who might need more assistance.

The most common intervention utilized in a CISM program is that of one-on-one support. Team members make a point of being available to anyone involved in a critical incident that needs individual support. The team members will also seek out anyone team members are concerned about and offer additional support. CISM teams provide enhanced support services when they reach out to the families of emergency personnel. People feel cared for themselves when they know that their families are being cared for properly. Efficient CISM teams make sure that they provide a wide range of follow-up services. On occasion, some people need a referral for psychotherapy. CISM teams can be instrumental in helping people find the best referral sources to suit their needs.

No CISM team can rely on only one tactic to accomplish its crisis intervention goals. It is not possible that any single tactic will be applicable to all people, under all circumstances, and at all times. The only way to properly manage critical incident stress is to have a comprehensive, systematic, and multicomponent program in place to serve the organization. A brief summary of the core components of a CISM program follows.

- Stress education and immunization training
- On-scene support services
  - Individual support
  - Advice to supervisors
  - Support to direct victims of the incident
- Demobilizations for disasters
- Defusing on the day of the incident
- Critical incident stress debriefing (CISD)
- Significant other support services
- Follow-up services
- Referrals for professional support and/or therapy

CISM is all about keeping healthy people healthy and functional people functional. CISM is simply good personnel management. Good management means taking good care of one's people. A primary goal of the CISM system is to take good care of people.

SUMMARY

An EMS system cannot function without a human element. Building on the tradition of early first aid providers, the prehospital provider of today is recognized as a trained and skilled provider of emergency care. National standard curriculums ensure consistency in the education of EMS personnel. The role of the prehospital provider is recognized through statewide certification and licensure requirements and legislation.

No matter how well trained or highly skilled, the prehospital provider alone cannot meet all the needs of the sick or injured. Prehospital providers work in coordination with hospital-based providers in a systems approach to the delivery of EMS. Hospital providers have a long tradition of EMS involvement both as providers, educators, and medical directors.

EMS providers come from varied backgrounds and work in a variety of system configurations. Some are dedicated volunteers while others are employed full-time in EMS. Regardless of their status, all EMS providers face numerous challenges working in the profession. This can lead to stress and in severe cases, traumatic stress. It is important for providers to be aware of their own well-being and to recognize when help is needed. In cases of traumatic stress, CISM is one means to assist the provider and maintain a healthy work force.

STUDENT STUDY QUESTIONS

1. What are the three levels of emergency medical technician (EMT) and how do they differ?

2. Name three hospital-based providers that are routinely involved in the EMS system.

3. How does a wilderness EMT differ from an EMT-B?

4. Defend the position that emergency medical dispatchers should be considered EMS providers.

5. List the various types of interventions provided by the CISM process.

BIBLIOGRAPHY

American Academy of Orthopaedic Surgeons. (1971). *Emergency care and transportation of the sick and injured* (1st ed.). Menasha, WI: George Banta Co.

American Society of Hospital Based Emergency Air Medical Services. (1988). *Air-medical crew national standard curriculum.* Pasadena, CA: Author.

Everly, G. S., & Mitchell, J. T. (1997). *Critical incident stress management (CISM): a new era and standard of care in crisis intervention.* Ellicott City, MD: Chevron Publishing.

National Academy of Sciences, National Research Council. (1966). *Accidental death and disability: The neglected disease of modern society* (p. 73). Washington, DC: Author.

National Highway Traffic Safety Administration. (1998). *Emergency medical technician—intermediate national standard curriculum.* Washington, DC: Author.

National Highway Traffic Safety Administration. (1998). *Emergency medical technician—paramedic national standard curriculum.* Washington, DC: Author.

National Highway Traffic Safety Administration and Health Resources and Services Administration. (2000). *EMS education agenda for the future: a systems approach.* Washington, DC: Authors.

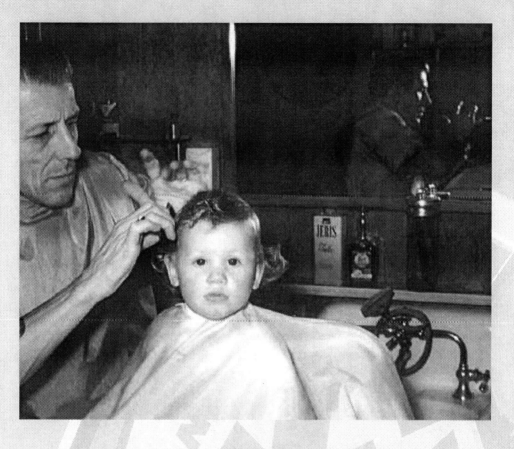

Case Study

The scene is a local barbershop.

"Good morning, Henry, how are you doing this morning?"

"Oh, a little stiff. I didn't sleep well last night with all that commotion up the street."

"What was the problem?"

"That new young couple that just moved in. Their kid fell and hit his head or some such thing. Would have thought the place was on fire with all the fire engines, ambulances, and police cars that responded. What ever happened to just getting an ambulance? Now you call and they send the whole fire department. No wonder taxes keep going up!"

"I know what you mean, Henry, I know what you mean."

CHAPTER 5

Transportation

Outline

Objectives

Upon completion of this chapter, the reader should be able to:

- Identify the various types of EMS service providers.
- Define and differentiate between fixed-post staffing and event-driven staffing.
- State the role of a chase vehicle in providing ALS response.
- Identify BLS staffing configurations.
- Identify ALS staffing configurations.
- Define mobile health care.
- State the purpose of the federal star of life ambulance specifications.
- Differentiate between type I, II, and III ambulance designs.
- State the advantages and disadvantages of air medical transport.

Key Terms

ALS intercept
Ambulance trust
Chase vehicle
Commercial providers
Event-driven resource
   deployment
Fixed-post staffing
High-performance EMS
   systems
Hospital based

KKK-A-1822
Medium duty ambulance
Mobile health care
Paramedic engine
   company
Pathway management
Peak hour
Peak load staffing
Posting plans
Public safety agency

Public utility model
Service providers
Star-of-life ambulance
System status
   management
Third service
Type I ambulance
Type II ambulance
Type III ambulance

THE TRANSPORTATION ATTRIBUTE

Fundamental to any emergency medical system is the need for efficient conveyance of the patient to definitive care. This is most often accomplished using an ambulance. Indeed, the term "ambulance driver" is still used to describe prehospital providers in general. However, given the advanced training of today's providers, this term could be considered demeaning. Nevertheless, some form of specialized vehicle staffed with trained prehospital providers is the basic component of EMS transportation. To fully understand the transportation attribute, it is necessary to look at it in three ways: who provides the service, how it is delivered, and how it is staffed.

Service Providers

Who provides EMS service varies greatly across the country and depends on the needs of a specific community. Although EMS is thought of as an important public service, it is not always provided as a governmental function. The relationship of EMS with other emergency **service providers** also varies from jurisdiction to jurisdiction. In most cases however, systems have evolved that best suit the needs of the community. Various approaches to the delivery of EMS are presented below.

Fire Service Perhaps the most traditional provider of EMS transportation is the fire service. Many fire departments took on the responsibility for ambulance service to provide support to their own personnel on the fire scene or as a public service when other providers ceased providing service. In many rural communities, the fire service was the natural choice because it already had in place a structure to deliver emergency services. In the early days of advanced life support (ALS) development, pioneering physicians such as Nagel in Miami and Cobb in Seattle saw the fire service as the ideal delivery system. The fire department already had trained personnel, strategically located stations, and response vehicles.

In the latter part of the twentieth century, the role and expectation of the American fire service changed. Budget issues, coupled with declining fire incidents, forced many communities to look at the role of the local fire service. Expanding the role of the fire service beyond fire suppression and prevention was seen as a means to increase efficiency. Today, the fire service is involved not only in EMS, but also hazardous materials response, urban search and rescue, and domestic terrorism response.

The fire service's embracing of EMS has not always been positive. As the role of the fire service began to change, and the integration of EMS brought new training, personnel, and response patterns, some departments were reluctant to accept what has been called the "stepchild of the fire service." Demand for EMS exceeds that of fire suppression. Stations with EMS units experienced increased alarms that disrupted traditional station routines. Personnel assigned to EMS units were often hired as EMTs and paramedics without fire training. This led to union membership issues, changes in labor standards, supervision conflicts, and promotion concerns. In some systems, engine company personnel were required to obtain EMS training as well as respond with an engine or truck company on critical EMS calls. Firefighters who had joined the fire department to fight fires soon found themselves spending most of a shift responding to EMS calls. Over time, however, the fire service accepted EMS as one of its prime missions. Major fire service organizations such as the International Association of Fire Chiefs (IAFC) and the International Association of Fire Fighters (IAFF), the predominant fire service union, have active EMS sections that support EMS in the fire service.

Commercial Service Since the early inception of ambulance service, for-profit or **commercial providers** have played a vital role as a source of transportation. Just as most communities have a fire department, they most likely have a funeral home as well. Although one may not like to consider the similarities, a hearse has much in common with an ambulance, especially the early Cadillac ambulances. These were ambulances built on luxury car chassis by Cadillac, Oldsmobile, and Buick. With a hearse, funeral directors could easily remove the rollers and retaining hardware for a coffin and replace it with a stretcher. A removable "red light" was stuck on the roof and the hearse became an ambulance. Equipment and training were minimal at best. Through this transformation, the funeral director was able to expand his services and revenue while providing a needed public service. In areas of high demand, some funeral directors actually established separate ambulance divisions or services.

When thinking of transport services, emergency, or 911 service is what most often comes to mind. However, there is a need to provide nonemergency or routine transports, that is, transfers of bedridden patients from hospital to hospital, hospital to nursing home, hospital to home, or nursing home to doctor's office and return. These transports are usually paid for by the patient's insurance. The need to provide such service has been the impetus behind the founding of many commercial ambulance companies. In urban areas where 911 service is provided by the fire department, commercial operators handle the interfacility transports. In suburban and rural areas, the fire department or rescue squad may also provide interfacility transport. However, as the demand for 911 service increases, and the availability of volunteers decreases, these services are forced to turn over this aspect of their operation to commercial providers. Often the need for an interfacility transport arises on short notice. This makes the task of finding a volunteer crew more difficult as well as ties up the crew and vehicle for an extended period of time. Thus many commercial operators are expanding their service areas.

Transport of patients by ambulance can be lucrative given the fact that such transports are billable to insurance companies as well as Medicare and Medicaid. Operators can also charge for expendable items, oxygen, mileage, and night differential in addition to the basic cost of the transport. Commercial operators often compete for exclusive contracts with hospitals, extended care facilities, and managed care organizations. Increasingly, commercial services are becoming involved in **pathway management**. This is the management of how a patient enters into the health care system. For instance, if a patient falls and injures her leg and cannot walk, she has a number of options. The traditional action would be to dial 911 and request an ambulance. If the injury is not too serious, the patient could be transported to the hospital emergency department by a private automobile. With pathway management, the injured patient would call her managed care organization utilizing a dedicated telephone number. A health care professional would interrogate the patient and advise the best course of action. If an ambulance is needed and the situation is not life-threatening, a commercial ambulance service would be dispatched. This service has a contract with the managed care organization to provide transport at an agreed upon rate that is less than the 911 service rate. They will also transport the patient to a hospital or urgent care facility that is part of the organization's plan. This also results in lower costs to the managed care organization. Such flexibility is not possible utilizing traditional 911 ambulance service.

In an effort to reduce cost, some municipalities and jurisdictions have abandoned public service ambulance service in favor of commercial service. Commercial operators bid on a governmental contract to provide 911 service. The contract often contains a performance clause that specifies the required response time and response coverage. Failure to meet these requirements will result in fines and possible loss of the contract. Because delivery of 911 service can be expensive, the commercial operator will often negotiate a clause in the contract giving the operator exclusive rights to nonemergency and interfacility transports within the service area.

As the demand for commercial ambulance service increased, the industry underwent a major change in the 1980s and 1990s. Small "mom and pop" ambulance services were bought out by large consolidators. This reduced local competition and increased the ability of commercial operators to compete with public service EMS systems. National consolidators also provided "one-stop-shopping" for managed care organizations interested in pathway management and interfacility transports at service locations across the country.

In addition to providing efficiency and economy of scale, commercial operators were not constrained by fixed-post locations and staffing patterns common with public service EMS systems, especially the fire service. This increased flexibility led to the development of posting strategies that are event driven. This concept will be discussed in more detail later in this chapter. The interest of the commercial ambulance industry is served by the American Ambulance Association.

Third Service The **third service** approach to EMS delivery involves the creation of a separate public safety service to deliver EMS. The term third service is derived from EMS being added to the traditional municipal services of police and fire. In a third service system, EMS is delivered by uniformed personnel who have their own vehicles, command structure, and in some cases their own stations. More often, EMS vehicles and personnel are posted to fire stations because the stations are already in place and have the necessary services. However, the EMS personnel are not part of the fire department. Some municipalities have aligned their third service with the police department rather than the fire department.

The third service concept solves many of the conflicts associated with the integration of personnel and services into a fire department. Often the personnel and services do not fit the department's traditional structure and mission. However, such a system adds additional expense by duplicating much of the infrastructure already present in the fire service.

Public Safety Agency Jurisdictions have traditionally provided fire and police protection for their citizens. With the addition of EMS, a jurisdiction now had to provide three services at the taxpayer's expense. A concept that has developed in a few jurisdictions is to combine all of the public safety functions into one agency. A department of public safety provides fire, police, and EMS services within one organizational structure. Public safety stations may serve as a fire station, EMS station, and a police station all in one. Jurisdictions that fully embrace this concept have public safety officers who are trained to provide all three levels of service.

As an example, if a fire alarm is received, a minimum crew responds the fire engine to the scene. Officers on police patrol respond along with EMS personnel to complete the crew and provide command. In a medical emergency, a police car may respond to the scene with a police officer–paramedic who can upgrade the ambulance to ALS. In other jurisdictions, there may be a single **public safety agency** that employs police, fire, and EMS personnel, but each service is a separate division within the agency.

The main advantage of the public service concept is that it utilizes personnel to their maximum efficiency. A crucial disadvantage is that it requires personnel to maintain proficiency in diverse areas. There is also the potential for resource conflicts between the different services comprising the public safety agency. Figures 5-1 and 5-2 show the structure of these systems.

Hospital Based Hospitals have a long tradition of providing ambulance service. As the community provider of medical care, ambulance service was a natural extension of the hospital's role in the community. Today, few hospitals provide ambulance service. Changes in hospital ownership, business practices, and federal regulations have limited **hospital-based** EMS systems. Those still functioning most often provide ALS or specialized transport service.

As advanced life support was developing, various delivery models were tried. Early on, hospital-based providers were used to move ALS into the field setting. Doctors and nurses were placed on ambulances to provide ALS. In smaller communities, an ambulance would respond to the hospital and pick up a nurse before responding to the scene of a cardiac emergency. In those systems that chose not to utilize paramedics exclusively, hospitals developed **chase vehicle** systems utilizing a nurse and paramedic combination. A hospital-based vehicle responds with the nurse and paramedic combination to upgrade a basic life support (BLS) ambulance. Based on local medical protocols, the nurse may be able to provide specialized interventions not normally permitted of paramedics. Having initiated treatment of the patient in the field, the hospital-based crew is able to continue this care in the emergency department. When not responding to calls, the nurse and paramedic are able to assist in the emergency department as additional staff.

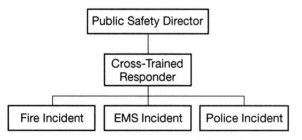

Figure 5-1 Consolidated Public Safety Organization

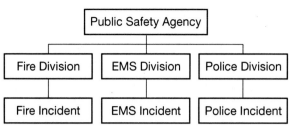

Figure 5-2 Public Safety Agency

Through regulation and/or competition, the services provided by hospitals in a geographical area may vary. This prevents hospitals in the same catchment area from duplicating services available at a nearby hospital, thus controlling cost. For example, in an urban area, only one hospital may perform open-heart surgery. Another would be authorized to provide high-risk obstetrical services. Because of this control, the necessity to transfer patients between health care facilities is increased.

To facilitate the transfer of patients, some hospitals have established specialized transport services. These services may be land based and/or air medical. Specialized vehicles, some as large as motor homes, are equipped to support patients during the transfer. Crew configuration varies, but as a minimum includes a critical care registered nurse (CCRN), a critical care transport paramedic, and a driver. For extremely critical patients, a physician is added to the crew. To avoid the cost and management of a fleet of vehicles and personnel, some hospitals have contracted with a commercial operator to provide transport service infrastructure.

First Responder The term *first responder* refers to the rapid response of trained personnel to the scene to provide life-sustaining care until the arrival of definitive care and transport. Although not technically a transport service, first responder service is an integral part of the EMS system in many areas. An example of such a service would be a fire engine crew responding to a medical emergency to provide immediate care such as airway management, oxygen, and vital signs. Even in areas where the fire department provides EMS service, it is not unusual for the closest emergency unit to be dispatched. In busy systems, the first responder unit can provide care until a transport unit arrives. Some jurisdictions have been creative in designating first responder units by utilizing police, public works personnel, and highway maintenance crews.

Ambulance Trust The **ambulance trust** combines aspects of private and governmental EMS systems. The trust is responsible for providing EMS service. A board of trustees oversees the operation of the service and manages its affairs. The prime advantage of the trust system is that it removes the provision of EMS from political influence and control. Such a system works well for multijurisdictional or regional systems that extend across political boundaries.

Public Utility Model The **public utility model** for delivery of EMS utilizes a governing strategy similar to that used to provide basic utility services such as electricity and gas. An EMS authority is established with responsibility for providing EMS. The authority contracts with a commercial provider to deliver services. To ensure continuity of service, the authority usually owns the EMS vehicles and equipment. By owning the system's equipment, the likelihood of the commercial contractor defaulting is limited. The authority also establishes performance standards for monitoring the performance of the commercial contractor.

Integrated Given the different configurations for EMS systems, it is possible to develop other systems that combine aspects of two or more systems. An example of an integrated system would be a commercial ambulance operator providing BLS level transport and the fire department providing ALS upgrade service. In such a system, the fire department responds with paramedics who provide ALS. The paramedic then accompanies the patient to the hospital in the commercial operator's BLS ambulance. A similar system would be ALS provided by a hospital with transport by the fire department or commercial operator. There are even systems that have two different entities providing BLS transport and ALS transport. Integrated systems allow localities to custom design EMS systems to best meet a community's unique needs.

Delivery Systems

Just as there are variations in who delivers EMS, there are also variations in how EMS is delivered. Variations are based on how to determine the number and type of ambulances available to respond.

Fixed-Post Staffing The traditional approach to the delivery of EMS has been for the provider, whether commercial or public safety, to respond from a fixed station to the incident scene. When a call is received, the dispatch center determines the closest available unit. Regardless of the demand for EMS service, the same number of units would be in-service at any given time. This is a **fixed-post staffing** delivery system.

Fixed-post staffing systems developed for one of two reasons. In the case of a commercial provider, the operator has one central location from which ambulances operate, usually the company's headquarters. This is where personnel report for work, restock units, bring units for maintenance, and return at the end of a shift. Some commercial operators covering large areas may have satellite centers that serve a similar function.

In the case of fire department EMS, ambulances were placed in the fire stations. For small communities, this may be a central location. In others, the fire department may have multiple stations. It is interesting to note that in many older urban centers the location of fire stations was determined by how far the horses that pulled steamer engines could run. Yet today the location of these same stations determines the placement of EMS units.

Most fixed-post systems do not take into consideration the changes in the demand for EMS service that occur over the course of a day or according to the day of the week. On average, the demand for EMS service decreases during the late evening and early morning hours and rises during the day, especially around dawn and during rush hour periods. Demand patterns also change between workdays and weekends. In a fixed-post system, the number of units in service remains constant. Thus some units are utilized more than others depending on the time of day and day of the week. For example, a unit located in a downtown urban area would be busiest during normal working hours. However, this same unit would be underutilized at night and on weekends. Fixed-post systems may temporarily transfer units to cover open areas, but this is done on an ad hoc basis.

Although the fixed-post system attempts to provide uniform coverage for a given area, the system does not necessarily do so in the most efficient manner. Maximum utilization of units and personnel is not usually obtained by such a system.

Event-Driven Staffing In contrast to fixed-post staffing, **event-driven resource deployment** matches an EMS system's resources to predicted demand using data on historical patterns. All **high-performance EMS systems**, that is EMS systems that produce clinical quality, response time reliability, customer satisfaction, and economic efficiency, simultaneously, use event-driven resource deployment. These techniques were first developed by Jack Stout, an EMS economist and consultant, in the late 1970s and early 1980s and tested initially in the EMS systems of Tulsa, Oklahoma, and Kansas City, Missouri. They are referred to as "advanced system status management." **System status management** is "the process of preparing the system to produce the best possible response to the next EMS call" (Stout, 1983).

The Center for Economic and Management Research at Oklahoma University found that demand for emergency medical services was similar to that of the electric utility industry (Stout, 1985). Demand for EMS fluctuates by the hour of the day and the day of the week just as the demand for electric power varies. There is more demand for EMS on Saturday night at 10:00 PM than there is on Monday morning at 4:00 AM. The center found that the geographic distribution of calls also varied by the hour of the day and the day of the week.

In recognition of these findings, high-performance providers use **peak load staffing** which means they add units to hours with predictably high demand and have fewer units when demand is low. Therefore, these systems do not use many 24-hour shifts. Instead they use a variety of shifts including 8-, 9-, 10-, 11-, 12-, 14-, and 16-hour shifts. These shifts also start at various times throughout the day so that the supply of units closely matches the demand for those units.

EMS demand also shows a geographic pattern. As people move through the day so does the demand for EMS. High-performance services study these geographic patterns and position their vehicles accordingly. They create **posting plans** for each hour of each day. These services use a process developed by Jack Stout in which a group of experienced dispatchers and field providers, using maps showing the distribution of calls for each hour of each day, determine the optimal location for their units. They start by determining where they would post one ambulance if there was only one unit available to the entire system, and then where they would post two units if that was all that was available, and so on. This is done for the number of units available for service during that one hour. After one hour is done the group goes to the next hour until posting plans for all 168 hours have been developed. This is a great deal of work. But once these plans are developed they must be explained to all of the providers so that all personnel understand the logic of the post locations and staffing levels.

High-performance providers maintain ambulance fleets that are 120% to 130% in excess of the maximum number of units that might be scheduled at the peak hour of coverage. The **peak hour** is the hour in which the most ambulances are scheduled to be on duty at one time. These providers also hire vehicle service technicians whose primary function is to wash and stock ambulances so that when a crew arrives at headquarters to report for duty, their ambulance is waiting for them, already washed, stocked, and prepared for service. The crew verifies the status of critical equipment and then advises the control center of their availability for service. Crews are dispatched to calls and to post locations throughout the day in response to the demand for service on that particular day.

Many high-performance systems are also full service systems and therefore the ambulance crews handle both emergency and nonemergency requests for service. As crews are assigned to calls, the remaining ambulances are repositioned so that the system is always configured to best respond to the next life-threatening emergency.

At the end of their shift, the crew returns the ambulance to the fleet facility where the vehicle is washed and restocked. Vehicles are being taken and returned throughout the day and it is only in rare circumstances that a vehicle will be immediately given to another crew. All units are frontline units and are fully equipped. Crews are not always assigned to the same ambulance on successive shifts but all the ambulances are configured identically. When there is a need for additional units they can be quickly added to the system. The extra capacity also makes it possible to schedule routine and preventive maintenance of vehicles without reducing the number of ambulances available to the system.

ALS Intercept The **ALS intercept** or chase vehicle delivery system combines fixed-post and event-driven systems. Chase vehicles, also known as "fly cars" or "chase cars," are most often used to provide ALS service. A nontransport vehicle staffed with ALS providers and equipment responds from a central location to upgrade a BLS transport unit (Figure 5-3). The chase vehicle can either respond to the scene or rendezvous with the ambulance en route to the hospital. Some systems staff the chase vehicle with two ALS providers and double equipment to allow the unit to return to service after transferring a provider and equipment to the transport unit.

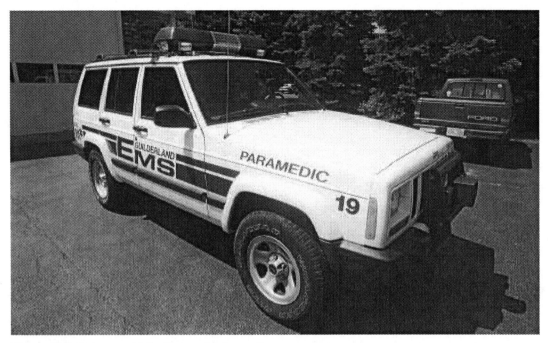

Figure 5-3 Advanced Life Support Intercept

The main advantage of a chase vehicle is that specialized services such as ALS can be provided to a large area with a minimum of staffing and equipment. A disadvantage is longer response times for ALS if the unit must cover a large geographical area. In some parts of the United States, police officers provide ALS chase vehicle service utilizing specially equipped police cars.

Staffing Configuration

Just as there are variations in delivery systems, there are also variations in EMS unit staffing. A minimum of two individuals are needed for a transport vehicle, one to drive and the other to provide patient care. This may seem logical, but prior to the modern era of EMS, some services responded only with a driver who loaded the patient in the back using a "one-man cot" and sped off to the hospital. This led to the term "ambulance driver" being used to refer to anyone who rode on an ambulance. The reader is cautioned that staffing configuration varies greatly among jurisdictions. The examples below represent the most common configurations.

BLS Staffing The staffing pattern for BLS units centers around an EMT-B providing patient care on the scene and en route to the hospital. Thus it is possible to have only one crew member trained in patient care. Although not an optimal arrangement, especially when two-person skills are required, this configuration reduces crew cost and provides greater availability of drivers. The availability of someone to drive the ambulance may be a critical issue in some volunteer organizations. It is also possible to utilize other public safety personnel such as first responders and firefighters as drivers.

The more common BLS crew configuration is EMT/EMT. This provides two trained personnel to provide patient care on the scene. Additionally, the crew members can take turns driving and providing patient care. In the event of a multipatient situation, both crew members can provide initial patient stabilization. For critical patients, it is possible for both providers to assist with patient care during transport with a first responder or firefighter enlisted to drive.

ALS Staffing Advanced life support staffing is more variable than BLS staffing. Possible staffing configurations include:

- EMT–Intermediate/EMT–Intermediate
- EMT–Intermediate/EMT–Basic
- EMT–Intermediate/other
- Paramedic/paramedic
- Paramedic/nurse
- Paramedic/EMT–Intermediate
- Paramedic/EMT-Basic
- Paramedic/other

Advanced life support staffing is dependent on the nature of the EMS system and the type of incident a unit responds to. In a single-tier system, an ALS unit will respond to both ALS and BLS calls. In a two-tier system, the ALS ambulance will only respond to ALS calls thus having two paramedics on board may be an advantage. Having a non-paramedic as the driver limits that individual to always driving and not practicing patient care skills. In rare instances, a driver with limited or no medical training may accompany a paramedic. Such an arrangement limits a unit's flexibility and places the total burden of patient care on the paramedic.

As a means to increase the utilization of fire suppression units and staff, some fire departments are assigning a paramedic to an engine or ladder company. The vehicle is equipped as an ALS upgrade vehicle. Similar to the chase car concept, the **paramedic engine company** responds to an incident and provides a paramedic and equipment. The engine company can remain in service as a fire suppression unit while the paramedic accompanies the patient in the transport unit. In the event of a fire call, the engine company would respond similarly to a regular engine company and the paramedic would function as a member of the crew. This configuration has the advantage of providing enhanced EMS response along with maintaining fire suppression capability. Likewise, the addition of a paramedic to the crew enhances unit staffing. Expensive fire trucks and crews are more fully utilized.

MOBILE HEALTH CARE

As managed care organizations search for new ways to provide lower cost health services, taking services to the patient seems a less expensive alternative than having the patient come to the hospital or clinic. This has led to the concept of **mobile health care**. Mobile health care will not only respond to less critical acute situations, but will also provide ongoing care for chronic medical problems as well as wellness and prevention activities. Given that EMS systems already have trained personnel and vehicles available, EMS was initially seen as the best source for this type of service. However, as more research is done, this may not prove to be the case given the clinical nature and volume associated with such services. The use of paramedics with expanded knowledge and skills, or the use of allied health professionals such as physician's assistants, is being investigated.

EMS VEHICLES

Having trained personnel respond to the scene of a medical or trauma emergency would not be effective if there were no means to transport the patient to definitive care. Thus a dedicated transport vehicle—an ambulance—is needed.

Ambulances have progressed from special chariots in ancient times to horse-drawn carriages during the Napoleonic period to motorized vehicles in the twentieth century.

In 1969, the National Research Council, National Academy of Sciences, published *Medical Requirements for Ambulance Design and Equipment* (NAS, 1969). From these general recommendations, the National Highway Traffic Safety Administration, in 1973, developed *Ambulance Design Criteria* (NHTSA, 1973). This document presented specific engineering criteria for ambulance design and construction. These specifications were adopted by the federal government and required for any ambulance vehicle purchased with federal funds. The General Services Administration specification for ambulances is known as **KKK-A-1822**. Ambulances designed to specification are called **star-of-life ambulance** because they are the only vehicles allowed to display the federally registered "star-of-life" emblem.

The purpose of the KKK specifications is to:

> . . . describe ambulances which are authorized to display the "Star of Life" symbol. It establishes minimum specifications, test parameters, and essential criteria for ambulance design, performance, equipment, appearance, and to provide a practical degree of standardization. The object is to provide ambulances that are nationally recognized, properly constructed, easily maintained, and, when professionally staffed and provisioned, will function reliably in pre-hospital or other mobile emergency medical service (General Services Administration, 1994).

The most significant aspect of the KKK standards is the designation of three types of ambulance designs. Each design has a configuration "A" for ALS and a configuration

"B" for BLS. Thus you may have a type IIB ambulance that is a van chassis designed for BLS transport.

Type I

The **type I ambulance** is designed as a "conventional, cab-chassis with modular ambulance body" (General Services Administration, 1994). Essentially, a type I is a pickup truck with an ambulance module in place of the truck bed (Figure 5-4). This unit is designed so that the ambulance module can be removed and placed on a new chassis as needed. Most type I ambulances do not have a means to go from the cab to the ambulance module, an arrangement known as a "walk-through."

Advantages of the type I include a more robust chassis and easy access to the engine compartment. Disadvantages are a harder ride, a greater height from street to floor in the patient compartment, and lack of a walk-through.

Type II

The **type II ambulance** is a van converted into an ambulance (Figure 5-5). The KKK specification is "standard van, forward control, integral cab-body ambulance" (General Services Administration, 1994). A standard commercial van is converted to provide more headroom by adding a raised roof. A divider panel equipped with a walk-through is installed to separate the cab from the patient compartment.

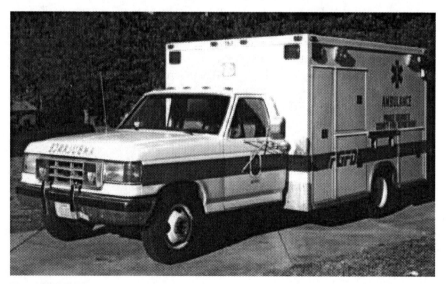

Figure 5-4 Type I Ambulance

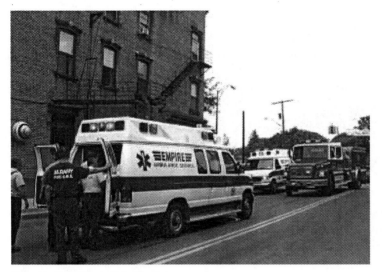

Figure 5-5 Type II Ambulance

The main advantage of a type II ambulance is cost. Of the three ambulance types, the type II is the least costly to produce. This makes it economical for BLS transport services that do not need a large patient compartment. The van is also more maneuverable. The main disadvantage is interior space. Because space is so limited, it is difficult to configure a type II ambulance for ALS even though type II ambulances are used for ALS. The van generally does not last as long as a type I and type III ambulances which have heavier chassis construction.

Type III

The **type III ambulance** combines the attributes of the type I and type II ambulance. It is the most common ambulance configuration in use today (Figure 5-6). A "specialty van, forward control and control integrated cab-body or combination containerized modular ambulance" (General Services Administration, 1994) describes the type III ambulance which has a van-style chassis with a modular ambulance body mounted similar to the type I configuration. The van chassis may be integral or connected directly to the modular body or it may be separate from the body. A walk-through is almost always provided.

Advantages of the type III include a heavier chassis than the type II, a walk-through, and increased maneuverability. Disadvantages include poor access to the engine compartment and greater wear on chassis components.

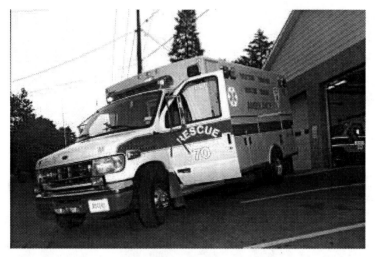

Figure 5-6 Type III Ambulance

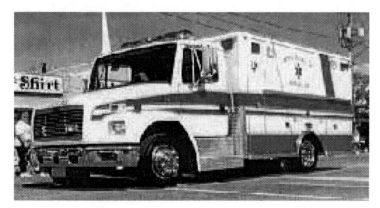

Figure 5-7 Medium Duty Ambulance

Medium Duty

Some type I ambulances are built on larger 1¼ ton chassis. These heavy-duty units are referred to as **medium duty** ambulances by some manufacturers (Figure 5-7). They are currently not specifically addressed in the KKK standards. The larger chassis provides heavier brake and power-train components as well as the ability to mount larger patient compartment modules. Disadvantages of the medium duty unit include decreased maneuverability with increased size and greater height from street level to patient compartment floor. Because this makes loading the ambulance stretcher difficult and unsafe, most medium duty units are equipped with air shocks that deflate on the scene to lower the back of the unit.

AIR MEDICAL TRANSPORT

Although the vast majority of patients are transported to definitive care by traditional ground ambulances, there are times when more rapid transport, or transport over long distances, requires other forms of transportation. Such transports are most often handled by air medical transport units. Air medical transport utilizes rotor wing (helicopter) or fixed wing (airplane) aircraft.

Advantages of air medical transport include:

- High speed
- Greater response area
- Not hindered by vehicle traffic
- Access to remote areas (rotor wing)
- Adequate patient compartment (fixed wing)

Disadvantages include:

- High cost
- Weather limits
- Increased training demand
- Increased danger to patient and crew
- Greater operational demand and control
- Greater logistic coordination (fixed wing)
- Fixed wing requires landing strip

Air medical transport can be used for on-scene response and transport or for interhospital transfers of critical patients. Crew configuration depends on the aircraft type and mission. The majority of helicopters are staffed with a paramedic and flight nurse. Fixed wing aircraft, which are used for long distance transfers, often carry a physician or critical care registered nurse. The National Association of Flight Paramedics has established a certification program for flight paramedics.

Regulation of air medical transport involves flight operations and medical control. Flight operations in the United States are under the jurisdiction of the Federal Aviation Administration (FAA). The FAA regulates aircraft airworthiness and flight crew certification as well as operational parameters. The Commission on Accreditation of Medical Transport Systems (CAMTS) provides voluntary accreditation for air medical services. Patient transfer regulations such as COBRA also apply to the transfer of patients by air.

AMBULANCE EQUIPMENT

Regardless of the type of ambulance configuration an EMS service utilizes, the vehicle alone would be of limited value if it were not properly equipped. Since 1961, the

Committee on Trauma of the American College of Surgeons has produced a list of essential equipment for ambulances. Starting in 1988, the American College of Emergency Physicians produced a similar list. In 2000, the two lists were combined.

Ambulance equipment can be grouped into two broad categories, equipment for basic level providers and equipment for advanced level providers (ACEP and ACS, 2000).

Basic Level Provider Essential Equipment

- *Ventilation and airway equipment.* Equipment for clearing and maintaining a patient's airway. Examples include suction apparatus, pocket mask, and bag-valve mask.
- *Monitoring and defibrillation.* Automatic external defibrillator (AED).
- *Immobilization devices.* Equipment for splinting suspected or broken bones. Examples include cervical collar, splints, and backboards.
- *Bandages.* Equipment for control of bleeding and care of soft tissue injuries. Examples include burn pack, gauze sponges, and roller gauze.
- *Communication equipment.* Equipment for two-way communications between provider, dispatch center, and medical direction.
- *Obstetrical delivery.* Equipment for management of childbirth.
- *Miscellaneous.* Equipment used for patient assessment and patient transfer. Examples include stethoscope, blood pressure cuff, and ambulance stretcher.
- *Infection control.* Includes equipment for body substance isolation including latex-free equipment.
- *Injury prevention equipment.* Safety equipment for crew and passengers including seat belts, helmets, eye protection, and fire extinguisher.

Advanced Level Provider Essential Equipment

- *Vascular access.* Equipment for initiation and maintenance of intravenous lines.
- *Airway and ventilation equipment.* Equipment for advanced management of the airway. Includes equipment for endotracheal intubation.
- *Cardiac.* Portable cardiac monitor/defibrillator/pacer.
- *Other advanced equipment.* Includes nebulizer, glucometer, and pulse oximeter.
- *Medications.* Medications required for advanced life support.
- *Optional advanced equipment.* Automated monitoring equipment and specialized equipment for advanced life support procedures.

SUMMARY

An EMS system would not be able to function if it did not provide a means for the transport of patients to definitive care. How transport is provided, and by whom, varies widely. Traditionally, public safety agencies such as the fire department have been the usual providers of EMS service. In other areas, commercial operators provide transportation often utilizing an event-driven deployment system, as opposed to the fixed-post staffing common of public safety agencies.

The vehicles used for EMS transportation have changed greatly over time. Through standardization developed by the federal government, ambulance vehicles are now built to a set standard based on one of three basic designs. For special, rapid transport, air medical transport utilizing rotor wing or fixed wing aircraft has proven effective.

STUDY QUESTIONS

1. Differentiate between an ambulance trust and a hospital-based EMS service provider.
2. What is meant by an integrated EMS service?
3. Discuss the advantages of event-driven staffing versus fixed-post staffing.
4. List the various types of ALS staffing.
5. Why are ambulances built to KKK-A-1822 referred to as star-of-life ambulances?
6. State a situation when air medical transport by rotor wing aircraft would be appropriate.

BIBLIOGRAPHY

American College of Emergency Physicians & American College of Surgeons. (2000). *Equipment for ambulances.* Dallas, TX: Author.

General Services Administration. (1994). *Federal specification for the star-of-life ambulance KKK-A-1822D* (GSA Publication AMBU-0001). General Services Administration: Washington, DC.

National Academy of Science. (1969). *Medical requirements for ambulance design and equipment.* Washington, DC: Author.

National Highway Traffic Safety Administration (1973). *Ambulance design criteria.* Committee on Ambulance Design Criteria and National Research Council: Washington, DC.

Stout, J. (1983). System status management: The strategy of ambulance placement. *Journal of Emergency Medical Services. 8*(9), 22–32.

Stout, J. (1985). Public utility model revisited: Part 1–origins. *Journal of Emergency Medical Services. 10*(2), 55.

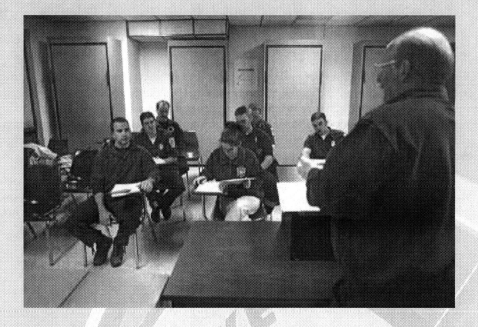

Case Study

The scene is a classroom at a municipal fire department training center. A captain assigned to EMS training is addressing a group of paramedics.

"Good morning and welcome to our annual recertification and quality review session for A and C shift paramedics. I'm glad to see that so many of you could attend on your day off. As I am sure you are aware, you will receive overtime pay for this session as required by your contract. Be sure to submit a form 22 to your station captain the next shift you work."

"To begin, I would like to introduce Dr. Stone, our medical director. I know that Dr. Stone is no stranger to you as he has ridden with most of you on calls, and you have seen him in the ED at Mercy. Dr. Stone."

"Thank you, Captain Simpson. It is indeed a pleasure to meet with all of you again. At least this meeting is a little calmer than some of the runs we have taken in the field. This morning I want to go over a few things with you. First, I want to update you on the stats from the EMS Quality Improvement Committee. Second, I want to talk about a couple of new drugs we may be seeing in the field. And finally, I want to review proper documentation of head injury patients. From my review of your run reports, this is an area that we can work together to improve. So, let's get started."

CHAPTER 6

Medical Oversight

Outline

Historical Background
Models of Medical Oversight
   Indirect Medical Oversight
      System Design
      Protocols

Education
   Quality Systems
  Direct Medical Oversight
Regulation and Legislation

Objectives

Upon completion of this chapter, the reader should be able to:

- State the role of medical oversight in EMS.
- Differentiate between medical control and medical oversight.
- Review the history of medical oversight in EMS.
- State the importance of regulation and legislation related to medical oversight.
- Describe models of medical oversight.
- Differentiate between indirect and direct medical oversight.
- State the primary roles of an EMS system medical director.
- Identify a national position paper related to medical oversight.
- Differentiate between a protocol and a standing order.

Key Terms

Algorithm
Continuous quality
  improvement (CQI)
Direct medical oversight
Indirect medical
  oversight

Medical
  command/medical
  direction
Medical director
Medical oversight
Off-line medical oversight

On-line medical oversight
Prospective
Protocol
Retrospective
Standing order
System medical oversight

HISTORICAL BACKGROUND

For many years, the term **medical direction** or **medical command** was used to describe physician involvement in EMS. The physician who took responsibility for the practice of medicine by prehospital providers was the **medical director**. Such terminology implied a rigid hierarchy of control with the physician at the top and the EMT at the bottom. As EMS systems developed and became more sophisticated, and physicians became more comfortable with their role in EMS, the concept of **medical oversight** replaced the rigidity of medical control. Oversight implies more of a quality of care approach to medical direction than just physician authorization for providers to function. This approach is more proactive and ongoing than reactive and prescriptive.

The history of medical direction and oversight parallels that of EMS system development. An early example of medical direction is the advice given to Napoleon by his physicians about evacuating injured soldiers. During the Civil War, physicians coordinated the treatment of battlefield casualties. World War II saw the introduction of trained "physician extenders" in the form of corpsmen.

In the 1960s and 1970s, the medical literature reported new advances in the resuscitation of sudden cardiac death victims. Recognizing time as an important aspect of these interventions, pioneering EMS physicians attempted to introduce techniques such as CPR, artificial ventilation, and defibrillation into the prehospital environment. In 1969, Dr. Eugene Nagel began to train members of the Miami Fire Department to provide advanced life support (ALS). As part of the training for these early paramedics, and to show support for nonphysician delivery of ALS, Dr. Nagel allowed students to intubate and ventilate him. This is perhaps the ultimate testament of physician advocacy!

Physician support for advanced life support in the field was not limited to urban areas. In the rural county of Haywood in the Great Smokies area of North Carolina, Dr. Ralph Feichter worked with the local rescue squad to develop an all-volunteer ALS team. Through support from the local medical society and hospital, Dr. Feichter trained 40 volunteers in advanced cardiac life support in the late 1960s.

The first medical directors were recruited as part-time volunteer advisors, sharing their EMS time with a career elsewhere in medicine. Momentum was developing to establish respect for the emergency medical physician's expertise in prehospital care. In parallel, legislative recognition was sought for the prehospital provider as a limited practitioner of medicine under physician oversight. By 1974, many states, local jurisdictions, or local medical societies were recognized in law as mandating medical direction for ALS providers. Although the earliest providers were very involved, the proliferation of ALS programs brought about by the availability of federal funding and the relative shortfall of available volunteer physicians led to a period of underemphasis of medical direction in EMS.

Through the 1980s, in some urban and suburban areas a "modern director" emerged, possessing special credentials and a more clearly defined role. These professionals, many of them with academic ties and teaching experience in emergency medicine, were able to apply clinical knowledge to EMS systems. The American College of Emergency Physicians (ACEP) embraced the EMS cause by publishing a position paper in 1989, *The Principles of EMS Systems* (Roush, 1989). This paper called for active participation and involvement of physicians in all aspects of EMS including design, implementation, evaluation, and system revision. General requirements for the physician in the role of medical director were also outlined. Further recognition of the activities of physicians in EMS as a unique vocation worthy of its own status led to the creation of the National Association of EMS Physicians (NAEMSP). The association became the lead physician society for prehospital emergency care. Recognizing the lack of a national standard or job description outlining the specific activities of a physician director, in 1998 the NAEMSP published a position paper containing a job description and checklist against which systems could compare their medical direction. This position paper highlighted the various duties by classifying them under many of the subsystems inherent in EMS (Table 6-1). The position paper also defined essential and desirable qualifications of directors, and makes a statement advocating appropriate support for directors by jurisdictions or agencies (Table 6-2).

The physician's role is seen as collaborative. An EMS system medical director is an advocate for the patient and public health as well as for the EMS system and the EMS

Table 6-1   Role of the Medical Director

- Dispatch
- Clinical Care, Including Continuous Quality Improvement (CQI)
- Physician Clinical Roles
- EMS Education
- Administrative Duties, Liaison Roles, Finance, and Legislation
- Public and Occupational Health Arena
- System Evaluation
- EMS Research

Table 6-2   Qualifications of the Medical Director

Essential Qualifications
- Licensed to practice medicine or osteopathy
- Familiar with local/regional EMS activity

Desirable Qualifications
- Board certification or board preparedness in emergency medicine
- Active clinical practice of emergency medicine
- Completion of an EMS fellowship

Acceptable Qualifications
- Board certification or board preparedness in a clinical specialty

---

provider. Physician involvement in EMS is not limited to medical practice issues but to all aspects of EMS. An effective EMS physician will be involved in processes before, during, and after the emergency incident.

Medical oversight has also been recognized as important for all levels of EMS provider. Traditionally, physician involvement was limited to providers delivering ALS. Now, with EMT-Bs authorized to assist patients with medications and perform more advanced techniques such as IV initiation and advanced airway control, the need for medical oversight is critical at all levels.

MODELS OF MEDICAL OVERSIGHT

With the advent of the modern EMS physician, as described by NAEMSP, the term **medical oversight** became preferable. Over the years, the definition of medical oversight has been refined. It has become a system of physician-directed quality assurance providing accountability for medical care in the prehospital setting. It is the implementation and supervision by a physician of the medical aspects of an EMS system designed to deliver emergency care in the prehospital setting.

Through medical oversight, the physician is primarily able to affect a system of care rather than each individual patient served. Second, the physician involved targets the quality of care delivered routinely and acts as a consultant for the medical aspects of delivery, which may involve each subsystem of EMS. The physician's understanding of the epidemiology of prehospital emergencies and the scientific basis for interventions drives the system's decision making. Medical direction provides and creates a line of medical accountability from patient through physician extender to physician. There are two aspects of medical oversight: indirect and direct.

Indirect Medical Oversight

Indirect, off-line, or **system medical oversight** implies physician input that is administrative, involving all facets, but remote from the patient encounter itself. By far the most relevant and comprehensive tasks for medical directors occur by indirect oversight. The basis for day-to-day care rests with the system medical director. Clearly in the United States, it has been established and accepted that physicians are not needed in the ambulance for the typical patient encounter. Rather, medical consultation is needed to help develop, and to refine, a system of care that is in place for any potential patient. As such, the medical director may have a variable role based on a system's structure. Although it would be ideal for the medical director to be involved full time, this is often not the case. At the minimum, the medical director serves as a legal means for a system and providers to function. The involvement of such directors is often limited to just signing forms, testing, and personnel approval. Some jurisdictions have primary oversight by a committee, with the medical director as a physician advisor. In others, the medical director is a primary part-time or full-time position, with a contract or job description that supports local duties and authority, and gives management status to the position. In this case, the director may be the sole ultimate authority, working with other leaders to make decisions that maintain or implement change in the system. Finally, the director may be a cabinet position directly accountable to a mayor or county executive, as would be the director of public health. In each model, there are specific areas of EMS where off-line medical direction has a place and a key role.

System Design The physician medical director brings a unique perspective to EMS system design. The physician can analyze the medical needs of a population, the available resources, the levels of providers, the geographic area, and hospital resources. The physician can then suggest design characteristics of a system that prioritizes calls, dispatches the most appropriate care in a timely manner, intervenes in a beneficial manner, and transports the client to the closest appropriate facility. This analysis may lead to system characteristics such as priority medical dispatch, tiered assignments, police or fire automatic external defibrillators (AED) first response, as well as specialty referral policies.

In addition to the system care delivered by advanced providers, the creation of EMT-B (see Chapter 4) and emergency medical dispatch (see Chapter 10) has added new practitioners and skills to the basic arena. Both the framers of the *EMS Agenda for the Future* (NHTSA, 1996) and creators of national dispatch systems advocate strong medical direction. As the design of a system calls for these levels, state agencies place the responsibility of supervision of all levels of care on physicians.

Protocols Many consider protocol development the most important off-line component of medical oversight. **Protocols** are a preauthorized set of instructions that guide patient care. Protocols often use a decision tree that flows from patient assessment to patient management. These flowcharts are called **algorithms**. A protocol consists of a series of algorithms for each of the medical and trauma situations a provider will encounter in the field. For example:

- Nontraumatic shock
- Cardiac arrest—nontraumatic (Figure 6-1)
- Trouble breathing
- Suspected myocardial infarction
- Limb amputation
- Allergic reaction

Depending on the level of medical supervision and communication capacity, system protocols may contain points at which the field provider must contact medical control for further treatment actions (Figure 6-2). This most often occurs for situations involving critical interventions or conditions that are hard to differentiate in the field.

Protocols are drafted to give the various levels of providers an appropriate amount of autonomy in intervening on a patient's behalf without immediate physician consultation. By definition, the protocols represent that part of EMS that truly parallels the practice of medicine. It stands to reason that the medical director's input into the planning, implementation, and revision of these documents is a key reason for the EMS physician's existence. Despite the need for medical expertise, diplomacy and humility dictate that the protocol development process involves managers, nurses, ED physicians, prehospital providers, and other interested professionals.

Another term that is often used synonymously with protocol is **standing order**. In some systems, a standing order refers to the ability of providers to initiate treatment on their own without direct medical control. The standing order is part of the system protocol. Others define a standing order as direct orders issued to a provider to deal with a specific patient situation. For example, a paramedic may request through direct medical control a drug order to give Valium to a seizure patient in the event the patient begins seizing. The physician's order to do so would be a standing order. However, the use of Valium in this situation is allowed under system protocol. Standing orders support protocols.

Education Emergency medical service education is a cornerstone of prospective off-line medical direction. **Prospective** refers to physician involvement while a process or activity is happening. The role of the medical director in EMS education includes academic instruction, curriculum review, setting standards for class performance, evaluation, and student counseling. In most systems, the physician must rely on qualified nonphysician EMS educators to train providers. Perhaps the ideal compromise is the physician who makes targeted appearances in the classroom, cadaver lab, megacode recertification and drills, or when new information in medicine would be best disseminated by a physician. Whenever possible, EMS students should complete a clinical rotation with the medical director in the ED.

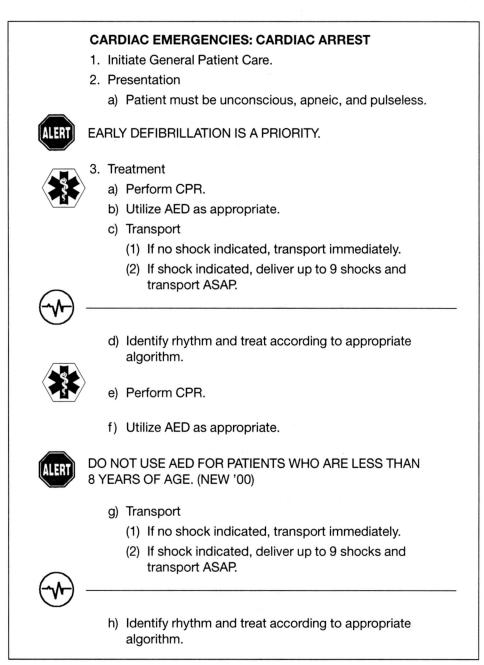

CARDIAC EMERGENCIES: CARDIAC ARREST

1. Initiate General Patient Care.
2. Presentation
   a) Patient must be unconscious, apneic, and pulseless.

ALERT EARLY DEFIBRILLATION IS A PRIORITY.

3. Treatment
   a) Perform CPR.
   b) Utilize AED as appropriate.
   c) Transport
      (1) If no shock indicated, transport immediately.
      (2) If shock indicated, deliver up to 9 shocks and transport ASAP.

   d) Identify rhythm and treat according to appropriate algorithm.
   e) Perform CPR.

   f) Utilize AED as appropriate.

ALERT DO NOT USE AED FOR PATIENTS WHO ARE LESS THAN 8 YEARS OF AGE. (NEW '00)

   g) Transport
      (1) If no shock indicated, transport immediately.
      (2) If shock indicated, deliver up to 9 shocks and transport ASAP.

   h) Identify rhythm and treat according to appropriate algorithm.

Figure 6-1 ALS Protocol Algorithm
(Reprinted with permission of the Maryland Institute of Emergency Medical Services Systems.)

CARDIAC EMERGENCIES: HYPERKALEMIA

1. Initiate General Patient Care.

2. Presentation

    a) Certain conditions may produce an elevated serum potassium level that can cause hemodynamic complications.

3. Treatment

    a) Patients must meet the following criteria:

       (1) Suspected hyperkalemia (e.g., crush syndrome) or renal dialysis patients **AND**

       (2) Hemodynamically unstable renal dialysis patients or patients suspected of having an elevated potassium with bradycardia and wide QRS complexes.

    b) Place patient in position of comfort.

    c) Assess and treat for shock, if indicated.

    d) Constantly monitor airway and reassess vital signs every 5 minutes

---

    e) Initiate IV LR KVO.

    f) Initiate Bradycardia protocol.

    g) **Administer calcium chloride 0.5–1.0 grams slow IVP over 2 minutes.**

ALERT **MAY BE MODIFIED BY MEDICAL CONSULTATION.**

    h) Place patient in position of comfort.

    i) Assess and treat for shock, if indicated.

    j) Constantly monitor airway and reassess vital signs every 5 minutes

Figure 6-2 ALS Protocol Algorithm Requiring Medical Consultation (Reprinted with permission of the Maryland Institute of Emergency Medical Services Systems.)

Quality Systems In the 1950s, one of the fathers of quality improvement (QI), W. E. Deming, brought his message to a limited number of American industries and to Japan, where he facilitated a dramatic turnaround in the quality of industrial processes and goals. By the 1980s, a renewal of interest in quality, management skills, and ultimate output brought Deming's efforts back to U.S. industries. He laid out his 14 points for the success of Western management, which include positive goals for training, communications, morale, and the elimination of traditional barriers such as workforce fear, arbitrary standards, and meaningless slogans.

Joseph Juran was a synergistic force in the area of quality management, with the development of a trilogy that describes a perpetual effort to maintain quality while looking for opportunities for improvement. In quality planning, one defines who the customers (recipients of products or services) are and their needs; determines the products that will serve those needs; and the key processes and methods of operation that will generate those products. In quality control, the processes are monitored to ensure that they maintain the appropriate output of quality products. In quality improvement, the waste or inefficiency of the process is identified as an opportunity for beneficial change. This change is implemented in the process, and a new, better zone of quality control is established.

Donabedian is one of the pioneers of quality systems with respect to health care. His well-known model focuses on three elements that are key to the delivery of services. The structure obviously determines the framework in which care can take place. The process implies the care itself, and the method of its delivery. The outcome refers to the effects of the care and the subsequent health status of patients.

All three of these concepts and their authors have relevance to EMS medical oversight. The EMS physician can advocate for education, good morale, communicating free of fear, and providing constructive feedback, consistent with Deming's principles. The director can identify patients as customers and focus on the system-wide response to needs as endorsed by Juran. The structure can parallel system design and equipment, the process relates to resources and protocols for all levels of provider and how they are educated, and the outcome may be determined through data collection mechanisms best sanctioned by a physician.

Quality of care is the ultimate goal of any health care service. Many medical directors feel that their primary role is to be the ultimate authority on quality. This emphasis on quality has led to the change in terminology from medical direction to medical oversight. Oversight infers a **continuous quality improvement (CQI)** approach to physician involvement in EMS systems.

Providers that see the medical director infrequently may view requests for information about care provided with concern and suspicion. Traditional quality assurance (QA) focuses on evaluating individual problem cases and may lead to affixing blame on providers. An EMS system and medical director who uses CQI shifts the focus away from blaming the individual provider toward studying and improving the system's process. Continuous quality improvement also uses a scientific process to collect and study data, in order to make decisions versus traditional system decision making with subjective opinions. The outcome may be determined through data collection mechanisms that are best sanctioned by physicians. The result of the medical director's commitment to CQI is an evaluation method that looks at and corrects system problems first, that promotes positive feedback using objective data, and that uses re-education to bring about cultural changes rather than encourage individual negative feedback.

In a system of CQI, there is still a place for **retrospective** review of care. Retrospective refers to the process of looking at or studying something after it has occurred, such as reviewing completed incident reports. Quality improvement takes place alongside QA and trends are identified that call for future re-education. CQI responds differently to these trends. This method is described as solving more than 80% of quality concerns. Only in very unusual cases, where educational feedback and remediation have failed, is disciplinary action the next best course. In implementing a quality management system, the physician's biggest challenge will be to find the data collection mechanism that captures long-term outcome parameters, which is often not available through the records of prehospital systems.

Direct Medical Oversight

Direct, or **on-line medical oversight** implies real-time physician involvement in a patient encounter with EMS providers. This entails communication by radio or telephone directed at obtaining advice in patient treatment. In some cases, physicians on-scene personally provided supervision. On-line medical direction is provided in several ways. First, it is most commonly described as an established consultation after the assessment of a patient and initiation of care until a decision point that requires physician input. In this model, through legislation or directly, the system director delegates the contact to other physicians who are on duty or available at the receiving hospital. Within such a system, several possibilities exist. The provider may call into an approved emergency department (ED) physician at the receiving facility. The on-line contact may be directed to a physician at a regional base station that serves more than one receiving facility. In some locals, such as the city of Pittsburgh, the on-duty EMS physician may carry a portable radio and provide consultation regardless of location while on duty. Finally, the medical director may monitor system operations and provide on-line direction to providers by radio or phone in special situations. In some locations, for instance California, specially trained allied health professionals provide on-line medical command. Nurses or paramedics answer consultations and consult with physicians for difficult or special cases.

In a less common scenario, direct medical oversight is accomplished by a physician on-scene. In this model, the medical director is most commonly involved. Some directors make a regular effort to ride in the field to monitor the process of care, as a mentorship program, to develop sensitivity to the provider's work, or to provide supervision. A physician may also be on-scene who is not part of the EMS system.

Such bystander physicians include office physicians or a physician who stops to render aid. The authority of a bystander physician to provide direct medical control varies. If a physician wishes to provide medical direction, she will often be required to accompany the patient to the receiving facility.

Although the advantage of on-line medical direction seems obvious to the casual observer, there remains true debate on the value of routine physician consultation. Indeed, the medical literature not only points to a lack of positive impact on patient care, but some studies suggest that routine on-line direction is counterproductive. However, consultation for specific, critical patient presentations or when providers desire assistance should be available.

REGULATION AND LEGISLATION

Because ALS care requires the practicing of medicine without a license, most states recognized the unique status of the paramedic. However, no state authorizes paramedics to function independently. Thus the medical director extends his medical license to the prehospital provider. The prehospital provider is practicing medicine under the medical director's license. Because of this, the medical director is responsible for the actions of the providers and incurs any liability associated with this relationship. It is this extension of licensure that the medical director most often uses to support his role in all aspects of an EMS system. The legal role of the physician in the provision of ALS is not always as clearly defined as that of the paramedic. Consequently, the physician's authority varies and is often open to interpretation.

In the early years of EMS, the development of EMS systems, especially the provision of ALS, was highly dependent on support from the local medical society. Often a local physician would become an advocate for EMS and champion its cause with the medical society and hospital. Some early EMS systems sought physician support and advocacy to institute ALS, whereas others were influenced by physicians to develop ALS. The willingness of a physician to place his license on the line was often the only form of official medical control and sanction for paramedics to perform ALS.

As ALS systems proliferated, the need for formal recognition of ALS providers and medical control was recognized. In 1970, California passed the Wedworth-Townsend Paramedic Act which legally recognized paramedics. This act served as a model for similar legislation nationwide. Maryland's early EMS laws governing the Cardiac Rescue Technician, the state's first ALS provider, mandated medical supervision starting in 1973. Other states followed this trend over time with some states not incorporating medical direction laws until after 1991. The nature of medical direction specified by state laws and regulation varies and is often open to interpretation.

Considered necessary for the delivery of ALS, medical direction has only recently been introduced for BLS services. This change was bought about by changes in the revised National Standard Curriculum for the EMT-B. States have had to change their EMS laws and regulations to expand the coverage of medical direction. Some states, such as California and New Jersey, require a designated medical director for each EMS service. In Maryland, providers can only be state certified as an EMT-B if they are affiliated with an agency that has established medical direction.

SUMMARY

Physicians play an important role in prehospital care. Since the advent of advanced life support, prehospital care has come to be accepted as the practice of medicine by physician extenders. Thus the delivery of care must be physician supervised. The nature of this supervision, which is now recognized as a quality assurance issue, has become known as medical oversight rather than the original approach of medical direction. In most states and jurisdictions, the role of the medical director is legally defined. The director is involved in system design, education, protocols, and quality management.

STUDY QUESTIONS

1. Define medical oversight.
2. State the role of CQI in system medical direction.
3. Differentiate between direct and indirect medical control.
4. Differentiate between prospective and retrospective medical oversight.
5. Briefly defend the need for the medical oversight of BLS providers.

BIBLIOGRAPHY

Alonso-Serra, H., Blanton, D., & O'Connor, R. E. (1997). *Physician medical direction in EMS*. Lenexa, KS: National Association of EMS Physicians.

Deming, W. E. *Out of the crisis*. 1986. Massachusetts Institute of Technology.

Donabedian, A. Exploration in quality assessment and monitoring (3 vols) 1980–1985. Health Administration Press.

Juran, J. M. *Juran on leadership for quality*. 1989. Free Press.

National Highway Traffic Safety Administration. (1996). *Emergency medical services: agenda for the future*. Washington, DC: Author.

Polsky, S. S., Krohmer, J., Maningas, P., McDowell, R., Benson, N., & Pons, P. (1993). Guidelines for medical direction of prehospital EMS. *Annals of Emergency Medicine. 22*, 742–744.

Roush, W. R. (Ed.). (1989). *Principles of EMS systems*. Dallas, TX: American College of Emergency Physicians.

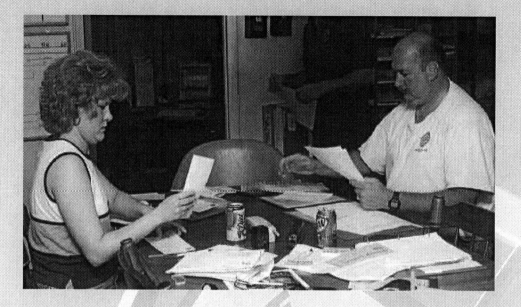

Case Study

The scene is the lounge at a community rescue squad. A group of squad members are engaged in informal conversation.

"Hey, Jim, did you see the notice on the board about the new paramedic program being offered by the community college?" asks Steve, a new member of the squad.

"Yeah, sounds pretty good. Too bad they didn't have that when I took paramedic," responds Steve, a senior member.

"How'd you get your paramedic?" asks Jim.

Steve responds "I went down to Raleigh and took it with the guys from the fire department. They offer it at the fire academy."

"You took paramedic at a fire academy?" Steve asks with a puzzled look on his face. "I thought you had to go to the hospital and stuff."

Jim replies "Yeah, we did that, too. I was able to do some of my clinical time here in town at Community."

"Well I think I'm going to apply for the college program. My dad says I should get a degree. He's probably right. But I want to make sure I do something I like and this will be perfect." Steve offers.

"You know" Jim explains, "after you get your AA degree, you can transfer to a university and complete a degree in emergency health services. Some of the colleges even have four-year paramedic programs."

"No kidding!" Steve remarks, "That could mean a lot for a person's future."

The tones sound and Jim and Steve head for the ambulance.

CHAPTER 7

Educational Systems

Outline

Objectives

Upon completion of this chapter, the reader should be able to:

- Outline the historical development of EMS education in the United States.
- State the purpose of a national standard curriculum.
- Identify the *National Emergency Medical Services Education and Practice Blueprint.*
- State the function of the National Registry of EMTs.
- List five settings for EMS education and training.
- Identify specialized courses developed to meet the needs of special clinical populations.
- State the role of continuing education in EMS provider recertification.
- State the role of accreditation in EMS education and training.

Key Terms

Academy
Accreditation
Articulation agreement
Asynchronous learning
Baccalaureate education
Certification
Clinical experience
Commission on Accreditation of Allied
 Health Education Programs (CAAHEP)
Committee on Accreditation of
 Educational Programs for the
 Emergency Medical Services
 Professions (CoAEMSP)
Continuing Education Coordinating
 Board for EMS (CECBEMS)
Continuing Education Unit (CEU)
Credit program
EMS Education Agenda for the Future:
 A Systems Approach

Field internship
Joint Review Committee on Educational
 Programs for the EMT–Paramedic
 (JRCEMT-P)
Licensure
National Emergency Medical Services
 Education and Practice Blueprint
National EMS Core Content
National EMS Education Standards
National EMS Scope of Practice Model
National Registry of Emergency Medical
 Technicians
National Standard Curriculum
Noncredit program
Reciprocity
Self-study
Site visit

HISTORICAL BACKGROUND

The education of prehospital providers in the United States can be traced back to the 1890s and the mining towns of Pennsylvania (see Chapter 2 for more detail). To provide care for injured miners, towns formed first aid clubs. Some of the original instruction was provided by members of the St. John's Ambulance Association of England as such training did not exist in the United States. As more and more towns developed first aid clubs, contests in first aid were held between the towns. In 1908, members of the executive committee of the American Red Cross (ARC) observed a first aid contest. This led to the organization of the American Red Cross First Aid Bureau. To assist the ARC in developing a national first aid course, Colonel Charles Lynch was detailed from the U. S. Army. In 1910, Lynch wrote the first in a long series of Red Cross first aid textbooks.

Until the early 1970s, ARC Advanced First Aid was the defacto standard for ambulance personnel. Although most personnel were trained to this level, there were no standards for ambulance crews so some services responded with personnel who had no formal training or had received minimum in-house training at the local rescue station. It is interesting to note that ARC first aid manuals from the 1960s state what should be done "until the ambulance arrives" yet these very manuals were the ones being used to train the ambulance personnel.

The publication of *Accidental Death and Disability: The Neglected Disease of Modern Society* (NAS/NRC, 1966) exposed the poor level of training for ambulance providers. The document stated:

> There are no generally accepted standards for the competence or training of ambulance attendants. Attendants range from unschooled apprentices lacking training even in elementary first aid to poorly paid employees, public-spirited volunteers, and specially trained full-time personnel of fire, police, or commercial ambulance companies.

The EMS Committee of the National Academy of Sciences, National Research Council (NAS/NRC), investigated the training of ambulance personnel. As a result, they published in 1969, *Training of Ambulance Personnel and Others Responsible for Emergency Care of the Sick and Injured at the Scene and During Transport*. This report outlined basic topics to be covered in a training program for ambulance personnel. The report also called for the establishment of a national training curriculum.

Concurrent with the work of the NAS/NRC, the United States Department of Transportation, as part of an initiative to reduce highway fatalities, released a request for proposals (RFP) to develop a national standard curriculum for emergency medical technicians. As a result of this federal involvement, an 81-hour national standard curriculum for training of EMTs was adopted in 1970. Revised over the years, this curriculum became the EMT–Basic National Standard Curriculum, last revised in 1994. Subsequent national standard curricula have been created for the EMT–Paramedic, EMT–Intermediate, and first responder.

CONTROVERSIES IN EMS EDUCATION

Acceptance of EMT and paramedic training was not universal and immediate. For years, ARC Advanced First Aid had been the standard. Many providers resisted EMT, viewing it as too complex and too long. A common refrain was "What are they trying to do, make us doctors?" This was especially true among ambulance providers in career departments, many of whom had been providing service for years, and were now required to return to the classroom to take new training from doctors and nurses. EMT training also required a more rigorous approach to testing including practical testing. This was in contrast to the less stringent requirements of many first aid courses. Even to this day, concern over the length of a course is often more of an issue than the course objectives or advantage to the patient.

Another controversy in EMS education is the importance of skills to define provider levels. Although the amount of knowledge increases as one moves from EMT to paramedic, many providers measure their increased responsibility in the number and nature of new skills that they can perform. One example is endotracheal intubation, a procedure used to secure a patient's airway. For years, this skill was the exclusive domain of the paramedic. With the revision of the EMT curriculum in 1994, intubation became an optional skill for basic level providers. Endotracheal intubation for EMT-Bs remains controversial for a number of reasons, but one significant reason is pressure from paramedics who fear loss of this exclusive skill. Controversy over skill level is also an issue surrounding the EMT-I level provider. Because the EMT-I can do almost all of the skills traditionally assigned to paramedics, some paramedics feel threatened. System managers and medical directors are also beginning to question the efficacy of having paramedics as the primary ALS provider when an EMT-I would suffice in most situations. What these groups fail to realize is that what truly sets a paramedic above an EMT-B or EMT-I is knowledge level. The paramedic has received a much broader education in the "what" and "why" of prehospital medicine, not just the "how."

Perhaps the greatest influence on EMS education has been the unfortunate situation of education guiding policy instead of the converse. In an ideal situation, education would serve to teach students system policy. Instead, education has been used as a tool to force system change and influence policy and protocols. It is not uncommon for students to learn techniques and medications that are not currently approved in their EMS system. Or to learn a certain protocol to pass a certifying examination and then have to "unlearn" it in order to function appropriately in their local system. This is frustrating to students and causes tension between educators and administrators. It is hoped that the educational process presented by the *EMS Education Agenda for the Future: A Systems Approach* (to be discussed later in this chapter) will eliminate this and other current controversies in EMS education.

NATIONAL STANDARD CURRICULUM

Due to federal involvement in the curriculum development process, a series of **national standard curriculums** were developed for EMS provider education. EMS is unique in that it is the only health profession to have a formalized, standard curriculum that is nationally accepted. In other areas of health care education, standards and/or guidelines exist for education and training. However, these standards are not an actual curriculum complete with learning objectives and lesson plans.

A national standard curriculum provides a basis for education. Because the curriculum is designed for national acceptance, it provides a foundation upon which states and regions can build local training programs. Many states have developed their own local training curriculums building on the national standard. Some states have even codified the national curriculum as part of their EMS legislation. The common foundation of a national curriculum, however, ensures some degree of commonality between training programs and provides a basis for national certification and **reciprocity** (acceptance of training and certification by another jurisdiction). However, because the curriculum is designed for national acceptance, it is in many ways a compromise. It is impossible to write a curriculum that will ideally serve every EMS jurisdiction. Because of this, the *EMS Education Agenda for the Future: A Systems Approach,* has replaced the national standard curriculum with a core content, practice model, and educational standards.

THE NATIONAL EMS EDUCATION AND PRACTICE BLUEPRINT

Although a national standard curriculum for EMS education exists, many states and regions have made changes and developed variations of the national curriculum. This has led to the existence of almost 40 different levels of recognized EMS providers throughout the nation.

In 1990, the National Highway Traffic Safety Administration convened a consensus workshop to review current issues in EMS, one being the need for a national "blueprint" to serve as the foundation for EMS education. A consensus work group met in May 1993 to review a draft blueprint that had been sent to a nationwide review team. Their deliberations produced the ***National Emergency Medical Services Education and Practice Blueprint***. The *Blueprint* is different from a national curriculum in that it is a guide for curriculum development and provider certification (NREMT, 1993).

The *Blueprint* identifies four levels of EMS provider—first responder, EMT–Basic, EMT–Intermediate, and EMT–Paramedic. It also identifies 16 core elements or areas germane to all four provider levels (see Table 7-1). For each core element, there are progressively increasing knowledge and skill objectives. It is the intention of the *Blueprint* that a prehospital provider could move upward through the various provider levels by building on knowledge and skills taught in previous levels. By identifying the knowledge and skills for each provider level, the *Blueprint* intended to standardize EMS provider training nationwide. The *Blueprint* remains an important component of EMS education and continues to provide the framework for the development of the National EMS Scope of Practice Model. What each level of EMS provider is capable and authorized to do can be traced directly back to the *Blueprint*.

Table 7-1   *National EMS Education and Practice Blueprint* Core Elements

- Patient Assessment
- Airway
- Breathing
- Circulation
- Musculoskeletal
- Children and OB/GYN
- Behavioral
- Medication Administration
- Neurological
- Environmental
- EMS Systems
- Ethical/Legal
- Communications
- Documentation
- Safety
- Triage and Transportation

EMS EDUCATION AGENDA FOR THE FUTURE

Education systems is one of the 14 attributes identified in the *EMS Agenda for the Future*. In keeping with the *Agenda* implementation plan of developing a specific agenda for each attribute, the ***EMS Education Agenda for the Future: A Systems Approach***, was developed. A task force of administrators, medical directors, regulators, educators, and providers worked together to develop the *EMS Agenda* that was accepted by the National Highway Traffic Safety Administration (NHTSA) in 2000. Full implementation of the *EMS Agenda* is projected for 2010. The five components below, covering curriculum, testing, and accreditation, make up the *EMS Agenda*.

National EMS Core Content

In the past, EMS providers were taught using a national standard curriculum based on the *Blueprint*. Now, the knowledge, skills, and attitudes needed for each provider level are broadly defined in the ***National EMS Core Content.*** The core content presents a broad overview of what an EMS provider must know and be able to do. It is broad in focus to allow for state-of-the-art changes as well as state and regional variations. It is also based on research and a practice analysis, neither of which was used significantly to develop the previous national standard curriculum. Because the core content is global in scope, individual provider levels can be defined as needed, building on the foundation of the *Blueprint*. Although new to EMS, the idea of a core content has been used in the education of other professions.

National EMS Scope of Practice Model

The ***National EMS Scope of Practice Model*** is developed from, and replaces, the *Blueprint*. It defines the levels of EMS providers, the knowledge and skills needed for each provider level, and the entry competencies for each level. The scope is the basis for state scopes of practice and reciprocity.

National EMS Education Standards

The core content and scope together form the basis for the education of EMS providers. The ***National EMS Education Standards*** identify the minimal terminal education objective for students completing training at each provider level. The standards are the closest of the five components to the former national standard curriculum. All educational programs are required to teach to the standards, but how they achieve the terminal objectives is not specified. Institutions and instructors may use any approach or technology they like as long as the end result of producing a competent student is met. This makes changes in both the core content and educational technology, as well as regional and state variations, easier to implement. However, this flexibility requires institutions and regulatory agencies to engage in continued evaluation of the educational process and student outcomes to ensure quality and compliance of the educational program.

National EMS Education Program Accreditation

The *EMS Agenda* calls for the national **accreditation** of all EMS training programs to ensure students and consumers that the education being provided meets national guidelines. Previously, educational program accreditation was voluntary except for a few states that require all paramedic education to be accredited by the Committee on Accreditation of Emergency Medical Services Professsions (CoAEMSP) (discussed in detail later in this chapter). National accreditation would provide for self-review and peer assessment of educational programs as a means to ensure quality and compliance with national guidelines. This remains an area of controversy in the implementation of the *EMS Agenda*. It is possible that some states may assume the role of the accreditation body. There is also a financial cost associated with the current accreditation process that may be burdensome to some small programs.

National EMS Certification

The authority to practice as an EMS provider at any level is granted by the states. This authorization is either in the form of certification or licensure. **Certification** is a means to identify persons who have demonstrated a minimally acceptable level of proficiency. **Licensure** is authorization from an agency to practice based on evidence of competency or certification. Certification may be obtained from states or recognized certification bodies. Currently, the National Registry of EMTs is the only national organization providing competency testing at a national level.

The *EMS Agenda* calls for the establishment of a single, independent, national testing agency providing national EMS certification. This agency would be accepted by all states as certifying minimal competency for all levels of providers. Only graduates of nationally accredited education programs would be permitted to participate in national testing. As with national accreditation, national testing remains controversial because of its impact on the role of states in the certification process and the acceptance of one, national testing agency.

THE NATIONAL REGISTRY OF EMTS

As emergency medical technician and paramedic training opportunities increased in the early 1970s, the need for a uniform means of evaluating EMTs and paramedics was recognized. Many states had not yet developed formal certification or licensure procedures. The formation of a national registration body served to increase the recognition of EMTs and aid their acceptance by the medical community. Thus the **National Registry of Emergency Medical Technicians** was formed in 1970 with support from the American Medical Association. The National Registry, as it is commonly known, is a not-for-profit, independent, nongovernmental agency. The National Registry develops standardized examinations for all levels of EMTs as well as standards for registration and reregistration.

Currently, the National Registry plays an important role in EMT and paramedic education and certification. National Registry registration is used by many states as a means to grant reciprocity. It is also gaining increased acceptance by states as a primary means of EMT and paramedic certification as well as moving to fill the role of a national certifying agency as specified in the *EMS Education Agenda for the Future: A Systems Approach*. Up-to-date information on states accepting National Registry can be obtained on the National Registry web site www.nremt.org. Representatives from the National Registry serve on various EMS-related boards and commissions as well as providing assistance in practice analysis and curriculum development.

CoAEMSP

As the number of institutions providing EMS education continued to grow, a means was needed to measure and ensure program quality. In 1975, paramedic was recognized by the American Medical Association (AMA) as an allied health occupation. In 1976, a number of national organizations developed educational standards for paramedic education programs. These standards, or essentials, were adopted by the Council on Medical Education of the AMA as the basis for accreditation of paramedic education programs. A **Joint Review Committee on Educational Programs for the EMT–Paramedic (JRCEMT-P)** was formed to review and recommend programs for accreditation.

In 1994, the JRCEMT-P became part of the **Commission on Accreditation of Allied Health Education Programs (CAAHEP)**, an organization formed following the withdrawal of the AMA from the allied health accreditation process. CAAHEP accredits 18 recognized allied health professions and is recognized by the Commission on Recognition of Postsecondary Accreditation (CORPA) and the U.S. Department of Education as a national accreditation body. In 2000, CAAHEP reorganized its accreditation bodies into Committees on Accreditation (CoA). The JRCEMT-P became the **Committee on Accreditation of Emergency Medical Services Professions (CoAEMSP)**. This name change also signaled the intention of the CoAEMSP to begin providing accreditation for all levels of EMS provider education programs, not just paramedic education. This was in anticipation of the call for a national accreditation contained in the *Education Agenda*.

To become accredited, a program must show compliance with the CoAEMSP guidelines. After completing a formal application, the applying institution completes an extensive **self-study**. A referee reviews the study and if found to be complete, a **site visit** is authorized. During the site visit, a program director and a medical director visit the site and verify compliance with the guidelines. If all reports are acceptable, the institution is granted accreditation for a five-year term. To remain accredited, the institution must reapply every five years and complete a new self-study and site visit.

Although useful as a means to recognize educational programs that meet a set of nationally accepted guidelines, accreditation has, for the most part, been voluntary. Some states and regions have developed their own accreditation programs similar to the national model.

SETTINGS FOR EMS EDUCATION

The delivery of EMS education takes place in a wide variety of venues including health care organizations, educational institutions, public safety agencies, and the military.

Hospitals

Hospitals have long been involved in providing EMS education. During the late 1960s and early 1970s, hospitals were the primary source of experienced health care professionals with an interest in EMS. Many hospitals had established nursing and allied health education programs that could provide the personnel and resources required to train EMTs and paramedics. The availability of a hospital in most communities meant that EMS education could be offered to a wide variety of EMS providers. It was in the best interest of hospitals to participate in EMS education as they were often the receiving site for patients treated by EMS personnel. In urban areas where hospital catchment areas overlapped, investing in EMS education could be a means to encourage EMTs to transport patients to a participating hospital thus directly affecting hospital revenue. Some hospitals even started their own EMS service.

Because of the requirement for clinical training in the advanced levels of EMT, hospitals have taken a more active role in this area. However, some institutions do provide classroom space for basic level EMT instruction which is provided by nonhospital affiliated instructors. Often, hospital-based EMS instruction is coordinated either through the hospital's existing training department or an EMS coordinator working for the emergency department. Hospitals have even developed paramedic training programs into self-supporting enterprises.

Fire Departments

The history of early EMS is filled with examples of fire departments taking a pioneering role in the development of EMS, especially in the area of ALS. One reason for this involvement was that fire departments were already in place as a means to provide emergency services. Likewise, they had an organizational and training structure that could easily be adapted to support EMS activities.

Fire departments have always placed great emphasis on training. Most fire departments have an identified training staff as well as a training facility. Often referred to as the **academy**, this facility is the focal point for training activities. It is the site for training new recruits, thus the common reference in the fire service of "having gone through the academy." As the fire service expanded its role into EMS, the academy has become the focal point for EMS training activities as well. Various models for the delivery of EMS training by fire academies have evolved. In some departments, EMS training is a division of the training staff. In others, EMS training is a function of the EMS division, but usually offered in conjunction with the academy staff.

In suburban and rural fire departments, often staffed fully or partially by volunteers, the provision of EMS training may take many forms. Local jurisdictions may have a centrally located training center that serves the needs of local fire departments. A dedicated training staff or coordinator may be employed, or part-time and volunteer instructors may staff the center. In some states, a statewide training agency provides extension or field courses in the local area, often at centrally located fire stations or training facilities. In rural or less organized locations, the provision of EMS training may be handled by the individual fire departments using internal company instructors or local resources.

Because of the unique nature of EMS training, fire departments often partner with other agencies to provide the necessary training and field experience. For example, a fire department may enlist the assistance of a nurse from the local hospital to provide instruction while utilizing the hospital as a clinical experience site. Other educational institutions such as community colleges or technical training centers may be partnered with the fire department to provide classroom and instructional infrastructure for effective EMS training.

Technical Centers

The development of EMS fostered the need to provide EMS training to individuals and organizations not traditionally associated with EMS delivery. This would include businesses, factories, industrial safety teams, organizations, and others who might need to provide on-site emergency care to special populations. Many of the traditional EMS training facilities were unable to meet the needs of such groups. Therefore, commercially operated technical training centers either developed for this purpose or an EMS curriculum was added at existing institutions. The rise of commercial providers of EMS also spawned the need for stand-alone EMS training operations.

In most states, the provision of technical training by private institutions is closely regulated and centers and programs are usually required to be accredited. The curriculum usually follows a national standard to provide students with the greatest potential for employment.

Community Colleges

Community, junior, and technical colleges play an important role in EMS education, especially at the higher levels of ALS training. Community college offerings fall into two broad categories, **credit** and **noncredit programs**. Students enrolled in a credit program not only complete course work leading to certification or licensure, but also receive college credit that can be applied toward a degree or certificate. Noncredit programs are often provided under contract with a fire department, hospital, or private provider as a means to provide training for their personnel. This approach eliminates the need for an agency to maintain a dedicated training staff and facility. Faculty for community college programs often come from the ranks of the agency or group for which the training is being offered.

The role of the community college in EMS education has increased over the years. With the development of a national standard paramedic curriculum that requires prerequisite instruction in areas such as anatomy and physiology, the community colleges are ideally suited to provide program instruction and coordination. The increasing sophistication of EMS education makes the community college an ideal setting for program delivery. In some states, such as Florida, paramedic education must take place at the community college level.

Colleges and Universities

A recent entry into the education of EMS providers has been four-year colleges and universities. Since 1980, the number of institutions providing **baccalaureate**

education in the emergency health services has grown to 17 nationwide. In addition, three graduate level programs are available.

The approach to EMS education in colleges can be grouped in three ways. One approach is to offer a strictly clinical curriculum leading to a paramedic certification. This is most common among programs offered in conjunction with medical schools and allied health programs. The second approach is a combination curriculum that provides clinical education along with administrative and management education. Such programs often have agreements with business or management departments to provide the required nonclinical course work. The third configuration is a nonclinical curriculum that does not lead to certification or licensure.

To facilitate the educational needs of paramedics who have received training outside of a college or university, some colleges provide the means to formally recognize this training. Enrolled students are able to challenge clinical courses for credit via written and practical testing. Students who have completed paramedic training at a site that is accredited by the Commission on Accreditation of Allied Health Education Programs (CAAHEP) may also receive academic credit directly from some institutions. Likewise, many public four-year colleges have "2 + 2" **articulation agreements** (two years of community college plus two years at a four-year college) with community colleges. This ensures graduates of community college programs admission into the program and allows them to enter with 60 credits toward a degree.

Military

The military has an obvious need to train personnel to serve as medics or corpsmen to provide immediate care to wounded personnel as well as to train personnel to staff aid stations, clearing stations, and field hospitals. Additionally, the military must provide basic EMS services to military, dependent, and civilian personnel at larger military installations worldwide.

The training of military personnel follows closely the provider levels in civilian EMS. Medics and corpsmen are trained as EMT-Bs with some receiving EMT-I and paramedic level training. Because military personnel are likely to be reassigned on a regular basis, it is not practical to have local certification or licensure. To address the need for certification, the military makes use of National Registry certification. The National Registry even provides special "military style" certification patches for uniforms. Because military personnel have had training equivalent to civilian EMS providers, the military is a ready source of trained providers both after personnel leave the military and while still on active duty. It is not uncommon for military personnel living in a civilian community to volunteer or work part-time for EMS services.

A current trend in military medical education and continuing education is the reduction of such training by the military and reliance on civilian training sources and contractors for general medical education. This is especially true for specialized courses

Table 7-2 Common Sites for EMS Provider Education

	Hospital	Fire Department	Technical Center	Community College	4-Year College	Military
EMT-P	X	X	X	X	X	X
EMT-I	X	X	X	X		X
EMT-B		X	X	X		X
First Responder		X				

commonly provided to civilian EMS personnel. The various sites for EMS provider education are summarized in Table 7-2.

PROVIDER COURSES

The current provider levels and what each entails are discussed in Chapter 4. This section provides an overview of the training course for each level.

First Responder

The first responder training course is a minimum of 40 hours in length. It is a mixture of knowledge and skill education with the emphasis on teaching basic, lifesaving skills to a student who has little, if any, exposure to EMS and health care. There are no prerequisites for entrance into the course. The use of specialized EMS equipment is minimal. The main goal of the course is to prepare individuals to provide lifesaving, stabilizing care until arrival of EMT-level trained personnel. The first responder would not routinely be involved in the transport of a patient to a medical facility.

Major divisions of the first responder course include:

- *Preparatory.* Including introduction to EMS, roles and responsibilities, well-being of the first responder, legal and ethical issues, overview of the human body, and lifting and moving patients.
- *Airway.* Basic techniques to maintain an airway, building on skills taught in CPR. May include use of supplemental oxygen if available to the first responder.
- *Patient assessment.* Scene size-up, initial assessment, physical examination, ongoing assessment, and vital signs.
- *Circulation.* CPR techniques for adults, infants, and children and AED (automatic external defibrillator) use.

- *Illness and injury.* Medical emergencies, bleeding and soft tissue injuries, injuries to muscles and bones, and splinting.

- *Children and childbirth.* Childbirth and common conditions associated with children and infants.

- *EMS operations.* Introduces the first responder to the EMS system.

Successful completion of the first responder courses requires passing a written and practical examination.

Emergency Medical Technician–Basic

The EMT-B is the entry level provider for transport based EMS. EMT-B training prepares the EMT-B to control life-threatening injuries, stabilize non-life threatening situations, and engage in related activities such as emergency vehicle driving and equipment maintenance. CPR is a required prerequisite for entry into EMT-B training. The EMT-B is taught to use an assessment-based approach to patient care along with specialized medical equipment such as suction devices and traction splints. EMT-B training is between 110 and 130 hours in length and may include an orientation clinic in a hospital emergency department and/or precepted patient care on an ambulance.

The EMT–Basic National Standard Curriculum Educational Model contains the following major divisions:

- *Preparation.* Introduction to EMS, well-being of the EMT-B, medical, legal, and ethical issues, the human body, vital signs, SAMPLE history, and techniques to lift and move patients.

- *Airway.* Basic techniques as well as airway management using advanced adjuncts.

- *Patient assessment.* Scene size-up, initial assessment, focused history and physical exam, detailed physical exam, ongoing assessment, communications, and documentation.

- *Medical.* General pharmacology, respiratory emergencies, cardiovascular emergencies, diabetic emergencies, allergic reactions, poisoning/overdose, environmental emergencies, behavioral emergencies, and obstetrics.

- *Trauma.* Bleeding and shock, soft tissue injuries, musculoskeletal care, and injuries to the head and spine.

- *Infants and children.* Medical and trauma emergencies related to infants and children.

- *Operations.* Ambulance operations, gaining access, hazardous materials, and multiple-casualty incidents.

Some states allow EMT-Bs to place endotracheal tubes and start intravenous lines as optional skills. Training in these areas can either be part of the basic course or an add-on module. Successful completion of EMT-B training requires passing a written and practical examination and may require clinical observation and/or ambulance ride-along time.

Emergency Medical Technician–Intermediate

Training of the EMT-I moves from the basic life support level to advanced life support. The EMT-I is intended to be a generalist who can respond to a wide variety of typical EMS incidents involving medical and trauma emergencies. Prerequisite for EMT-I is EMT-B.

A typical EMT-I course is 300 to 400 hours in length consisting of 175 to 225 classroom and laboratory hours, 50 to 75 clinical hours, and 75 to 100 hours of field internship. EMT-I training differs from EMT-B in that the student must participate in a **clinical experience**, most often in a hospital emergency room, and a **field internship** during which the student manages actual EMS incidents under the supervision of a field preceptor. The student learns to use advanced equipment, administer medications, and perform invasive procedures. Because the EMT-I course covers a wide variety of topics, it is not uncommon to have more than one course instructor.

The EMT-Intermediate National Standard Curriculum Educational Model contains the following major divisions:

- *Preparatory.* Foundations of EMT-I, overview of human systems, emergency pharmacology, venous access, and medication administration.
- *Airway management and ventilation.* Airway anatomy, basic airway procedures, endotracheal intubation, and suctioning.
- *Patient assessment.* History taking, techniques of physical examination, patient assessment, clinical decision making, communications, and documentation.
- *Medical.* Respiratory emergencies, cardiovascular emergencies, diabetic emergencies, allergic reactions, poisoning/overdose, neurological emergencies, nontraumatic abdominal emergencies, environmental emergencies, behavioral emergencies, gynecological emergencies.
- *Trauma.* Trauma systems, mechanism of injury, hemorrhage and shock, burns, thoracic trauma, and trauma patient laboratory.
- *Special considerations.* Obstetric emergencies, neonatal emergencies, pediatrics, geriatrics.
- *Assessment-based management.* An integration of assessment and patient care techniques.

As with the EMT-B, final certification requires passing a written and practical examination. In addition, the student must have completed all required clinical experience and the field internship.

Emergency Medical Technician–Paramedic

As the most complex level of prehospital provider, education of the EMT-P can take many forms and occur at a variety of locations. Prerequisites for paramedic training include EMT-B (the student does not have to be an EMT-I) and a course, or courses, in anatomy and physiology.

Training programs can be structured as one continuous course, broken into modules, or offered as college level courses following a semester schedule. Because of variations in student preparation and experience, a typical paramedic course will run between 1000 and 1200 hours of instruction. It is more difficult to arrive at a set number of hours for an EMT-P course because of the clinical and field internship requirements. These activities specify a set number of patient encounters, not a minimum number of hours. Thus one student may encounter a variety of patients in a short period of time while another may have to wait for a specific encounter.

Instruction of the EMT-P course almost always requires multiple instructors with expertise in different clinical and medical areas. It would be quite a challenge for one person to teach an entire paramedic course. In addition to a course instructor, assistant instructors are often needed for laboratory and practice sessions, and guest lecturers are used to present a particular topic, skill, or clinical area. Paramedic training programs, especially those preparing students for National Registry testing and/or accredited by CoAEMSP, will also have a designated physician medical director.

The EMT-P course, like EMT-I, requires clinical experience and a field internship. In addition, the student may participate in special training experiences such as cadaver lab and pediatric airway practical. The field internship is designed to be a capstone experience that brings together all the knowledge, skills, and attitudes learned by the student throughout the class. Thus the internship is most often the last activity in which the student participates.

Course completion is based on successful completion of a written and practical test, completion of clinical patient encounters, and a successful evaluation of the field internship experience by a preceptor(s). Some programs also require review and final approval by the educational program medical director.

The EMT–Paramedic National Standard Curriculum Educational Model contains the following major divisions:

- *Preparatory.* EMS systems, roles and responsibilities, well-being of the paramedic, illness and injury prevention, medical/legal/ethical issues, general principles of pathophysiology, pharmacology, venous access and medication administration, therapeutic communications, and life span development.
- *Airway management and ventilation.* Basic and advanced airway procedures including nasotracheal intubation and surgical airway.
- *Patient assessment.* History taking, techniques of physical examination, patient assessment, clinical decision making, communications, and documentation.

- *Medical.* Pulmonary, cardiology, neurology, endocrinology, allergies and anaphylaxis, gastroenterology, renal/urology, toxicology, hematology, environmental conditions, infectious and communicable diseases, behavioral and psychiatric disorders, gynecology, and obstetrics.

- *Trauma.* Trauma systems, mechanism of injury, hemorrhage and shock, soft tissue trauma, burns, head and facial trauma, spinal trauma, thoracic trauma, abdominal trauma, and musculoskeletal trauma.

- *Special considerations.* Neonatology, pediatrics, geriatrics, abuse and assault, patients with special challenges, and acute interventions for the chronic care patient.

- *Assessment-based management.* Same as for the EMT-I.

- *Operations.* Ambulance operations, medical incident command, rescue awareness and operations, hazardous materials incidents, and crime scene awareness.

SPECIALIZED COURSES

Although EMS education is centered around a national core content and educational standards, the need has been shown for specialized courses that focus on a particular patient population. Stand-alone courses to address the needs of the trauma victim, cardiac victim, and pediatric patient have been developed. These "alphabet soup" courses are presented in an intense format usually designed around a weekend program of 16 hours. Textbooks, instructional materials, and instructor training are provided by the sponsoring agency. Students are required to pass a written and/or practical test to receive a certificate of successful completion. Until about five years ago, students successfully completing courses received "certification" but this is no longer done due to legal concerns. Table 7-3 lists common specialized courses and sponsoring agencies.

CONTINUING EDUCATION AND REFRESHER TRAINING

Prehospital provider education exposes the student to a vast body of knowledge and a variety of skills. The comprehensive nature of EMS requires that the student possess a basic knowledge of a wide variety of medical conditions and complications. However, the length of EMS training programs is insufficient to develop competency in all areas. Additionally, the case mix seen by the average field provider does not provide an opportunity for practice in all areas of EMS. Thus over time, the provider is inclined to forget rarely used knowledge and skills. This natural decay of proficiency is one reason continuing education and refresher training is required of most certified or licensed prehospital providers.

Table 7-3 Specialized Provider Courses*

American Heart Association (www.americanheart.org)
Advanced Cardiac Life Support (ACLS)
Advanced Cardiac Life Support—Experienced Provider (ACLS-EP)
Pediatric Advanced Life Support (PALS)
Neonatal Advanced Life Support (NALS)

BTLS International (www.btls.org)
Basic Trauma Life Support—Basic (BTLS-Basic)
Basic Trauma Life Support—Advanced (BTLS-Advanced)
Basic Trauma Life Support—Access (BTLS-Access)
Basic Trauma Life Support—Pediatric (BTLS-Pediatric)

National Association of Emergency Medical Technicians (www.naemt.org)
Advanced Medical Life Support (AMLS)
Prehospital Trauma Life Support—Basic (PhTLS-Basic)
Prehospital Trauma Life Support—Advanced (PhTLS-Advanced)

University of Maryland, Baltimore County (www.ehs.umbc.edu)
Critical Care Transport (CCEMTP)
Pediatric and Neonatal Critical Care Transport (PNCTT)

American Academy of Pediatrics (www.aap.org)
Pediatric Education for Prehospital Providers (PEPP)

Wilderness Medical Associates (www.wildmed.com)
Wilderness EMT
Wilderness Advanced Life Support (WALS)

Alfred State College (www.farmedic.com)
Farmedic

American Burn Association (www.ameriburn.org)
Advanced Burn Life Support (ABLS)

*This list is not intended to be all-inclusive; new courses are developed on a regular basis.

The field of medicine in general, and EMS in particular, is constantly changing. New approaches, procedures, drugs, and equipment continually appear. Each new addition requires that the field provider receive training in the new intervention. In order to keep current professionally, the field provider must participate in continuing education. Continuing education also provides a means for reviewing areas identified through quality assurance assessments as needing attention.

Continuing education for EMS providers is often part of recertification or relicensure requirements. Providers are required to complete a minimum number of hours, often in specified topic areas or a formalized refresher course. Additional hours in area(s) of the provider's choosing may be required to meet the total hour requirement. Run sheet reviews, case presentations, and rounds are examples of other approaches to continuing education.

Because of the varied nature of continuing education, a means is needed to "collect" continuing education credits and to standardize the value of a continuing education experience. This is provided by the use of **continuing education units** (CEU). One CEU is awarded for participation in a set number of hours of continuing education. The term *continuing medical education* (CME) is commonly used for physician continuing education. The value of a CEU and approval for a program to offer CEUs is determined by the various professional and regulatory agencies in the EMS field. To provide standardization in EMS education, a national group made up of representatives from EMS organizations was formed, **Continuing Education Coordinating Board for EMS (CECBEMS)**. The board approves continuing education programs and assigns the number of CEUs to be awarded.

For continuing education to be effective, it must be available to providers in a convenient form. Providers wishing to participate in continuing education may do so through any of the following activities:

Conferences and expositions

Local training programs

Regional or state training programs

Magazine articles in trade journals

Subscription videotapes

Satellite and cable broadcasts

Commercial training enterprises

In contrast to continuing education, refresher training implies a formal, structured educational activity. Participation in a refresher program is often mandated for recertification or relicensure. Typical refresher programs run 24 to 48 hours in length and provide an overview of the entire curriculum as well as important skills. A written and/or practical test may be associated with this training. The national standard curriculums recommend biannual refresher training.

TECHNOLOGY IN EDUCATION

There was a time in EMS education when an instructor would just show up at an ambulance station, set up some tables and chairs, pull a few items off the ambulance for demonstration, and be all set to teach. That rarely is the case today. Advances in educational technology as well as the sophistication of prehospital care have changed our approach to education. Longer course length, more required training, and increased responses are placing greater demands on EMS providers. Any time spent for training must be used efficiently.

Technology plays two major roles in EMS education. First, it assists the instructor in producing course materials and instructional aids. For centuries, teachers wrote on blackboards with chalk. Now, this process seems archaic. The availability of word-processing programs, color laser printers, scanners, multimedia production programs, streaming video, and computer projection allow the instructor to make audiovisual productions that only 10 years ago would have required production by a graphics studio. When computer generated audiovisual material is coupled with the Internet, the possibilities are almost endless. Instructors who do not use the latest technology are almost considered inferior by students even if the knowledge they impart is sound.

The second role of technology is in the area of skills instruction. Many of the techniques used in EMS are invasive, requiring insertion of a needle or cannula into the body. It is not always practical or ethical to have students perform these skills on each other or patients who do not have a clear medical need. It is also not possible to present every type of patient or pathology to a student. The alternative is simulation.

Simulation has been used in medical and EMS education for years. Many a student learned to give an intramuscular injection using an orange. And the history of medical education contains numerous accounts of students and physicians "robbing graves" to acquire cadavers for experimentation and learning (see Chapter 2). One of the earliest examples of simulation in EMS was the development of the CPR manikin by Asmund S. Laerdal in 1960. It was Mr. Laerdal's belief that a realistic looking manikin would help people learn CPR (Laerdal, 2000). Now, the inanimate CPR manikin has been connected to a computer that not only gives feedback of student performance, but also allows the manikin itself to respond in different ways. As advanced as this may seem, the potential of virtual reality will surely replace this analogue model with an educational experience as real and intense as actual CPR. The future of technology in EMS education is only limited by computer and virtual technology and by our ability to apply it to an educational experience.

ASYNCHRONOUS LEARNING

The traditional approach to education is to have students come to the instructor in an environment designed for learning. In EMS education, this approach has been slightly modified with the ability of the instructor to come to a physical location where a group of students is clustered. Now, it is no longer a requirement for students and instructor to assemble in one physical location. Computer and data transmission technology have provided the means to bring instruction to any student, at any place, at any time. This concept is known by a number of different names including distance learning, distance education, distributed learning, technology enhanced learning, and **asynchronous learning**. The learning is asynchronous in that the participants do not have to be temporally or geographically synchronized, i.e., in the same place at the same time.

Asynchronous learning has great potential in EMS education. Many EMS providers are shift workers, making it difficult to have each provider in the same classroom at the same time. Asynchronous learning provides a means to present educational materials to each shift or individual provider at a time most convenient to them. This eliminates the need for overtime shifts and allows for the rapid dissemination of information. Likewise, the student residing in an area not served by an EMS educational site would be able to receive training she would otherwise not have access to. Students are not the only ones who benefit from asynchronous learning; instructors and experts can now be available to students around the world to provide the best in EMS and medical education.

SUMMARY

The provision of education for prehospital providers takes many forms and occurs in a variety of settings. To ensure consistency in the delivery of prehospital education, the *EMS Education Agenda for the Future: A Systems Approach* has been adopted. This consensus document calls for the establishment of a core content and practice mode to support national education standards. Programs teaching EMS will be accredited and participate in national testing. Additionally, technology and asynchronous learning will shape and change the future of EMS education.

STUDY QUESTIONS

1. List, in chronological order, the major events that led to the development of a national standard curriculum for the EMT.

2. What is the purpose of a national standard curriculum?

3. Which document serves as a guide for curriculum development and provider certification?

4. Which organization provides a means for EMTs and paramedics to obtain reciprocity between states?

5. List six settings for EMS education and training.

6. Define asynchronous learning.

7. How is skills competency ensured once a prehospital provider is initially certified?

8. Briefly describe the CAAHEP accreditation process.

BIBLIOGRAPHY

Laerdal. (2000). Available: www.laerdal.com/html/annepop/html

National Academy of Sciences, National Research Council. (1969). *Training of ambulance personnel and others responsible for emergency care of the sick and injured at the scene and during transport*. Washington, DC: National Academy Press.

National Academy of Sciences, National Research Council. (1966). *Accidental death and disability: The neglected disease of modern society*. Washington, DC: Author.

National Highway Traffic Safety Administration. (2000). *Emergency medical services education agenda for the future: A systems approach*. Washington, DC: U.S. Government Printing Office.

National Registry of Emergency Medical Technicians. (1993). *National emergency medical services education and practice blueprint*. Columbus, OH: Author.

Pickett, S. E. (1923). *The American National Red Cross: Its origins, purpose, and service*. New York: The Century Co.

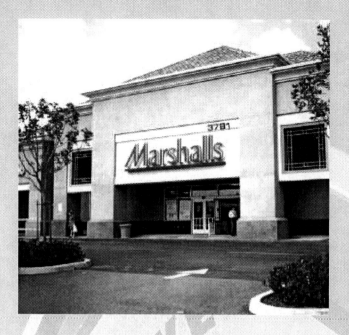

Case Study

The scene is a local shopping center.

"Good morning, my name is Tina and I'm an EMT with the rescue squad. Would you like to have your blood pressure checked?" she asks a middle age woman walking by.

"I'm in a bit of a hurry." responds the woman.

"I understand," says Tina. "Here is some information about the rescue squad. If you have any questions please contact us."

The woman takes the information and glances at the pamphlet cover. "You people are volunteers?" she asks.

Tina responds enthusiastically, "Yes, we are an all-volunteer organization."

The woman responds: "You mean if my family needs an ambulance only volunteers will come? I had no idea. Where we used to live the firemen ran the ambulance. Do you have training and equipment like they did?"

Tina replies, "Oh yes. We are all certified by the state and are nationally registered. And the state inspects our ambulance and equipment every year. You and your family should stop by the squad. We'd love to tell you more about us and answer any questions."

"I'll mention it to my husband." The woman begins to walk away, then pauses, "If you people are volunteers, then what do I get for my tax dollars?"

Tina begins to explain support for the rescue squad. The woman remains attentive and finally continues on her way, thanking Tina for the information.

CHAPTER 8

Public Education

Outline

Objectives

Upon completion of this chapter, the reader should be able to:

- State the role of public education in EMS.
- Define PIER and list its components.
- State the general goals of any PIER activity.
- List the stages of the public education process.
- Identify activities related to the three components of PIER.
- Describe the benefits to the EMS organization, the patient and public, and EMS providers of public education.
- Value the role of PSAs in public education.
- State the importance of technology in the delivery of public education.

Key Terms

Public education

Public information

Public information, education, and
   relations (PIER)

Public information officer (PIO)

Public relations

Public service announcement (PSA)

PUBLIC EDUCATION

The provision of EMS is a public service. As such, EMS must effectively communicate with the public it serves. This communication can take many forms and serve a variety of purposes. For instance, an EMS service may want to inform residents about a new level of service being offered, or the importance of using 911 to call for assistance. A system may also utilize public education to gain community support. Many EMS services are tax funded so maintaining public support is important.

Another, more contemporary form of public education in which EMS is becoming involved is wellness and injury prevention. Preventing illness and injury has not traditionally been seen as a concern of EMS. However, changes in both health care delivery and in attitudes within EMS have focused attention on this area. This idea will be discussed in more detail in Chapter 9. However, public education is an integral part of any prevention strategy. To be effective at preventing illness and injury you must have a well-informed public.

Many EMS services are already actively involved in some form of public education. This is especially true of volunteer organizations that rely on the public for direct financial support. Some common examples include:

- Signs and billboards at the EMS or fire station
- Newspaper articles
- Direct mailings
- Door-to-door solicitation
- Blood pressure checks at shopping areas and malls
- Participation in community events
- Station open house
- Visits to schools and day care facilities
- Presentations to civic organizations
- Reports to governmental boards and councils

Forms of Public Education

As seen from the list above, public education can take many forms. A common acronym to describe these activities is **PIER—public information, education, and**

relations. PIER was developed by the National Highway Traffic Safety Administration (NHTSA, 1994) and the Federal Emergency Management Agency (FEMA) to assist EMS agencies in effectively interacting with the public.

Public Information Public information activities involve informing the public about an event or incident. It is "news." When a reporter arrives at an incident scene, information provided by EMS is **public information**. Public information may also include announcements of upcoming events, fundraisers, membership drives, awards presented to members, etc. Public information is anything a service wants to tell the public about. Many services have a **public information officer (PIO)** who is responsible for public information activities and who serve as a focal point for the news media.

Public Education Changing the public's knowledge or skills is the goal of **public education**. It is the process of educating the public about an issue of importance to EMS. A community CPR class would be an example of public education. The class is designed to teach the public the skill of CPR.

Public Relations Of the three components of PIER, public relations is probably the hardest and most overlooked. **Public relations** is the process of shaping public opinion. It is the activities an organization engages in to convey a particular image or change the public's perception. For instance, if the local government is planning to cut taxes, the rescue squad may try to convince the public that this is bad because it will reduce funding for EMS. The squad will use public information and public education to garner support for their position.

Public relations is something an EMS organization must be constantly concerned about. Everything an organization does is subject to public scrutiny. And how the public perceives something may not be the reality of a situation. Take for instance the simple act of a duty crew taking an ambulance to the local ice cream shop for a snack while on duty. Some members of the public may see this as unnecessary vehicle wear and tear or fuel usage. They don't see this as an incentive for personnel to be at the station and available for emergency response. It is important for EMS systems to constantly be aware of how their actions will be viewed and interpreted by the lay public.

Benefits of Public Education

Engaging in public education and the broader PIER activities benefits not only the EMS system, but also the people served by the system and the individual EMS provider. The benefits of PIER to EMS are listed in Table 8-1.

PUBLIC EDUCATION PROCESS

Public education activities can take many forms. However, all such efforts involve the same basic steps. For public education to be effective, an EMS service must target programs for a specific community need and thus reach the right people. But most

Table 8-1   Benefits of PIER to EMS

Benefits to EMS

- Increases efficient use of existing resources by educating the public to prevent or properly respond to emergencies
- Increases political exposure and support
- Increases public support for additional resources
- Increases service membership and retention of current members
- Improves morale through positive public and internal recognition

Benefits to the Patient/Society

- Reduces the number of deaths and disabilities by educating the public on self-care, first response, and bystander care
- Reduces costs (for both the patient and health care in general)
- Reduces emotional trauma
- Improves EMS response
- Increases community pride, which aids in recruiting new businesses and residents

Benefits to Providers

- Increases recognition and rewards for community service
- Increases job security and ability to move up in ranks
- Increases personal satisfaction
- Improves the working environment

From National Highway Traffic Safety Administration and Federal Emergency Management Agency. (1994). *EMS PIER Manual: Public Information, Education and Relations in Emergency Medical Services* (FA-151). Washington, DC: U.S. Government Printing Office.

importantly, all public education must provide a consistent message. And, like all activities, it is important to constantly evaluate the effectiveness of every program and activity.

Delivery of a public education program begins first with planning. Planning will allow for the identification of program goals and objectives. It is important to consider a community's most critical need when planning public education activities. Planning will also help to identify the resources needed to carry out the educational activity. How to measure success must also be identified during the planning process. Evaluation should be planned and not something that is done after the activity has occurred.

As an example, an EMS service recognizes that bystanders are frequently removing young children involved in car crashes from car safety seats prior to the arrival of EMS. To address this problem, the EMS service plans a public education program. During the planning process, a working group of interested members would identify the specific problem to be addressed, in this case removing children from car seats. Next they would set a goal for their educational effort. This should be obtainable and measurable. A realistic goal might be to reduce the number of children removed from car safety seats by 50% within six months. Now that a goal has been set, the working group decides on a strategy, or strategies, as presented in Table 8-2, to reach their goal. They also decide that they will measure attainment of the goal by reviewing EMS incident reports for six months after initiation of public education activities.

The scope of a public education activity may be such that the EMS system alone cannot support it, or that it must reach members of the public not routinely impacted by EMS. This will require the development of partnerships and creative alliances to effectively deliver the proper message. Examples include working with civic organizations, church groups, special needs populations, social clubs, or other government agencies. The local news media should not be overlooked as a source of assistance. The media already has an established delivery system. Working with the media will help to develop a positive relationship that can lead to "more favorable press."

Using the child safety seat example, the EMS service realizes that they alone cannot get the message out to the general public. The working group meets with representatives of the local print media and radio stations. Together, they develop a PSA (see Figure 8-1) to be printed and aired over the next two months.

Evaluation of a public education activity must consider all aspects of the activity. Because an activity may be designed to change public behavior, immediate success cannot always be determined. For example, a three-month campaign educating the public about when to call EMS may not give immediate results. However, after reviewing and comparing a year's worth of run statistics, it may be seen that the number of inappropriate calls has declined. Evaluation should address issues of program planning, program monitoring, impact assessment, and resource utilization. In simpler terms, did you target the right population, reach that population, achieve your goal(s), and do so cost effectively? Regardless of the success or failure of a program, it is important to share the results with other EMS systems, public safety organizations, and community groups. By exchanging information, EMS systems and community organizations can work together to more effectively educate the public.

Public Service Announcements (PSA)

It is beyond the scope of this chapter to present and discuss all the methods available to reach the public. But one approach that is commonly associated with the emergency services is the **public service announcement (PSA)**. These are free spots on broadcast media or ads in print media. Broadcast stations are required to engage in

Table 8-2   Targeted PIER Strategies

EMS Organization Members
- Newsletters
- In-house communication pieces
- Recruitment materials
- Presentations
- Classes/courses
- Recognition programs
- Customer service training

Medical Community, First Responders, Nursing Homes, etc.
- Direct mail brochures
- Print or public broadcasts
- EMS system access materials
- Articles in local and national trade magazines
- Press kits
- Newsletters
- Audiovisual lectures and presentations
- Mock disaster exercises
- Support and assistance with other medical community programs
- Presentations

Local Government / EMS Regulators
- Newsletters
- Press kits
- Community service projects
- Presentations
- Brochures and reports
- Information and professional EMS lobbyists

General Public
- Community education programs and certifiable EMS training
- Community involvement—health fairs and civic organizations
- Public information through the media
- Public safety campaigns

From National Highway Traffic Safety Administration and Federal Emergency Management Agency. (1994) *EMS PIER Manual: Public Information, Education, and Relations in Emergency Medical Services* (FA-151). Washington, DC: U.S. Government Printing Office.

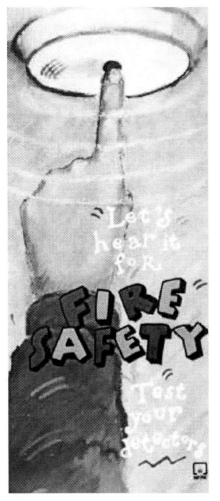

Figure 8-1 Sample Public Service Announcement (PSA)

some form of public service by the Federal Communications Commission (FCC). Stations often meet this requirement by providing free airtime to public safety and civic organizations. Stations will often assist with the scripting and production of PSAs. State or national EMS organizations may make prerecorded PSAs available to local EMS services for broadcast in their area. A common example would be announcements supporting local EMS during National EMS Week. State EMS agencies may produce PSAs to support EMS in general statewide. Broadcast PSAs typically run in 15 to 10 second spots. For newspapers and magazines, professionally developed ad copy is available. Some copy can be altered to include the name of the local EMS agency.

Although not a true PSA, many civic organizations will sell community calendars. Local residents can pay to have a birthday or anniversary listed. Meeting and fundraising dates are frequently included for public safety agencies free of charge as well as fire and safety messages. An example of this approach that has been especially helpful is PSAs reminding people to change the batteries in their smoke detectors.

Public Education and Technology

Changes in the technology of communication will affect the delivery of public education. Integration of the traditional telephone with cable television and the computer have led to new possibilities for information exchange. As the Internet becomes as common as the newspaper for communications, some EMS services have already embraced this technology. It is becoming common for EMS services to have web pages. Sites on the web provide information on practically every topic of interest to the public. EMS systems must be aware of new opportunities to reach the public and have the resources to effectively communicate in new and emerging media.

SUMMARY

The exchange of information with the public is essential to the operation of any EMS system. Such exchange is not limited to the traditional form of newspaper articles on annual service events, but must encompass all means of communications. Services use public education for both organizational and preventive aspects of EMS. Through a combination of public information, public education, and public relations (PIER) EMS systems extend their message and image to the community. Development of effective PIER programs involves planning, resources, and evaluation to reach the right people with the right message to bring about planned change. How services conduct public education is changing with technology and to remain effective, services must adapt to this technology as well.

STUDY QUESTIONS

1. Define PIER.

2. List three examples of activities associated with each component of PIER.

3. List the general goals of any public education activity.

4. Discuss how a community CPR program can benefit an EMS system, the general public, and EMS providers.

5. Briefly describe a PSA related to EMS or public safety that you have seen in the media.

6. Select a current communications technology and describe how it can be used to provide public education.

BIBLIOGRAPHY

National Highway Traffic Safety Administration and Federal Emergency Management Agency. (1994). *EMS PIER Manual: Public Information, Education and Relations in Emergency Medical Services* (FA-151). Washington, DC: U.S. Government Printing Office.

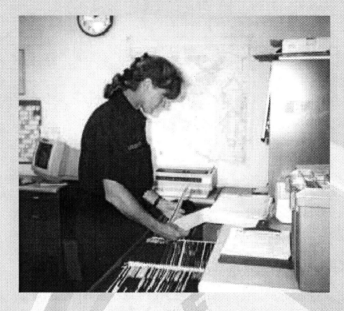

Case Study

While analyzing patient care reports during an ongoing quality assurance program members of a local EMS system identify a consistently large number of elderly individuals who suffer from falls in their homes. When further examined it is determined from the narrative on the report that the patients appeared to have tripped, causing them to fall. A program is designed to educate elderly members of the community on how to safely move about their homes. Included in the program are safe ways to go up and down stairs, the use of nightlights, and education about reducing floor hazards, such as throw rugs that can be tripped over. The program also includes a home safety checklist and a voluntary home inspection program to be performed by the EMS providers during off peak hours. The program is implemented, with community lectures hosted by off-duty EMS providers, the home safety list and home inspections advertised in the local newspaper, and EMS providers distributing information packets to elderly fall victims and their families to reduce future falls. Several months after the implementation of the fall prevention program, an examination of calls for elderly fall patients reveals that the incidence of falls has decreased.

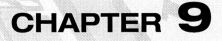

CHAPTER 9

Prevention

Outline

Injury Process
The Injury Event
Injury Types
  Falls
  Drowning
  Poisonings
  Violence
  Motor Vehicles
  Bicycles

Injury Prevention Concepts
  Interventions
  Surveillance
EMS and Injury Prevention
  Developing an Injury Prevention
Program

Objectives

Upon completion of this chapter, the reader should be able to:

- Identify the magnitude of the injury problem.

- Identify the components of the injury event.

- Differentiate between intentional and unintentional injuries.

- Discuss traffic-related injuries.

- Describe countermeasures against injury.

- Be familiar with the interpretation of Haddon's matrix.

- Identify the three E's of injury prevention.

- State the role of EMS in injury prevention.

Key Terms

Agent	Mortality	Three E's of injury
Environment	Prevention	prevention
Haddon's matrix	Primary prevention	Unintentional injuries
Host	Secondary injury	Vector
Injury	prevention	Years of Potential Life Lost
Intentional injuries	Surveillance	(YPLL)
Morbidity	Tertiary injury prevention	

INJURY PROCESS

Injury is the single greatest killer of Americans between the ages of 1 and 44. Every year, nonfatal injuries cause one in three of us to seek medical attention or render us unable to perform normal activities (National Research Council, 1985). The cost of injury is estimated to be over $180 billion annually. This number is more than twice the cost of cardiovascular disease and cancer combined (Campbell, 1998). Injury is the third leading cause of death and disability in all age groups and accounts for more **years of potential life lost (YPLL)** than any other health problem. (Baker et al., 1992). YPLL is a measure of the impact that injury and illness have on a society.

The modern view of injury began in the early to mid-1900s with the idea that some personal responsibility should be taken for injury. Motor vehicle crashes, house fires, drownings, assaults, and all the other ways in which injuries occur are not, as we used to think, accidents—random, uncontrollable acts of fate. They are understandable, predictable, and preventable. Injury is a public health problem that needs to be addressed by all health care personnel because it has consequences for the health of all Americans. Traffic injuries alone have produced more fatalities than all the wars in which the United States has fought, combined (National Committee for Injury Prevention and Control 1989).

THE INJURY EVENT

An injury is any unintentional or intentional damage to the body resulting from acute exposure to thermal, mechanical, electrical, chemical, or radiating energy or from the absence of such essentials such as heat or oxygen (National Committee for Injury Prevention and Control, 1989). Examples of the various types of injury relating to energy are found in Table 9-1.

Table 9-1   Injuries Relating to Energy

Energy Type	Explanation	Example
Thermal	Results from contact with source of heat or cold.	Burns, frostbite, heatstroke, hypothermia, etc.
Mechanical	Most common (motion) of all injury-causing energy types. Involves transfer of force between two moving objects.	Motor vehicle crashes, falls, penetrating injuries, etc.
Electrical	Involves the human body being subjected to an electrical field or current.	Lightning strike, contact with source of live electric current
Chemical	Involves the introduction of a chemical to the human body. This includes the ingestion of drugs.	Industrial incidents, HAZMAT spills, poisoning, overdose, chemical burns
Radiating	Exposure to radioactive isotopes which cause cellular mutation, illness, etc.	Nuclear incidents, industrial incidents, military actions

In this chapter, injuries will be discussed utilizing an epidemiological model to examine injuries and the injury process. It is often helpful to view an injury from an epidemiological perspective, because injuries have elements similar to those of other diseases and include a host, agent, vector, and environment. Injury events are also classified as occurring preevent, event, and postevent. In addition, injuries can also be characterized by epidemic episodes, seasonal variation, long-term trends, and demographic distribution.

The **host** is the person injured. The actual **agent** of injury is energy, and the mechanism by which that energy is transferred is the **vector**. For example, an automobile can be a vector for physical energy in a car crash, just as a faulty appliance can be a vector for electrical energy. In some cases, however, injury may also result from a lack of essential elements such as oxygen or heat. The **environment** is the surroundings in which an injury occurs. The environment provides an opportunity for the agent to be transferred to the host. For example, the environment may be a poorly lit road on a rainy night that contributed to a car crash (Gordan, 1949; Gibson, 1961; Haddon, 1963). Table 9-2 identifies the relationships between the injury, host, agent, vector,

Table 9-2   Relationship Between the Injury, Host, Agent, Vector, and Environment

Disease/ Injury	Host	Agent	Vector	Environment
Fall	Human	Mechanical (kinetic) energy	Flight of stairs	Poorly lit stairwell with no handrails
Poisoning	Human	Chemical energy	Toxic substance	Chemicals in nonchild-proof containers
West Nile Virus	Human	Flaviviridae	Mosquito bite	Areas with mosquito carriers present

and environment. Note that the third example compares the components of the injury event to a classic infection.

INJURY TYPES

Throughout history, injury has been a major cause of premature death. In modern America, injury takes a high toll on the lives of our citizens and is the leading killer of our children, teenagers, and young adults. Nearly 19,000 children and teenagers under age 20 died from injuries in 1997 in the U.S. Of these, 8,130 died of injuries related to motor vehicles; 3,749 were murdered; and 2,109 were suicides. Injuries such as falls and fires caused the other 4,802 deaths. In 1997, almost 150,000 Americans died because of injuries, and every year hundreds of thousands of Americans are nonfatally injured. Many suffer permanent disabilities (CDC, 2000).

Injuries are often classified by the behaviors and events that preceded them and the intent of the people involved. The commonly used major subdivisions of injuries include intentional and unintentional injuries. **Intentional injuries**, those caused with the desire to induce harm upon someone, include homicides, suicides, and assaults. **Unintentional injuries**, those caused without an intent to do harm, may include falls, motor vehicle crashes, and drowning. Although the events leading to intentional and unintentional injuries may be different, the mechanisms of injury and the injuries themselves are usually similar. For example, ingesting a toxic substance produces the same outcome even though the spectrum of behavior can range from completely unintentional, as when a person is not aware of the presence or nature of a drug or its potential effect, to overtly suicidal self-poisoning.

Falls

In the United States, one of every three adults 65 years old or older falls each year (Tinetti, Speechley, & Ginter 1988; Sattin, 1992). Falls are the leading cause of injury deaths among people 65 years and older. Fall-related death rates are higher among men than women and differ by race. White men have the highest death rate, followed by white women, black men, and black women (Hoyert, Kochanek, & Murphy, 1999). For adults 65 years old or older, 60% of fatal falls happen at home, 30% occur in public places, and 10% occur in health care institutions (Sorock, 1988). Of all fractures from falls, hip fractures cause the greatest number of deaths and lead to the most severe health problems (Barancik, Chatterjee, & Greene, 1983). Women sustain 75% to 80% of all hip fractures (Melton & Riggs, 1983). Half of all older adults hospitalized for hip fractures cannot return home or live independently after their injuries (Melton & Riggs, 1983; Scott, 1990).

Factors that contribute to falls include problems with gait and balance, neurological and musculoskeletal disabilities, psychoactive medication use, dementia, and visual impairment (Judge, Lindsey, & Underwood, 1993). Environmental hazards such as slippery surfaces, uneven floors, poor lighting, loose rugs, unstable furniture, and objects on floors may also play a role (Tinetti, Speechley, & Ginter, 1988).

Falls from heights have also been a significant source of injury. Falls from heights include from open windows, off roofs, from maintenance equipment, etc. In large cities, as well as communities with multiple story dwellings, falls from open windows are a serious problem. Cities such as New York have taken steps through building and fire code modification to ensure that windows cannot be opened wide enough for a child to conceivably fall from. Many occupational related falls from heights have been prevented by regulations imposed through the Occupational Safety and Health Administration (OSHA). OSHA provides safety regulations for individuals working in hazardous environments. Their role in injury prevention has saved countless lives.

Drowning

In 1997, 4,051 people drowned, including 964 children younger than 15 years old. Drowning is the second leading cause of injury-related death for children (aged 1 through 14 years), accounting for 905 deaths in 1997. In 1997, drowning rates were at least three times greater for males than for females for almost every age group (National Center for Health Statistics, 1998). Most children drown in swimming pools. According to the U.S. Consumer Product Safety Commission (CPSC), emergency departments reported that among children younger than 5 years old, about 320 fatal drownings in 1991 and nearly 2,300 nonfatal near-drownings in 1993 occurred in residential swimming pools (U.S. Consumer Product Safety Commission Clearinghouse, 1995).

Poisonings

Most poisonings happen in the home and involve children. In 1998, 92% of all poisonings occurred in the home and 53% involved children under the age of six years. Common household items such as pain relievers and cleaning substances are often the cause (Litovitz et al., 1999).

Poison control centers help millions of people each year and are extremely cost effective, ensuring that poisonings are treated rapidly and correctly. Three-fourths of these cases were managed at home over the telephone with the help of specialists trained in providing poison information (Litovitz et al., 1999). For every $1 spent on poison control centers, an estimated $7 is saved in medical care costs. By helping people manage emergencies at home, these centers prevent about 50,000 hospitalizations and 400,000 doctor's visits each year (Miller & Lestina, 1997).

Violence

Violence is defined most broadly as the use of physical force with the intent to inflict injury or death upon oneself or another. From a public health perspective, the fact that acts of violence may result in physical injury is the primary motivation for involvement. Violence or intentional injury manifests itself in many forms. From blunt to penetrating trauma, violence affects everyone, everywhere. One of public health's most significant contributions to violence prevention has been the use of a model of injury resulting from interactions among the host, agent, and environment. This model examines the importance of victim-offender relationships, and provides a framework through which these relationships can be understood and analyzed (National Committee for Injury Prevention and Control, 1989).

Motor Vehicles

Motor-vehicle crashes are the leading cause of injury-related deaths in the United States. In 1997, nearly 42,000 people died on the nation's roads and highways, and another 3.5 million suffered nonfatal injuries. Such crashes are the leading cause of death for Americans ages 1 to 34. However, the number of deaths on our highways has been declining because of the tremendous efforts of many groups over the last 30 years, advances in the design of vehicles and roads, laws requiring and regulating the use of lifesaving devices such as safety belts, and changes in societal attitudes toward destructive behaviors such as drinking and driving (CDC, 2000).

Seat-belt use increased from 11% in 1981 to 68% in 1997. In 1988, 60% of young drivers involved in fatal motor-vehicle crashes were not using restraints, but by 1995 the percentage had dropped to 46%. Alcohol was a factor in 32% of fatal motor-vehicle crashes among young drivers in 1988 and in 22% in 1997 (CDC, 2000).

Bicycles

In 1997, 813 bicyclists were killed in crashes with motor vehicles, an increase of 7% over the previous year (NHTSA, 1998). Of these, 31% were riders younger than 16 years old and 97% were not wearing helmets (IIHS, 1997). In the event of a crash, wearing a bicycle helmet reduces the risk of serious head injury by as much as 85% and the risk for brain injury by as much as 88% (Thompson, Rivera, & Thompson,

1989). In fact, if each rider wore a helmet, an estimated 500 bicycle-related fatalities and 151,000 nonfatal head injuries would be prevented each year—that's one death per day and one injury every four minutes (Sacks, Kresnov, Houston, & Russell, 1996).

The most common complaints of children and adolescents are that helmets are not fashionable, or "cool," their friends do not wear them, and/or they are uncomfortable (usually too hot). Riders also convey that they do not think about the importance of bike helmets, nor about the need to protect themselves from injury, particularly if they are not riding in traffic. By early 1998, 15 states and more than 65 local governments had enacted some form of bicycle helmet legislation. Most of these laws pertain to children and adolescents (Federal Register, 1998).

INJURY PREVENTION CONCEPTS

Prevention provides an opportunity to realize significant reductions in human **morbidity** (measurement of sickness or disease in a particular population) and **mortality** (measurement of death in a particular population) with a manageable investment. As a whole, the health care system is evolving from an emphasis on providing highly technologic, curative care to improving health through prevention and wellness. The objective is to prevent people from ever requiring costly medical care (NHTSA, 1996). Engaging in prevention activities is the responsibility of every health care practitioner, including those involved with the provision of EMS (NHTSA, 1996).

The goal of **primary prevention** is to prevent injury from occurring in the first place. Examples may include wearing a seat belt or helmet and installing smoke detectors. Strategies that attempt to minimize further injury or death after the initial trauma or injury event has occurred are called **secondary injury prevention**. Medical treatment such as securing the airway or C-spine immobilization are included in **tertiary injury prevention**.

Injury prevention and control is the process of using knowledge about the injury event to design prevention programs and evaluate their success. Perhaps the most important principle of injury prevention and control is that injury is a disease, which can be prevented or modified by changing the transmission of energy (such as force) to an individual (host).

The components of the injury process (host, agent, vector) described earlier may be used to develop preventive measures for injuries. Before prevention measures can be developed, it is helpful to first identify the factors affecting the extent of the injury before, during, and after an injury to decrease morbidity and mortality. These components are examined pre-event, during the injury event, and postevent. This concept was developed by Dr. William Haddon and uses **Haddon's matrix** to illustrate the idea. The matrix can be used to identify factors affecting the extent of injury, from which prevention strategies or interventions may be designed.

Table 9-3 is a matrix taken from an injury prevention program targeted at reducing commercial fishing fatalities in Alaska, where the occupational fatality rate was more than twenty times the national average (NIOSH, 1997). Identification of factors affecting the extent of an injury during a specific phase event, and developing a program targeted at changing or modifying these factors, is crucial in creating a successful injury prevention program.

Interventions

Injury prevention interventions are generally classified into three groups, known as the three E's. **The three E's of injury prevention** include engineering, enforcement, and education. These interventions are methods used to identify injury prevention and control methods. For example, a program to decrease head injuries from bicycling may incorporate the three E's by designing helmets that cover more of the head (engineering), enforcing/lobbying for helmet laws (enforcement), and teaching children about bicycle safety (education).

Table 9-3   Injury Prevention Program Matrix

Phase	Host/Human	Agent/Vehicle	Environment
Pre-event	Captain and crew fatigue Stress Prescription or illegal drugs/alcohol Inadequate training/ exposure	Unstable vessel Unstable work platform Complex machinery and operations	High winds Large waves Icing Short daylight Limited fishing seasons Vessels far apart
Injury Event	Captain and crew reaction to emergency PFD not available/ not working	Listing or capsized vessel Delayed abandonment Emergency circumstance not understood Man overboard (MOB)	High winds Large waves Darkness Poor radio communications Cold water
Postevent	Poor use of available emergency equipment Hypothermia Drowning Lost at sea	Vessel sinking Poor crew response to MOB	High winds Large waves Cold water

Surveillance

Lastly, **surveillance**, or the collection of information, may be used. Surveillance tells us how big the injury problem is, where it is, and who is affected. This information allows decision makers to allocate programs and resources where they are most needed. For example, prehospital care providers play a crucial role in the documentation of the mechanism of injury in great detail. Surveillance data also tell us how well we are doing over time, where to shift resources, or to set a different direction.

EMS AND INJURY PREVENTION

The 1966 report "Accidental Death and Disability: The Neglected Disease of Modern Society" released by the National Academy of Sciences/National Research Council recognized injury as a disease that could be treated and prevented. This document, along with others, spurred the involvement of emergency medical services in the prevention of injuries.

Over the past thirty years our society has come to expect that EMS will be there when we need it. EMS has progressed from fifty years ago when a hearse took the acutely ill and injured to the hospital between funeral runs, to high-tech EMS systems employing the latest tools to save lives. As highly evolved as today's EMS systems may be, one crucial flaw in the paradigm of EMS delivery still exists, that is, the primary function of an EMS system is reactive—responding after something has happened, rather than proactive—preventing the incident from happening at all. Many of today's EMS system leaders believe that the future of EMS will be as much proactive as it is reactive. The question that always comes to mind is what injuries can be prevented? In this section we will examine the role that an EMS system can have in the injury prevention process.

EMS providers are the first members of the health care community to respond to most injuries and illnesses and are ideal individuals to lead injury prevention campaigns. Given the unique perspectives EMS providers possess of injuries, they are invaluable advocates, prevention program designers, and public educators capable of preventing injuries from occurring. In essence, their dedication to primary prevention will position EMS professionals as key leaders in community health, and establish or improve relationships with other agencies and community organizations (EMSC, 1998).

To help reaffirm this commitment to primary prevention, in 1996 a group of EMS professionals and injury prevention experts developed the *Consensus Statement on the EMS Role in Primary Injury Prevention*. This document states:

> Emergency medical services (EMS) organizations and individual providers must participate in primary injury prevention activities. This participation will benefit patients, communities, and the EMS system . . . implementation of primary injury prevention activities is an effective way to reduce death, disabilities, and health care costs. EMS has an obligation to actively participate in primary injury prevention activities. (USDOT, 1996).

Through developing this statement, the consensus committee identified key primary injury prevention activities for the leaders, decision makers, and individual providers from EMS systems across the nation to carry out. The following recommendations can be used in developing injury prevention strategies:

Essential activities for EMS leaders and decision makers:

- Protecting individual EMS providers from injury
- Providing education to EMS providers in the fundamentals of primary injury prevention
- Supporting and promoting the collection and utilization of injury data
- Obtaining support and resources for primary injury prevention activities
- Networking with other injury prevention organizations
- Empowering individuals to conduct primary injury prevention activities in the local community
- Interacting with the media to promote injury prevention
- Participating in injury prevention interventions in the community

Essential injury prevention knowledge areas for individual EMS providers are:

- Principles of primary prevention
- Personal injury prevention and role modeling
- Safe emergency vehicle operation
- Injury risk identification
- Documentation of injury data
- One-on-one safety education

The *EMS Agenda for the Future* (NHTSA, 1996) identified 14 key areas in emergency medical services that are in need of further development. Prevention was one of them. The agenda identifies that prevention is a worthwhile investment, providing significant reduction in mortality and morbidity. It recognizes that prevention activities are the responsibility of every member of the health care community. Divided into three sections, the agenda describes current status, goals, and direction on how to attain the goals.

The current status described is reflective of the shift in health care management paradigms. One of the key shifts that has taken place is the concept of improving health through prevention and wellness, thus reducing or even eliminating a medical condition from occurring. This is a significant change from the idea of waiting for an incident to occur requiring high-tech, high-cost medical intervention. The ultimate goal is clear—"to prevent people from ever requiring costly medical care". (EMS Agenda, p. 39). Also identified in the current status is that injury is the third leading cause of death and disability in all age groups, accounting for more years of potential life lost than any other health problem.

Supporting evidence for highly effective public safety driven prevention programs is also presented. Such evidence includes the fire service's efforts to affect engineering, enforcement, and education related to fire safety, which has led to significant reductions in the numbers of fire-related injuries and deaths. An example of this is the "stop, drop, and roll" campaign if your clothes catch fire. Law enforcement agencies have also played a significant role in injury prevention. Through programs such as these geared at aggressive enforcement of impaired driving laws, significant reductions in traffic-related deaths and injuries secondary to impaired driving have been observed. EMS agencies themselves have proven their own ability to effectively reduce preventable injuries. Programs in New York to prevent falls from height, and drowning programs in Pinellas County, Florida, and Tucson, Arizona, have demonstrated that EMS can have an impact. Unified efforts are underway, though still early in development. An example of this is the Safe Communities concept, which involves a systematic approach to address all injuries and emphasizes the need for coordination among prevention, acute care, and rehabilitation efforts. EMS systems can provide crucial injury-related data pertinent to the study of injuries and design of risk reduction strategies.

The goals for injury prevention programs focus on EMS programs incorporating prevention into their everyday practice. Ideally, EMS systems and providers will be continuously engaged in injury and illness prevention programs. Prevention programs should be developed based on system-specific needs, identifying injury and illness patterns prone to that service delivery area. Promotion of prevention-oriented environments throughout the EMS system (both internally within the system and externally in the community) is paramount. Continuing education will convey the very prevention principles discussed in this chapter to all providers in the system, providing an understanding of how prevention activities relate to providers themselves as well as outreach activities.

Attaining these goals requires EMS systems to work with other community agencies as well as health care providers who possess expertise and interest in prevention activities (e.g., other public safety agencies, safety councils, public health departments, etc.). The purpose of a multiagency approach is to identify appropriate targets for prevention as well as to share the implementation of the programs. The agenda stresses the importance of EMS systems in identifying potential roles within partnerships to prevent injury and illness. Also included is EMS acting as an advocate for legislation geared toward injury and illness prevention. Prevention principles and their role in improving both individual and community health need to be incorporated into the core contents of EMS provider training programs. Lastly, EMS must continue to document the incidence of injury and illness along with specific circumstances and convey this information to others.

Developing an Injury Prevention Program

As stated above, EMS can play a critical role in injury prevention. This does not mean, however, that EMS must develop and implement prevention programs. Many agencies exist that can provide assistance in developing and implementing an injury or illness prevention program. Several approaches to prevention programs already exist (EMSC, 1998).

- Support an already developed activity
- Provide leadership and advocacy for another agency's work
- Develop a new injury prevention program in collaboration with other agencies

The most effective prevention strategies use a collaborative, systems-based approach which incorporates all allied health care disciplines and the appropriate agencies. See Appendix C for a guide for developing or expanding an injury prevention effort. Remember that every state has unique issues and resources, so carefully review all available information associated with injury and injury prevention in your state. This will be the most important action you will take.

SUMMARY

Traditionally injury prevention has not been associated with EMS. However, as EMS expands its role and moves more in line with current focuses in health care, injury prevention becomes an important component for EMS. As a major source of trauma and death, injuries are in most cases preventable. By understanding the nature and cause of injury, EMS can use its unique position in the community to foster injury prevention both for its constituents as well as EMS providers.

STUDY QUESTIONS

1. Cite examples of common causes of injury in the United States.

2. Diagram the relationship between the components of the injury event.

3. Cite at least five examples of intentional and unintentional injuries.

4. Describe the role of the three levels of injury countermeasures.

5. Discuss the use of the Haddon's matrix as an injury prevention tool.

6. Discuss how the three E's of injury prevention can be used to reduce injuries.

7. Discuss the role of EMS in injury prevention.

BIBLIOGRAPHY

Baker, S. P., O'Neill, B., Ginsburg, M. J., & Guohua, L. (1992). *The injury fact book* (2nd ed.). New York: Oxford University Press.

Barancik, J. I., Chatterjee, B. F., & Greene, Y. C. (1983). Northeastern Ohio trauma study: I. Magnitude of the problem. *American Journal of Public Health, 73,* 746–751.

Campbell, J. E. (1998). *Basic trauma life support for paramedics and advanced EMS providers* (3rd ed.). Upper Saddle River, NJ: Prentice Hall.

Centers for Disease Control and Prevention, National Institute for Injury Prevention and Control. (2000). *Fact book 2000.* Washington, DC: U.S. Government Printing Office.

Emergency Medical Services for Children Resource Center. (1998). *Preventing childhood emergencies: A guide to developing effective injury prevention initiatives* (2nd ed.). Washington, DC: Author.

Federal Register. U.S. Consumer Product Safety Commission. Safety standard for bicycle helmets; Final rule. FR Doc. 98-4214, February 13, 1998.

Gibson, J. J. (1961). The contribution of experimental psychology to the formulation of the problem of safety: A brief for basic research. Reprinted from: *Behavioral approaches to accident research.* New York: New York Association for the Aid of Crippled Children.

Gordan, J. E. (1949). The epidemiology of accidents. *American Journal of Public Health, 39,* 504–515.

Haddon, W. (1963). A note concerning accident theory and research with special reference to motor vehicle accidents. *Annals of the New York Academy of Science, 107,* 635–646.

Hoyert, D. L., Kochanek, K. D., & Murphy, S. L. (1999). Deaths: Final data for 1997. *National vital statistics reports, 47*(19).

Insurance Institute for Highway Safety. (1997). *Fatality Facts: Bicycles*. Arlington, VA: Author.

Judge, J. O., Lindsey, C., & Underwood, M., (1993). Balance improvements in older women: Effects of exercise training. *Physical Therapy, 73,* 254–265.

Litovitz, T. L., Klein-Schwartz, W., Caravati, E. M., Youniss, J., Crouch, B., Lee, S. (1999). 1998 annual report of the American Association of Poison Control Centers toxic exposure surveillance system. *American Journal of Emergency Medicine,* 17, 435–87.

Melton, L. J., III., Riggs, B. L. (1983). Epidemiology of age-related fractures. In L. V. Avioli (Ed.), *The osteoporotic syndrome* (pp. 45–72). New York: Grune & Stratton.

Miller, T. R., & Lestina, D. C. (1997). Costs of poisoning in the United States and savings from poison control centers: A benefit-cost analysis. *Annals of Emergency Medicine, 29,* 239–245.

National Center for Health Statistics. (1998). *National Mortality Data, 1997.* Hyattsville, MD: Author.

National Committee for Injury Prevention and Control. (1989). *Injury prevention: Meeting the challenge.* New York: Oxford University Press.

National Highway Transportation Safety Administration. (1998). *Traffic safety facts, 1997: Bicyclists.* Washington, DC: Author.

National Highway Traffic Safety Administration. (1996). *EMS agenda for the future.* Washington, DC: Author.

National Institute of Occupational Safety and Health. (1997). *Commercial fishing fatalities in Alaska: Risk factors and prevention strategies.* Washington, DC: United States Department of Health and Human Services.

National Research Council. (1985). *Injury in America: A continuing public health problem.* Washington, DC: National Academy Press.

Sacks, J. J., Kresnow, M., Houston, B., & Russell, J. (1996). Bicycle helmet use among American children, 1994. *Injury Prevention, 2,* 258–262.

Sattin, R. W. (1992). Falls among older persons: A public health perspective. *Annual Review of Public Health, 13,* 489–508.

Scott, J. C. (1990). Osteoporosis and hip fractures. *Rheumatic Diseases Clinics of North America, 16,* 717–40.

Sorock, G. S. (1988). Falls among the elderly: Epidemiology and prevention. *American Journal of Preventive Medicine, 4,* 282–288.

Thompson, R. S., Rivara, F. P., & Thompson, D. C. (1989). A case-control study of the effectiveness of bicycle safety helmets. *New England Journal of Medicine, 320,* 1361–1367.

Tinetti, M. E., Speechley, M., & Ginter, S. F. (1988). Risk factors for falls among elderly persons living in the community. *New England Journal of Medicine, 319,* 1701–1707.

How to Plan for the Unexpected: Preventing Child Drownings United States Consumer Product Safety Commission Clearinghouse. Washington, DC. Pub. No. 359, 1995.

United States Department of Transportation. (1996). *Consensus statement on the EMS role in primary injury prevention.* Washington, DC: Author.

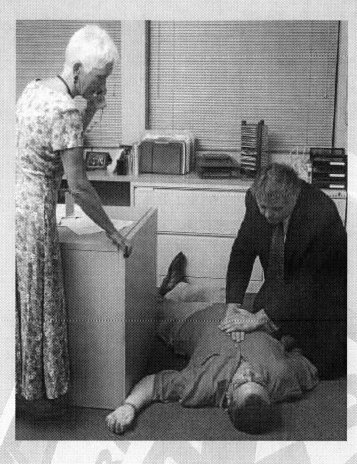

Case Study

"Bridget, call the paramedics! Chris was having chest pains and he has collapsed at his desk! Dial 911! Hurry!", exclaims Shane to his coworker. He runs back into Chris' office. Bridget dials 911.

"Madison County 911. What is your emergency?" asks the 911 call taker.

"A coworker has collapsed. He was having chest pains. We need an ambulance and paramedics, fast!"

"Miss, are you calling from 905 Kingsbridge Terrace, the Universal Investment Company?"

"Yes, that's correct. Suite 104."

"I show the phone number as 555-549-6721. Is that correct and is there an extension?"

"Extension 10. Please hurry and send the paramedics."

(continues)

CHAPTER 10

Public Access

Outline

Objectives

Upon completion of this chapter, the reader should be able to:

- Identify the universal access number in the United States.

- Review the development of 911 as the universal access number.

- State the role and function of a PSAP.

- Describe what happens when a person calls 911.

- State the role of nonemergency access numbers such as 311.

- List the two major components of pathway management.

- State the importance of public education in the efficient operation of a 911 system.

Case Study (continued)

After confirming the caller information displayed on the enhanced 911 system screen, the call taker electronically transfers the information and call nature to the EMS dispatcher. The closest ALS unit is alerted to respond.

"They have been dispatched miss. Will there be any problem with them gaining access to your office?"

"No, the front door is right in front of the building entrance."

As Bridget gives this information, the call taker enters it and passes it to the dispatch for relay to the responding unit.

"Miss, I need you to remain on the line. I'm transferring you to another dispatcher who will ask you some more questions and provide assistance until EMS arrives. Please stay on the line."

At this point, Bridget is transferred to an emergency medical dispatcher who provides prearrival instructions for Shane and Bridget to assist their coworker until the ambulance arrives.

Key Terms

Automatic location
  information (ALI)
Automatic number
  identification (ANI)
Basic 911
Call taker
Chain of survival
Computer-aided dispatch
  (CAD)

Dispatch center
Dispatch life support
  (DLS)
Emergency medical
  dispatch
Enhanced 911
Nonemergency access
  number

Pathway management
Prearrival instructions
Priority dispatching
Public access
Public safety answering
  point (PSAP)
Telecommunicator
Universal access number

PUBLIC ACCESS

A community could have the most sophisticated EMS system, staffed with highly trained paramedics responding in modern ambulances, but if the public does not have a simple and effective means of activating the system, it is worthless. The American Heart Association, in the **chain of survival**, has recognized the importance of

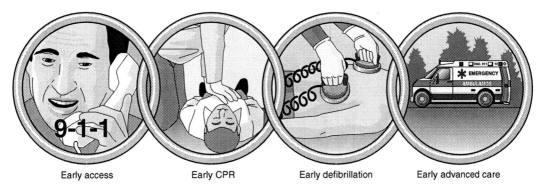

Early access   Early CPR   Early defibrillation   Early advanced care

Figure 10-1 Chain of Survival
(From the American Heart Association)

public access in EMS response (Figure 10-1). The chain links early access, early CPR, early defibrillation, and early advanced cardiac care together in a chain of survival for the victim of out-of-hospital acute coronary syndromes (AHA, 2000).

Public access is also important in noncardiac related events such as trauma and severe respiratory distress. Because emergency medical systems exist to serve the public, access to the system is as important as the system components themselves. **Public access** is more than just having the capability to call 911. Public access involves the ability of an EMS system to respond appropriately to a caller's needs regardless of the callers socioeconomic status, age, or perceived need. An effective EMS system will have the ability to provide differing levels of response depending on the caller's needs. An appropriate response may not be the dispatch of a traditional ambulance, but referral to another agency or response network.

Emergency medical services systems have traditionally functioned independent of other community health resources, both public and private. However, the integration of health care systems within a community and the effects of managed care are changing the role of EMS. Emergency medical services systems can no longer remain isolated. As a focal point for entry into the health care system, they must be responsive not only to the patient's needs, but also to the needs and concerns of the total community health care system.

911

When one thinks of public access, the **universal access number** 911 most often comes to mind. 911 is available to almost 93% of the U.S. population (www.nena.org). Prior to 1968, however, a person needing emergency assistance either dialed a seven-digit number or "O" for the operator. In those areas of the country not covered by 911, a caller must still dial a seven-digit number to request assistance.

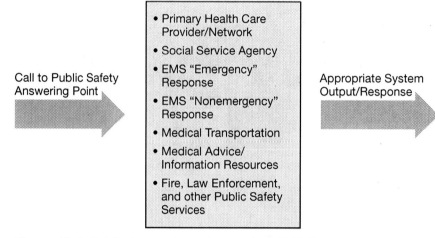

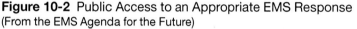

Figure 10-2 Public Access to an Appropriate EMS Response
(From the EMS Agenda for the Future)

The development of 911 was encouraged by fire and EMS services. In 1957, the first suggestion for a universal number for access came from the National Association of Fire Chiefs. The need for such a number to provide quick access for law enforcement emergencies was recognized by the President's Commission on Law Enforcement and Administration of Justice in 1967. Responding to these concerns, the Federal Communications Commission (FCC) approached American Telephone and Telegraph (AT&T) in 1967 to see if such a number was possible. In 1968, AT&T introduced 911 as the universal emergency access number. It should be noted that prior to the early 1970s, telephone service in the United States was provided by one system, the Bell Telephone System, part of AT&T. Thus action by AT&T was nationwide and covered all phone systems in the United States. To further the development of 911, the U.S. Congress passed legislation supporting implementation of 911 nationwide and in 1973 the White House Office of Telecommunications issued a national policy statement on the advantages of 911. The first 911 call was made on February 16, 1968, in Haleyville, Alabama. Advantages of the digits 911 include:

- Easily dialed, especially for rotary dial phones that were common in the 1960s
- Easily remembered
- Unique number, having never been assigned as an area code or service code
- Only one number for people to remember
- Same number for people traveling through different areas
- Reduced problems in contacting proper emergency agency
- Ability of pay or restricted phones to accept 911 calls

911 Operation The main purpose of the number 911 is to connect a caller with an emergency to a **public safety answering point (PSAP)**. Once connected to a PSAP, the caller can be routed to the proper emergency services dispatching agency. Depending on the sophistication of the local PSAP, the person answering the 911 call may also be the emergency dispatcher. However, the ideal situation is for the PSAP to be staffed with **call takers** whose primary responsibility is answering 911 calls and forwarding the caller to the proper agency.

In addition to providing easy access to emergency services, 911 also provides basic information important for call dispatching. Such information includes the caller's telephone number and location of the caller's phone. The first 911 system, known as **basic 911**, provided limited information about the caller. With the introduction of a digital database of phone number information, a more sophisticated 911 was possible. **Enhanced 911** provides **automatic number identification (ANI)** and **automatic location information (ALI)**. When a person dials 911, ANI gives the calling number and ALI provides the street address for the phone. Enhanced 911 also has automated call routing that ensures that an emergency call is directed to the proper PSAP. This feature is important because telephone service areas usually do not follow city or county boundaries.

A developing service being integrated with 911 is geographic information systems (GIS) and global positioning system (GPS) technology. Such integration will allow better location of incidents as well as specific routing of emergency responders to the scene. This is especially important in remote rural areas where traditional addressing information such as house numbers and street signs are not readily available or accessible. An example of such a system is the "On-Star Alarm System" available in some automobiles. The driver or passenger need only push a button to summon medical or police assistance. Sensors in the car relay the vehicle's position via GPS to a central monitoring station that contacts the appropriate PSAP. Similar systems are capable of detecting a vehicle crash and initiating a call without input from the vehicle passengers.

An expanding technology that has had a profound effect on 911 notification and locating is the cellular telephone. The FCC requires that all cellular phones, even those without a service contract, be capable of connecting to a 911 system nationwide. Because cellular telephones do not operate from a fixed location, dialing 911 will provide only the phone's number, not its location. Routing of the call to a PSAP is in some cases dependent on the location where the phone service was initiated or the service area of the phone's number, not the actual location of the phone. Cellular phones utilize "cells" as part of the trunking system. Like phone service areas, cells may not follow jurisdictional boundaries, or a caller may move between cells while on the line. Unless a caller is familiar with an area, it may be difficult to pinpoint the location of an incident. To eliminate this problem, various public safety groups have persuaded the FCC to require all digital cellular phones manufactured after 2001 to have either GPS capability or some other means to identify the caller's location. Thus when a cellular 911 call is received, the PSAP will have the latitude and longitude of the phone making the call. This technology is known as wireless enhanced 911.

Public Safety Answering Point (PSAP)

The public safety answering point (PSAP), also sometime called a public safety access point, is also an integral part of public access. PSAPs have evolved over the years from a single dispatcher who answered the phone as well as determined the running assignment and dispatched the call, to multilayer, multifunction central communication centers. The PSAP serves as the answering point for 911 calls. Once a **telecommunicator** or call taker determines the nature of the caller's emergency, information needed to dispatch the proper emergency service is transferred to that service's dispatch center. Depending on the incident, the call taker may remain on the line, transfer the caller, or hang up. If the call is a medical emergency, the caller will be transferred to an emergency medical dispatcher who will provide prearrival instructions. Simultaneously the service dispatcher will be alerting and directing the necessary units to the incident scene.

Although the staffing and complexity of a PSAP will vary, all PSAPs serve as a focal point for public access to emergency services. By being a centralized point of contact, the PSAP is able to obtain necessary information and direct the caller to the proper response agency. If a PSAP were not part of the public access system, callers would need to know which service they needed when dialing 911. Prior to the establishment of PSAPs, the 911 operator would answer "police, fire, ambulance." The caller would have to pick which one they needed and then be transferred. Now, the PSAP telecommunicator will answer "911, what is your emergency?" and direct the call appropriately.

CALL PROCESSING

When a person calls 911, all they know is that the phone is answered in a timely manner and the proper emergency services unit arrives to help. Although this process may seem simple, it involves a number of interrelated steps, all of which must work together seamlessly to provide efficient access to emergency services.

Call Taking

When 911 is dialed, the caller is connected to the PSAP and a person who answers the 911 line. Regardless of the ultimate responsibility and other duties of the person answering the call, at this point they function as a call taker. What happens next depends on the sophistication of the PSAP and the communications system.

In the simplest system, the call taker is the only person to handle the entire incident (Figure 10-3A). They may be the only person working at the PSAP. Once the information necessary for dispatching the call has been acquired from the caller and the 911 system, the caller is disconnected and the call taker assumes the role of a dispatcher.

In larger systems, the call taker may transfer the call to a dispatcher who then determines the response package, type and number of units needed to handle the call, and alerts the indicated units (Figure 10-3B). The caller may either remain on the line or be disconnected. If the caller remains on the line, she is given either to an emergency medical dispatcher, who provides prearrival instructions, or remains with the incident dispatcher who provides prearrival instructions.

In the most sophisticated PSAPs, the 911 call takers are a separate group of dispatchers who just answer 911 lines (Figure 10-3C). They then transfer the calls to the respective agencies, police, fire, and EMS. The 911 answering center may not even be located in the same building or area of the service dispatch centers. This arrangement is common in most major metropolitan areas.

Dispatch Center

The **dispatch center** is responsible for receiving the 911 information, processing the call, and coordinating communications. The center may be service specific or it may handle dispatch for multiple services (e.g., fire and police). Because the dispatch center must constantly know the status of all response units in the service, and select the

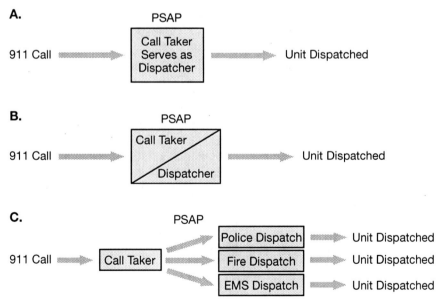

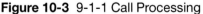

Figure 10-3 9-1-1 Call Processing
A. Minimal Configuration; B. Separate Call Taker—Dispatcher; C. PSAP with Separate Dispatch Center

most appropriate combination of units to handle a call, many centers utilize **computer-aided dispatch**, commonly called CAD. A CAD system is special software that tracks units status and automatically recommends the proper response package for a given geographic location and incident type. Some CAD systems are capable of alerting units and sending location and incident information directly to the units electronically. Units may be equipped with automatic tracking and status notification that continually updates the CAD system via radio. The main advantage of a CAD system is speed and accuracy. Location information can be transferred directly into the CAD from an E-911 (enhanced) system. Location-specific information can also be stored such as information about a handicapped person on premises or special hazards. The CAD will always assemble the correct response package based on preprogrammed parameters and unit status. This eliminates the dispatcher having to enter information or manually select units to respond. In dispatch centers not equipped with a CAD, a card system is used. The term is derived from the practice of either using a paper card to record incident information and/or having cards for different geographical areas and special locations. The dispatcher must select the right card that lists the units due to respond for each type of emergency incident. This process is time-consuming and subject to error and interpretation.

In addition to incident dispatch and coordination, the dispatch center may also serve as the notification agency for hospitals and other resources as well as the coordinating center for medical communications (see Chapter 11). The center also handles communications between the dispatch centers of the various emergency services and their units. For instance, if an ambulance crew needs police assistance, the request would be forwarded to the police dispatch center via the EMS center.

Dispatch Life Support

Dispatch life support (DLS) is a term used to encompass emergency medical dispatching, priority dispatching, and prearrival instructions. More and more dispatch centers are utilizing DLS as a means to provide increased services and better public access to EMS systems. The concepts of DLS have their roots in work done by Jeff Clawson, an emergency physician and fire department medical director from Salt Lake City, who began the concept of emergency medical dispatch in 1977. The importance of DLS was recognized by the National Association of EMS Physicians (www.naemsp.org) in 1989 with the publication of a position paper supporting emergency medical dispatching. The NAEMSP called for, among other things, recognition of the emergency medical dispatcher as an integral part of the EMS system. The paper also encouraged dispatch centers nationwide to adopt DLS.

If a dispatch center utilizes DLS, the 911 caller will not merely confirm the incident location and nature, but will be quickly interrogated using priority dispatch to determine the appropriate level of response (BLS versus ALS). Once the priority dispatch information has been obtained, the dispatcher may provide prearrival instruction. Depending on the complexity of the dispatch center, prearrival instructions may be

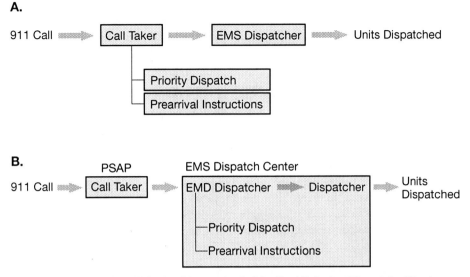

Figure 10-4 Medical Priority Dispatch. A. Medical Priority Dispatch, Single Dispatch Center; B. Medical Priority Dispatch, Separate Dispatch Center

provided by yet another telecommunicator (Figure 10-4). Most likely, the original dispatcher will remain on the line and unit dispatch handled by another dispatcher. Transfer of all the information between the various dispatchers is via the CAD system. As new information is provided, or changes in the patient's condition are noted, the EMD dispatcher will pass this information on to the responding units. Arrival of EMS personnel at the patient's side ends the EMD phase of the incident.

Emergency Medical Dispatch Emergency medical dispatch, commonly called EMD, is the process of sending the right units to the right location with the right resources. It would be a waste to send an ambulance staffed with two paramedics to a call for a broken toe. Unless the dispatcher knows the true nature of the incident, this cannot be avoided. Emergency medical dispatch allows the dispatcher not only to function as a member of the EMS response team, but also to more efficiently manage system resources. This is accomplished through the use of priority dispatch.

Priority Dispatching Priority dispatching is the process of using a scripted series of questions to interrogate the caller and determine the proper level of EMS system response. The emergency medical dispatcher asks a series of initial questions to clarify the nature and severity of the incident. After this quick interview, units are dispatched.

Prearrival Instructions Prearrival instructions are a means to provide first aid instructions via phone. Instead of disconnecting the caller after the initial interrogation, the caller has the option of remaining on the line and receiving instructions on how to care either for themselves or the patient. The dispatcher follows a set sequence of questions and provides instructions based on the caller's answers. Instructions for complex activities such as CPR and childbirth can be given over the phone.

NONEMERGENCY ACCESS NUMBERS

As 911 became known as the most direct means to reach police and emergency services, people began using it as a general number for any type of governmental assistance. Callers have dialed 911 to ask directions, inquire about garbage pickup, complain about rodent control, or find the correct time. All of these inappropriate calls place a strain on the PSAP, especially in populated urban areas. Public education programs, such as "Make the Right Call" (see chapter 8), have helped to educate the public, but have not eliminated the problem. In major urban areas, the demand on the 911 service can become so severe that callers will receive a busy signal or recording when calling during peak times.

Looking for a way to reduce inappropriate 911 calls, a number of cities are implementing **nonemergency access numbers**. The most common is 311. The first use of 311 occurred in 1996 in Baltimore, Maryland. The city developed a 311 system with support from the Department of Justice Office of Community Oriented Policing Services (COPS). The slogan "Where there is an urgency, but no emergency" was used to promote the number. After implementation of 311, Baltimore experienced a significant improvement in 911 system efficiency and responsiveness.

Because of the possibility of a real emergency being reported via 311, such services should be part of the PSAP operation. 311 systems should also have ANI and ALI capability to ensure proper handling of emergency calls. The number 311 must also be a local, nontoll call just like 911.

PATHWAYS MANAGEMENT

Public access deals with the means by which a person enters into the EMS system. Entry into EMS is also a pathway for entry into the broader health care system. When people perceive that they have an emergency situation, they dial 911 for assistance. EMS is dispatched and, in most cases, the person is transported to a hospital. After the event is over, the patient submits the bills to the insurance company for payment. In this situation, the insurance company has no control over the patient's decision to call 911, the EMS treatment provided, or the medical facility the patient is transported to. If the patient's perceived problem turns out not to be an emergency, the insurance company is still obligated to cover the costs. If the insurance company or managed care organization (MCO) could control the patient's entry into the medical system, they could potentially reduce false calls or inappropriate use, thus saving money. The means by which MCOs have attempted to control access is through pathway management.

Pathway management is a process whereby a MCO subscriber calls a central number and speaks with a health care professional, usually a nurse. Using a set of algorithms, the call taker evaluates the caller's complaint and decides on the appropriate course of action (Figure 10-5A). This may include calling 911, calling a physician, seeing a physician, or self-treatment. Through the use of telephone triage, the MCO is able to control patient entry into the health care system and ensure that the patient accesses an appropriate level of care.

The concept of pathway management can also be applied to 911 service. By screening calls for EMS assistance, a call taker can reduce the number of inappropriate requests for EMS service, thus reducing EMS system demand (Figure 10-5B). Some systems even go as far as calling a taxi to assist callers not in need of emergency services. To screen calls, 911 systems utilize field paramedics assigned to a rotation in dispatch.

A comprehensive pathway management system operating through a PSAP must include two main components. The first is a means to triage emergency calls. This is accomplished through the use of emergency medical dispatch (EMD). EMD utilizes a series of set questions and algorithms to interrogate the caller and determine the appropriate level of EMS response. The second is nonemergency triage. This process involves interrogating patients whose condition does not require an EMS response. Nonemergency triage is the same process as described above for MCO subscribers.

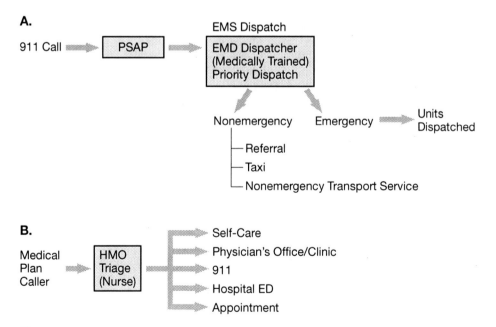

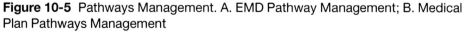

Figure 10-5 Pathways Management. A. EMD Pathway Management; B. Medical Plan Pathways Management

How best to provide these two services to the public remains controversial. Should they be handled through a public safety PSAP or is nonemergency triage outside the scope of public safety? Would a combined public-private venture better serve the public? These questions will only be answered as the EMS community gains more experience with pathway management.

PUBLIC EDUCATION

To be effective as a means to serve the public, EMS must take steps to ensure that the public knows how and when to call 911. As entry into the health care system becomes more controlled through such processes as pathway management and preauthorization, it is critical for the general public to know how to get the help they need. Public education as a function of an EMS system is discussed in Chapter 8.

A program to educate the public about appropriate use of 911 is "Make the Right Call." Sponsored by the National Highway Traffic Safety Administration, "Make the Right Call" is a media campaign designed to educate the public. A newer version of the program is "Children Make the Right Call to EMS." This version is designed to educate children, especially those old enough to be left alone, about when to call EMS as well as providing safety prevention information.

SUMMARY

When an individual needs emergency assistance, there must exist a means to access such assistance. Without easy access to EMS, even the best EMS system would be ineffective. To facilitate quick contact, the universal access number 911 was developed to connect the public with a PSAP. As demand for EMS and other emergency services has grown, the 911 system has evolved to include nonemergency numbers and pathway management.

STUDY QUESTIONS

1. Define public access.
2. What is the purpose of 911?
3. What is a PSAP?
4. Why were nonemergency access numbers developed?
5. What are the two main components of pathway management?
6. Why is public education an important part of public access?

BIBLIOGRAPHY

Breneiser, C. S. (1998, May–June). Enhanced E9-1-1: Products that give Enhanced 9-1-1 even more. *9-1-1 Magazine,* 14.

Clawson, J. J. (1989, October–December). Emergency medical dispatching. *Prehospital and Disaster Medicine,* p. 125–52.

Davis, C. (1998, May–June). Touring America's PSAPs: An Aussie's vacation among US communications centers. *9-1-1 Magazine,* 52.

Gilbert, S. (1998, July–August). Pathway management—back to the basics. *9-1-1 Magazine,* 64.

Gilbert, S. (1998, September–October). Pathway management implementation models. *9-1-1 Magazine,* 56.

National Emergency Number Association. (1999). How 9-1-1 works [On-line]. Available: www.nena9-1-1.org/History%20of%20NENA%20and%20911/history4.html

American Heart Association. Circulation, 2000; 102: Suppl. 1.

National Emergency Number Association. (1999). The development of 9-1-1 [On-line]. Available: www.nena9-1-1.org/History%20of%20NENA%20and%20911/history3.html

National Emergency Number Association. (2000). The development of 9-1-1 [On-line]. Available: www.nena.org/PressRoom Publications/9-1-1 facts.html.

Wilson, C. A. (1998, May/June). Wherefore 9-1-1?. *9-1-1 Magazine,* 46.

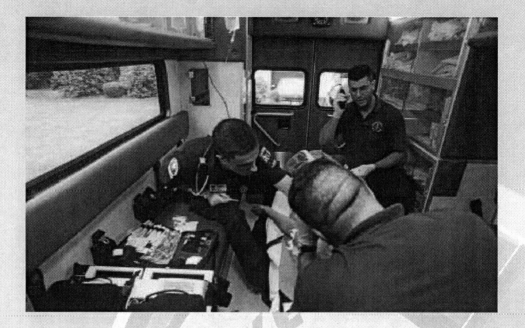

Case Study

The scene is the back of an ALS ambulance en route to the hospital. The paramedic is attempting consultation with the receiving hospital:

Paramedic 19: Paramedic 19 to EMRC on call one.

EMRC: Paramedic 19 EMRC.

Paramedic 19: EMRC, this is Carroll County Paramedic 19 en route to CCGH. I have a priority one cardiac requesting a med channel with CCGH and physician consultation.

EMRC: Carroll 19 switch to Med 4, Med 4 and standby.

(After a brief pause . . .)

EMRC: Carroll 19 you have CCGH on the line.

Paramedic 19: CCGH this is Paramedic 19. We are en route to your location with a priority one cardiac. ETA 17 minutes. Requesting a physician online for a drug order. Do you copy?

CCGH: Paramedic 19 this is Dr. Moore. We copy. Go ahead.

Paramedic 19: We are presently en route to your location with a 63-year-old male, chief complaint heavy, constant, substernal chest pain, onset 1 hour ago while at rest. Patient is conscious and alert but uncomfortable

(continues)

CHAPTER 11

Communications

Outline

Objectives

Upon completion of this chapter, the reader should be able to:

- State the importance of communications in an EMS system.
- Identify communications as one of the original 15 EMS system components.
- Identify the components of an EMS incident.

due to chest pain. We are following chest pain protocol. Vital signs are pulse 82 and regular, BP 162/82, and respirations 21. 12-lead ECG indicates inferior MI. Do you copy so far?

CCGH: We copy, go ahead.

Paramedic 19: OK CCGH. Given the patient's discomfort and apprehension, I would like permission to administer up to 4 mg of morphine as needed for pain control. Patient has no reported allergies. Do you concur?

CCGH: Yes 19, go ahead and give up to 4 mg morphine as needed for pain control. Advise if there is any change in the patient's condition en route.

Paramedic 19: OK, confirming up to 4 mg morphine for pain control. We'll see you in about 14 minutes. Do you have a bed assignment?

CCGH: Standby, I'll check with nursing.

(After a brief pause . . .)

CCGH: Paramedic 19 take your patient to bed 2, do you copy?

Paramedic 19: Copy bed 2, see you in about 12. Paramedic 19 clear.

- List the roles of communications in an EMS system.
- Differentiate between system and medical communications.
- Identify the EMS telecommunicator as a member of the EMS response team.
- List the roles of the EMS telecommunicator.
- List the functions of the EMS telecommunicator.
- Identify means of training telecommunicators.
- State the importance of prearrival instructions.
- Define a systems communication system.
- Define a medical communication system.
- Define biotelemetry.
- State the role of telemedicine in the future of medical communications.

Key Terms

800 MHz	Global satellite positioning	Portable
Base station	systems (GPS)	Prearrival medical
Biotelemetry	Med channels	instructions
Cellular	Medical communications	Systems communications
Computer-aided dispatch	Mobile unit	Telecommunicators
(CAD)	National EMS Radio	Telemedicine
Dispatcher	System	Trunked system
Duplex	Personal data assistant	Ultra high frequency range
Frequency	(PDA)	(UHF)

COMMUNICATIONS

An EMS system is made up of various components which must be able to effectively and efficiently work together. This coordination is accomplished through communications. Communication occurs at all levels of the system and takes various forms. Everything from a yearly briefing of constituent groups by a local EMS director, to the on-line medical consultation by an ambulance in the field, to the exchange of information by physicians in the emergency department are all examples of EMS communications. However, this chapter will focus on the use of communications to coordinate the emergency response to a citizen's call for help and the system and medical communications associated with such a call.

Communications was one of the original 15 EMS system components and remains one of the 14 system attributes as defined in the *EMS Agenda for the Future*. The EMS Systems Act of 1973 called for a system of communications that addresses each of the following:

*   The personnel, facilities, and equipment of the system will be joined by a central communications system.
*   Calls for EMS will be handled by a central communications center.
*   Incoming calls will be medically screened.
*   911 will be utilized as the universal access number.
*   The system will allow "direct communication connection and interconnections" with all parts of the EMS system and with other EMS systems.

"We can talk to astronauts on the moon, but an ambulance can't talk with a hospital ER" was a common statement during the early days of EMS. The statement acknowledged the availability of technology to improve EMS communications, but also identified the poor state, or lack, of operational EMS communications. Ambulances either did not have radios or utilized citizen band (CB) channels and commercial frequencies that were often shared with other users. It was not uncommon for ambulances to just show up at the emergency room without any prior notification. A system for on-line medical direction did not exist. If EMS was going to advance, ambulances, para-medics, hospitals, and regional centers all needed the capability to connect to each other.

Role of Communications

As the "glue" that ties an EMS system together, communications serve a variety of roles in EMS. These include:

- Contact between person needing help and dispatcher
- Contact between dispatch and responding EMS providers
- Contact between field providers and receiving hospital
- Contact between field providers and medical control
- Contact between field providers and other responders/units

Effective EMS system communications provide for:

- System control and administration
- Scene control and coordination
- Medical direction

Perhaps the most important thing to remember regarding communications is that system personnel function as members of a team. The team can only function as efficiently as its communications. The typical EMS event can be broken down into a series of communication phases. These include:

- Occurrence
- Detection
- Notification
- Dispatch
- Prearrival instructions
- Response
- Scene communications
- Medical communications
- Transport
- Hospital arrival
- Return to service

Occurrence Not all EMS events are as vivid as an auto crash. Some are very subtle and sensed only by the victim, such as a person with chest pain or trouble breathing. Even then, not everyone will appreciate the significance of symptoms. For some, denial will influence their decision-making process and delay movement to the second phase, detection.

Detection Someone must perceive that an event has taken place and recognize the need for EMS. An individual might see someone lying in a field. Is there a need for EMS, or is the person just sleeping? A person with chest pain needs to communicate, either verbally or through actions, that they are in distress. Others must be able to recognize the communication as a call for help.

Notification Once the need for EMS has been established, the system must be called into action. This is most commonly accomplished by using the universal access number 911. The victim or third party contacts the public safety access point (PSAP) requesting help. Once the nature of the call is understood by the call taker, proper units can be dispatched.

Dispatch In order to help the victim, the proper services must be alerted to respond. Dispatch is the process of putting together the proper response package and alerting units to respond. It also involves passing necessary response information to the responding providers such as location, map coordinates, and nature of the call.

Prearrival Instructions After dispatching the call, some dispatch centers may provide assistance to the victim or caller by providing **prearrival medical instructions**. Using a set of standardized criteria, the dispatcher interrogates the caller and provides instructions on how to provide immediate, lifesaving care. Prearrival instructions are given while responding units are en route to the scene.

Response Having determined the nature of the call, the dispatcher selects the appropriate unit or units and alerts either the unit's station or the unit itself to respond. If more information about the incident is determined, it is passed on to responding units.

Scene Communications Communications to and from the scene can be the most crucial of all incident communications. In addition to advising the dispatch center of arrival and departure from the scene, scene communications may also include requests for additional resources, police assistance, updated call status, cancelling of responding units, and scene command and coordination.

Medical Communications Once contact with the patient has been made, EMS personnel need to communicate with the receiving facility. If medical control orders are needed, personnel are put in contact with a medical command physician. Medical command is most often contacted via the medical radio system. Cellular telephones are also being used increasingly to conduct medical consultations.

Transport Once a transport destination has been determined, the EMS crew needs to advise the receiving hospital that they are en route. Notification can be made via the operational radio system or via a dedicated medical control radio system, depending on the EMS service's operating procedures.

Hospital Arrival In addition to advising the dispatch center that the unit has arrived at the hospital, EMS personnel must also communicate their patient assessment and treatment to the emergency department staff. Even if the crew has notified the hospital via radio or phone, updated information and patient response to treatment needs to be conveyed. In some hospitals, this is accomplished during a patient status report.

Return to Service Once the unit is restocked and ready to handle another call, the dispatch center is notified that the unit is available for response. Depending on service procedures, the unit may not make any further contact with the dispatch center until alerted for another call. In fixed-base systems, the unit may advise when it has returned to its quarters.

ROLE OF THE DISPATCHER

In order for effective communications to occur, there must be coordination between all parties involved in the incident and the EMS system. If units and personnel simply got on the radio and started talking, chaos would quickly follow and the EMS system would not be able to function. To prevent this from happening, EMS system communications are coordinated through a central dispatch center. The center may be the public safety access point (PSAP) or it may be an agency-specific center that receives 911 call transfers. Center staff consists of emergency service **telecommunicators** commonly known as **dispatchers**.

The role and place of the dispatcher in emergency incidents has changed over time. For many years, the dispatcher was looked on with disdain by responders. Early dispatchers lacked formal training, close supervision, and often were in jobs they didn't want. It was not uncommon for a firefighter or policeman who was unable to work in the field to be assigned to communications duty. No consideration was given for the employee's interest or ability as a dispatcher. In some small communities, the local dispatcher was a housewife who was home during the day and thus able to answer the phone and alert the local fire department or rescue squad. Once the station was alerted, the job of the dispatcher was often considered finished.

Now, the dispatcher is a formal member of the emergency response team. Dispatchers and dispatch centers do more than just receive 911 calls and alert units. They provide services that are just as important as those provided by EMS personnel responding to the scene. Advances in technology have played a significant role in bringing about this change.

The role of the EMS dispatcher in an EMS event includes:

- Being a recognized part of the EMS team
- Serving as the public's first point of contact with EMS
- Coordination of response
- Coordination of communications

- Prevision of prearrival instructions
- Incident data collection

The functions of an EMS dispatcher during an EMS event include:

- Call taking
- Alerting and directing response
- Monitoring and coordinating communications
- Prearrival medical instructions
- Maintaining incident record

Dispatcher Training

Preparing individuals to serve as dispatchers can be as varied as completion of a national certification course to just on-the-job training. Prior to beginning training, a selection process is used. Approaches to dispatcher selection include:

- Formal application with structured selection process
- Entrance testing
- Required experience and training (prior field experience; certification as a paramedic)
- Knowledge of the response area
- Assignment or detailing of personnel (some systems require rotation through dispatch for field personnel)

SYSTEMS COMMUNICATIONS TECHNOLOGY

Communications within an EMS system can be divided into two broad groups—systems communications and medical communications. **Systems communications** involves the communications necessary for operating and coordinating an EMS system. The main functions of systems communications are alerting and dispatching units and coordinating unit status. **Medical communications** are used to provide on-line medical control with a physician and notification of receiving facilities. Often, the two functions are integrated into one central communications system.

Systems Communications

The backbone of systems communications is the two-way radio. Radios have been used in fire and EMS vehicles since the 1930s. Technology developed in World War II made mobile radios more practical. War surplus and civil defense equipment also provided a source of radios for emergency vehicles. Development of the transistor in the 1950s made mobile communications equipment smaller and more reliable as well as reduced the power needs of such units. This led to the development of "lunch box"

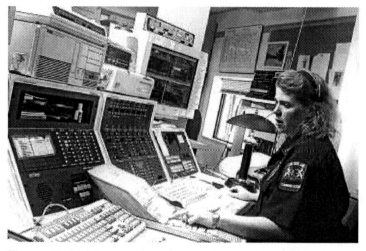

Figure 11-1 Often the dispatch center serves as the base station for EMS systems.

type **portable** units which eventually evolved into handheld portables or "walkie-talkies."

The basic components of a communications system consist of two parts. Messages are sent out to field units via a central **base station**. The base station is traditionally located at the dispatch or control center (Figure 11-1), which is a high-power unit capable of radiating a signal over the entire service area. Often, the base transmitter is located on a hill or mountain top to increase coverage as reception is line-of-sight. The dispatch center utilizes a remote base that is connected to the transmitter site by telephone lines or a microwave link. Depending on the **frequency** of the radio system, additional transmitter sites may be provided to improve coverage.

The second component of the radio system is the **mobile unit**. This is a radio unit located in a vehicle (Figure 11-2). Powered by the vehicle electrical system, the mobile unit allows contact with the base station or with other mobile units provided they are within range. To improve communications among vehicles, some systems utilize repeaters. Repeaters are transmitters that receive the weak signal from the mobile unit and rebroadcast it through the base station. Thus a mobile unit is able to talk to other units that normally would be out of range.

Because regular radio systems are limited to the power of the transmitter as well as the availability of frequencies on which to operate, a new system has been developed similar to that used for cellular phones. In a **trunked system**, the coverage area is divided into a series of cells. Each cell has its own transmitter and repeater. When a mobile or handheld unit in a cell transmits, the cell site receives the signal, repeats it back to the cell, and sends it by wire or microwave link to the other cells in the sys-

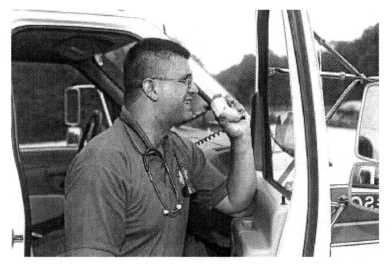

Figure 11-2 The mobile radio unit is in the emergency response vehicle.

tem where it is also rebroadcast. Thus a unit needs only enough power to reach the local site, but can communicate with any other unit within the cell system because the cells are linked or trunked. In addition to the cell trunking, trunked systems also use computer technology to shift radio units to an unused frequency each time the unit transmits. This allows many users to talk without interfering with one another and uses only a limited number of frequencies. This makes more effective use of the limited radio spectrum. It also allows units to be assigned to common groups for intergroup communications. For example, at a major rescue call, all EMS units could be on one talk group while the fire services would be on another and the police still another. Each group could talk among itself without interfering with the other groups. A common talk group would allow all units or group command officers to talk to each other when needed. Trunked systems utilize radio frequencies in the 800 to 900 MHz range, thus the popular term **800 megahertz** radio system. Computer control of such systems also allows for special functions and more sophisticated communication devices.

To speed up the communications process and to eliminate errors common to voice communications, radio systems are now incorporating direct computer-to-computer communications. Information received at the dispatch center is entered into the **CAD** or **computer-aided dispatch** computer. Computer-aided dispatch integrates location information, unit status, and other factors to determine the optimal dispatch package to send to an incident. This information is transmitted directly from the center's computer-aided dispatch computer to field units and displayed on a mobile data terminal. Two-way linkage also allows providers in the field to communicate via the vehicle computer with the dispatch center or other site for in-field information. In addition to call information, vehicle and crew status can also be transmitted. Linking mobile computers with vehicle **global satellite positioning systems (GPS)** allows dispatch personnel to monitor vehicle movements in real time. GPS system integration also provides mapping and travel route information directly to the vehicle crew. Continued evolution of the computer into the radio system will result in direct links between prehospital providers and the dispatch center via **personal data assistant (PDA)** type devices. These PDAs will integrate voice, data, and GPS functions in a single handheld or worn device.

Medical Communications

Paralleling the system communications system is medical communications. This can be a completely separate system or integrated into system communications. The medical communications system allows the prehospital provider to consult with medical control, pass patient information to a receiving facility, transmit **biotelemetry** (patient physiological parameters such as ECG), and monitor the diversion status of facilities.

In the formative years of paramedic service, it was thought that paramedics would routinely transmit the patient's ECG to the base hospital for confirmation. On-line medical consultation would also be needed during the treatment of serious medical and trauma cases. To facilitate this increased communications need, the Federal Communications Commission (FCC) designed a set of frequencies in the **ultra high frequency range (UHF)** for exclusive use nationwide by EMS known as the **national EMS radio system**. At the time, UHF was an emerging radio technology much as 800 MHz and cellular systems are today. Also, transmission of biotelemetry was not allowed on lower frequency radio systems commonly in use at the time. The FCC designated 10 pairs of frequencies. One frequency of each pair was for transmission from a base station to units and the other for units back to the base station. This is known as a **duplex** radio system. Two pairs of frequencies were for dispatch and system control and the other eight were designated **med channels** for communications of patient information and biotelemetry (Figure 11-3). Because UHF is line of sight, these same frequencies could be used nationwide with limited interference from neighboring systems. Tone codes or channel guards were also used to limit reception of unwanted transmissions among contiguous radio networks. These same 10 frequency pairs are still in use today.

As paramedic practice became established, the need for transmission of ECGs to the base hospital for interpretation decreased. Paramedics proved their ability to accurately interpret ECGs in the field. Likewise, standing orders and protocols allowed paramedics to treat most patients without having to obtain on-line medical direction. Thus the use and nature of medical communications in many EMS systems changed. The system is now used more for notification and transfer of patient medical information than for on-line medical control. Some EMS systems no longer possess the ability to transmit ECGs from the field.

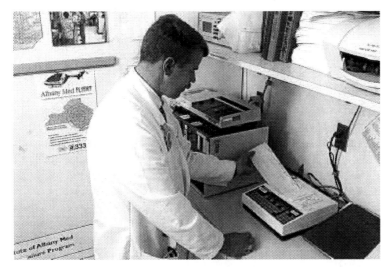

Figure 11-3 Biotelemetry allows an ECG to be received by the hospital while the EMS crew is en route.

Cellular Communications

The **cellular** telephone has become a complement for both system and medical communications. Because cellular communication is so ubiquitous nationwide, the technology has found a role in EMS communications. The development of digital cellular communications with its inherent privacy lends itself to the transmission of sensitive patient information. In addition, the bandwidth, or ability to transmit a broad spectrum of frequencies, of a cellular telephone is greater than that of most EMS radio systems. This makes cellular an ideal medium for the transmission of biotelemetry, most notably the 12-lead ECG.

Some services provide supervisors or personnel with cellular phones as a means to facilitate administrative communications and thus not tie up the regular communications system. This works well for field level administrators and special personnel such as PIOs, health and safety officers, and fleet maintenance.

The one major disadvantage of cellular communications is the potential for a cell site to become overloaded in the event of a major incident or disaster. Cellular communications rely on a series of overlapping cells, hence the name cellular, that act as individual radio systems tied together by a central computer. The computer assigns, transmits, and receives frequencies as they become available and coordinates the hand off of a phone call as it moves among the cells. If a large number of cellular phones are used at once in a cell, the cell can become overloaded resulting in a lack of service. Because the cell cannot differentiate between phones, a phone being used by an emergency responder would be treated the same as one used by a business executive. Thus there is the potential for less reliable service than through a dedicated radio system.

TELEMEDICINE

Although the transmission of ECGs from the field has decreased, new technology may reverse this trend. Biomedical monitoring devices being developed by civilian and military researchers are providing increasing amounts of real time patient data. Coupled with faster and more reliable communications networks, it is possible for field providers to utilize these devices to send increasing amounts of information to physicians and hospitals directly from the field. It is now possible for a physician at a distant location to assess and treat a patient without even physically seeing or touching him. Trauma centers and EDs can be better prepared to quickly treat patients upon arrival based on medical data relayed directly from the field. This new area of medical assessment and treatment is known as **telemedicine**. As computers and radios continue to be integrated, and miniaturization evolves, the future role of the prehospital provider may be that of sensor technician.

SUMMARY

Communications play a vital role in all phases of an EMS incident. The efficiency of an EMS system depends on the coordination of system and medical communications. As technology advances, the role of communications and electronic devices integrating sensors, computers, and communications will change the way EMS providers and physicians interact with patients in the field and during transport.

STUDY QUESTIONS

1. Communications in an effective EMS system provide three functions. List them.
2. List in order the communications phases of an EMS incident.
3. Describe the role of the dispatcher in an EMS event.
4. Differentiate between system communications and medical communications.
5. What purpose do the "med channels" serve in medical communications?
6. List two uses of cellular communications in EMS.

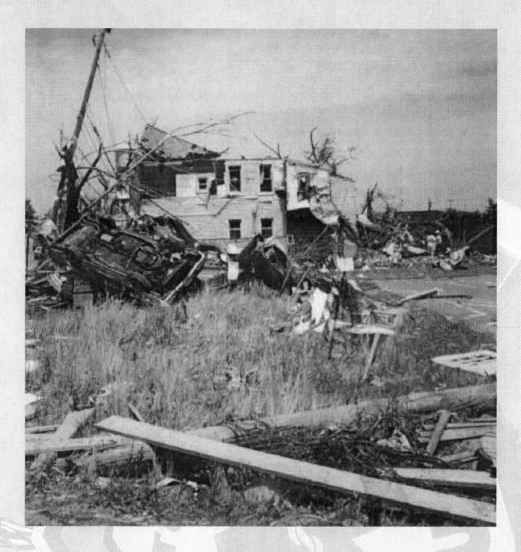

Case Study

Rescue Team Workers
Demonstrate Skills at Open House

THEOLA S. LABBE Staff writer

Colonie: In the aftermath of the vicious May 1998 tornado, a Mechanicville [NY] woman told rescue worker Warren Carr she heard a baby's cry from a home nearby. Carr, a member of the Capital District Urban Technical Search Team, readied the pole cameras and electronic listening equipment, gathered a few other team members and walked through the house, checking every closet and cranny of a home practically torn apart by the storm.

Two years of simulated building collapses and search-and-rescue trial runs had led up to that moment. The team, founded on a directive from Gov. Pataki

(continues)

CHAPTER 12

Disasters

Outline

Objectives

Upon completion of this chapter, the reader should be able to:

- State the importance of disaster planning for an EMS organization.
- Define disaster.
- Differentiate between types of disasters based on magnitude and cause.
- Identify disasters as either natural or technological.
- List the four key phases of disaster management and define each.
- Describe a hazard analysis.

in 1996 as a result of national disasters like the Oklahoma City bombing, includes firefighters and emergency workers from around the Capital Region. Before the tornado, the group had never put their expertise to use in a real-life situation.

The trapped infant turned out to be a false alarm. But over the next two days, the team spent more than 36 hours navigating tornado-ravaged homes to rescue people and pets, and worked with local fire officials in classifying homes and buildings as unsafe. A few months later, the team had their skills tested again when they assisted in the rescue of a construction worker buried in a Menands trench.

About two dozen team members practiced their rescue skills Saturday at an open house at the unit's base in an Albany International Airport hangar. Team members took turns dropping from the ceiling on a thick rope to demonstrate an air rescue, while others demonstrated an electronic machine called the "Life Detector," which can detect the faintest human movement or sound within a decimated structure.

Trained to perform with crisp efficiency in life-and-death circumstances, the group is a kind of local version of Federal Emergency Management Agency, which mobilizes in times of a national disaster. There is a FEMA team based in New York City, but "FEMA is not going to come to a trench rescue in Menands," said Michael Della Rocco, 48, who leads one of four squads in the rescue team.

Made up of volunteer and full-time firefighters and emergency workers, the 110 members of the search-and-rescue squad have taken classes in rope rescue, farm-related accidents, and building-collapse and water rescue, giving them more technical know-how than local firefighters, but not quite putting them on par with the federal emergency workers.

"Our whole purpose is to fill the gap in those medium kinds of circumstances," said Richard French, a team leader.

The team, funded by the state Office of Fire Prevention and Control, must be requested by a local fire department in order to respond in an emergency situation.

Labbe, T. S. (1999, October) Rescue Team Workers Demonstrate Skills at Open House. *Times Union*, p. D6.

- State the role of EMS in disaster mitigation.
- State the role of EMS in disaster preparedness.
- State the role of EMS in disaster response.
- Define ICS and list the key components of ICS.
- State the role of EMS in disaster recovery.
- Recognize the federal role in disasters.

Key Terms

Catastrophe	Individual resources	Recovery
Critical incident stress management (CISM)	Large-scale disaster	Response
	Location	Risk
Disaster	Major disaster	Section
Exposure	Manageable span of	Sector
Federal Emergency	control	Strategy
Management Agency	Mass casualty incident	Strike team
(FEMA)	Mitigation	Tactics
Hazard	Multiple casualty incident	Task force
Hazard analysis	Multiple patient incident	Technological disaster
Incident command system	Natural disaster	Vulnerability
(ICS)	Preparedness	

DISASTERS

A **disaster** is any destructive, dangerous or life-threatening situation that overwhelms the resources of a community. A disaster, sometimes in only a matter of minutes, places enormous strain on any EMS system. The 1993 World Trade Center bombing in New York City, for instance, generated over 1500 wounded people. Many of these sustained relatively minor wounds and ran out of every possible exit of the bombed building into the streets around the gigantic building. They expected immediate medical evaluation, treatment, and emergency transport to hospitals. The more seriously wounded people remained in the building and awaited rescue. They were unable to help themselves because of the severity of their wounds or because they were trapped in the wreckage. The EMS system had to respond quickly and efficiently or lives could have been lost and injuries compounded. Their efforts had to be carefully coordinated with fire, rescue, law enforcement, and other emergency operations agencies that were working at the scene. Procedures utilized in everyday, routine situations had to be drastically modified or the EMS system would have failed in its primary mission.

Some EMS systems managers believe that their programs are too small to need to plan for a disaster. They take on the attitude that it will never happen here and ignore the issue of preparing for a disaster or only give it cursory attention. They forget that some of the worst disasters in history occurred in small, isolated areas that have very limited resources. The Hinton railroad disaster occurred in a remote part of Alberta, Canada. Swiss Air flight 111 crashed in the Atlantic Ocean just off the coast from Peggy's Cove, a tiny community in Nova Scotia. Another tiny town called Barneveld, Wisconsin, was virtually wiped off the map when a tornado struck in 1984. The casualty count was 9 dead and 55 seriously wounded. Many others received minor wounds. Overall, the town sustained a 42% casualty rate!

Every EMS system, regardless of its size, is vulnerable to a disaster. EMS systems that have thought about their response to disaster situations and have developed disaster plans and practiced the procedures outlined in those plans have been far more successful in responding to a disaster than those systems that have not done so. Understanding disasters, planning for them, and training and drilling in advance ultimately saves lives, limits disabilities and hastens recovery of the victims of tragedies. Every community has the responsibility to actively participate in disaster planning and preparation. Every effort needs to be made to ensure that EMS plans are linked to those of fire, rescue, and law enforcement services. Disasters are everybody's business. This is especially so for EMS and other emergency services agencies.

The purpose of this chapter is to provide an introduction to disaster planning and disaster response for EMS students. This chapter does not provide comprehensive coverage of the disaster topic. Whole books have been written on disaster planning or response. Instead of attempting to be comprehensive, this chapter simply outlines the core concepts that are required for EMS systems personnel to understand and appropriately respond to one of the greatest operational challenges an EMS system can face—the disaster.

WHAT IS A DISASTER?

Every day, EMS systems around the world handle many thousands of illnesses, accidents, and incidents that threaten life, cause destruction, and may even produce death. Yet, these are not considered "disasters." They are called "emergencies" and they require immediate attention to reduce the threat of life loss, to save property, or to maintain public health and ensure safety. They are not called disasters because they are *within* the capabilities of local resources to effectively manage these situations.

A disaster, on the other hand, overwhelms an organization's or a community's ability to manage the situation alone with its own resources. A disaster is any situation that causes severe property damage, deaths, and/or multiple injuries and is *beyond* the capabilities of local resources.

Capabilities may include, but are not limited to:

- Personnel
- Facilities
- Communications
- Equipment
- Transportation resources
- Support services
- Security
- Specialized resources
- Finances

- Fuel
- Supplies
- Other

A **large scale disaster** is one in which the local resources are overwhelmed and an effective response requires state level resources such as the National Guard or the state's environmental protection agency. A **major disaster** is any disaster regardless of the cause, which, in the determination of the President of the United States, has caused damage of sufficient severity and magnitude to warrant major disaster assistance from the federal government to alleviate damage, loss, hardship, or suffering. A **catastrophe** is a disaster of extreme proportions and terribly overwhelming impact.

Some disasters produce no direct casualties. That is, there are no human deaths or wounded people as an immediate result of the disaster. Examples would be droughts that kill crops or oil spills that soil the environment and kill fish and other forms of wildlife. There may be horrific economic or environmental effects, but there are no direct human deaths or injuries. EMS systems would obviously have a limited or perhaps no role in such a disaster. The cleanup or restoration after such events, however, still requires state or federal resources that are beyond the capabilities of the local community and is therefore still considered a disaster.

Other disasters produce various levels of human loss and specific terms have been developed for those situations. A disaster with between 2 and 10 victims is called a **multiple patient incident**. A disaster situation in which 11 to 100 direct victims are generated is called a **multiple casualty incident**. Any disaster situation in which there are over 100 direct victims is called a **mass casualty incident**.

Natural Disasters

The word "disaster" comes from the ancient Latin language and meant "sick star." The Romans and other ancient peoples believed that when someone saw a "falling" or "shooting" star in the sky, it was a sign that a horrible catastrophe was about to happen. Early astronomers were often soothsayers and prophets who predicted that the gods were sending catastrophes upon the earth to express their displeasure with human beings or simply to show their power. The catastrophes were usually associated with some natural event such as an earthquake, a volcanic eruption, or a terrible storm.

Today we know that the movements of stars cannot accurately predict natural phenomena such as storms and earthquakes. The prediction of disasters is still quite inaccurate even with the most scientific equipment and procedures currently available. Emergency personnel, in particular, are not very good at predicting the future. They are better trained to react after an event has occurred. Knowledge of the natural phenomena that occur most commonly in one's area of operation, however, can help emergency personnel to meet the challenges presented by natural disasters.

A **natural disaster** is any disaster produced by the forces of nature—that is, those forces associated with earth, air, fire, and water. A list of natural disasters includes:

- Earthquakes
- Thunder storms
- Lightning
- Floods
- Tornadoes
- Hurricanes
- Tsunamis
- Freezes
- Blizzards
- Ice storms
- Heat
- Drought
- Fire
- Volcanoes
- Wind storms
- Dust storms
- Avalanches
- Other natural phenomena

Technological Disasters

Technological disasters are the second major group of disaster situations. A technological disaster is any disaster produced by mankind or by the things human beings make or use. Examples of technological disasters include:

- Hazardous materials
- Nuclear energy leaks
- Utility failures
- Pollution
- Epidemics
- Explosions
- Transportation incidents
- Fires
- Accidents
- Civil disturbance/riots

- War
- Terrorism
- Strikes/work slow downs
- Demonstrations
- Prison breaks/riots
- Energy shortages
- Material shortages
- Price wars
- Embargoes
- Attacks
- Nuclear attack
- Biological attack
- Chemical attack
- Limited conventional attacks

There is an important reason for dividing the types of disasters into natural and technological disasters. Technological disasters, more often than natural disasters, have additional dangers associated with them such as the presence of toxins or explosive conditions. Emergency personnel might be faced with violence, hostage situations, deliberately set secondary explosions, communicable diseases, or other dangerous conditions. When such potential dangers are present, the response of emergency personnel to a disaster must be modified and more carefully controlled to protect the emergency personnel. Rushing into volatile situations can be deadly to emergency operations personnel. At the very least, operations personnel can make a bad situation worse if they are not aware of the dangers. They need to be cautious when deployed to any disaster situation. Deployment to a technological disaster, however, requires a greater degree of caution because of the additional dangers to the operations personnel.

It is, of course, possible to have a combination of natural and technological disasters. An example would be an earthquake that causes a dam to burst. A flood may then result that, in turn, reaches a town and kills or injures the inhabitants. Or that same earthquake might cause a chemical leak at a manufacturing plant. The chemical leak can then threaten lives in the plant and possibly even in the community. It is important that responding personnel know the type of disaster they are responding to and its potential dangers. A full assessment of each disaster situation is essential before units are deployed and personnel are assigned to work within a disaster zone.

DISASTER MANAGEMENT

A well-organized and efficient disaster management program is no accident. Communities and their emergency medical services systems must sharpen their disaster management capabilities by planning and practice over a long period of time. It takes time, money, commitment, planning, education, coordination, practice, evaluation, and refinement to build an effective disaster management system.

The **Federal Emergency Management Agency (FEMA)** is the federal agency that is responsible for disaster management in the United States. It has summarized the various aspects of disaster management into four key phases. When communities follow the federal guidelines for disaster management in those four phases, they can develop comprehensive and consistent programs that match up with other community disaster programs. Then, when one community has to call upon other communities for assistance, they are able to work together more efficiently because their plans and procedures are very similar. FEMA has identified four major phases for developing disaster programs:

1. Mitigation
2. Preparedness
3. Response
4. Recovery

Mitigation

Mitigation refers to any efforts to identify, classify, and eliminate hazards and reduce the potential that they might produce a disaster. Mitigation also refers to efforts to reduce the damages encountered if a disaster cannot be prevented. Labeling hazardous materials, or erecting fences and warning signs to keep people out of danger zones are just a few of the many methods to lessen the potential for a disaster to occur. A community is also mitigating the destructiveness of a potential danger when it prohibits people from building on earthquake fault lines or within flood plains.

EMS Role EMS systems play significant roles in each of the four phases of disaster planning and management. EMS personnel need to be part of the mitigation phase because it would be more dangerous for them to be deployed into disaster situations when they do not know very much about the hazards they are likely to encounter. They should know the potential hazards in their areas. They should be able to see potentially dangerous environments marked on a community map. EMS personnel should join with fire service personnel when building inspections or site visits are made. They need to know what is manufactured or stored or what tasks are performed in specific areas and how dangerous the materials in a particular setting are.

Furthermore, EMS personnel should be on committees that evaluate hazards and threats to health and safety. Every possible effort should be made to rank the hazards from the most serious to the least serious. Then every effort must be made to eliminate or mitigate those hazards. And, when specific hazards cannot be eliminated, steps need to be taken to shield the public from exposure to the dangers. EMS expertise in emergency medical practices and procedures can be extremely helpful to the community disaster committee. Other emergency services groups such as the fire department and law enforcement agencies do not have the same level of expertise. EMS personnel should be active in making recommendations that mitigate the potential for an emergency or a disaster. It would be foolish and irresponsible for them to follow the temptation to abandon their responsibilities to assist in disaster mitigation and leave those efforts up to others. First, that would cause their community's mitigation efforts to be incomplete. Second, they would greatly increase threats to their personal safety by not participating in disaster mitigation efforts. It is certainly possible that they would be the first on the scene of a disaster and could easily become victims if not prepared for what they might encounter.

Preparedness

Preparedness has to do with resource identification and allocation as well as the training and drilling of disaster personnel. Planning, coordination, education, and practice are the mainstays of this particular area. FEMA runs intensive training courses for disaster management personnel. It helps communities to develop disaster response plans. It prepositions disaster response equipment. Every time a community runs a disaster drill it is participating in a preparedness program.

EMS Role The EMS role continues in disaster management by actively participating in the community's disaster planning process. Once the hazards in a community have been identified, evaluated, and labeled on a map, policies need to be established and plans need to be developed.

A policy is a statement by a government of a principle, an objective, or a procedure that is used to guide its activities to help to achieve its goals. For example, a city or county government might write a policy that states its emergency services organizations will work in a united and coordinated manner to manage a disaster. This policy requires a unified command structure should a disaster occur in that community. Failure to work together without appropriate justification would violate the stated policy and department or agency leaders could be reprimanded or even fired for their failure to cooperate with another agency during a disaster.

Another example of a policy is that a specific office within the government will act as an official spokesperson to the news media. No one else would be permitted to speak officially for the government. This type of policy clarifies areas of responsibility and field leaders know who to refer the media to when they begin to ask questions. The existence of a clear policy helps to eliminate confusion and saves time and energy during a disaster situation.

Some policies are set up in advance of a disaster and they allow emergency personnel to immediately perform the tasks of rescue and treatment of victims. Other policies need to be established as the needs of particular situations arise. Usually during a disaster, governmental leaders convene to monitor the situation. Once informed of changing circumstances in the field, they can review existing policies and make new ones if necessary to allow emergency personnel to do their work in and around the disaster site. For instance, routine policies may only allow ten hours of overtime a week in a particular community. During a disaster, governmental officials might have to amend the routine policy and authorize additional overtime hours if such a waiver had never been written into the original policies.

Once policies have been written, then plans can be prepared. Disaster committees need to plan for command and control functions, communications, utilization of special resources, and involvement of resources outside of the community. Plans should also anticipate:

- Incident command system (ICS)
- Evacuation of populations
- Shelters
- Coordination with disaster intervention groups
- Need for specialized emergency equipment and procedures
- Alterations to procedures in the event of terrorism
- Safety and security of response personnel
- Perimeter control
- Response priorities
- Triage
- Treatment in the field
- Transportation
- Public information needs
- Debris removal
- Responder personal needs
- Management of an influx of volunteers
- Management of the media
- Security and other law enforcement issues

Plans should be brief. It has been found that plans longer than seven pages are almost never read and rarely ever used in an actual disaster. Plans are only guidelines and actual situations may demand alterations to the plan under field conditions. Plans, therefore, need to be somewhat flexible. Plans that are not practiced before disasters occur are essentially useless.

Preparedness goes well beyond policy and plan development. Preparedness also includes education, training, and practice. The organizations that have been the most successful in managing disasters are those that have spent a great deal of time educating and training their personnel and drilling them in the steps to take in an actual disaster. It is also important to train field officers on how to be innovative and improvise when plans become unworkable under field conditions or when communications with upper level command fails. If captains and lieutenants were not able to be innovative, the Normandy invasion on June 6, 1944 would have been an abysmal failure. Communications with the upper level command was cut off and the actions on the ground were not going according to plan. The weather conditions had pushed the invasion forces off course and off schedule. Enemy resistance was greater than what had been anticipated. This was particularly so on Omaha Beach. Individual commanders had to make quick and innovative decisions to save both the situation and the lives of many of their soldiers.

Planning, education, training, preparation, practice, and refinement of procedures pay off in the long run. Lives are saved, injury rates are lessened, and damages are limited. EMS systems cannot afford to be excluded from the preparedness functions in disaster management. No one could be expected to perform well in a situation for which they have not prepared.

Response

The **response** phase of disaster activity addresses the immediate and short-term effect of an emergency or disaster. Any actions that are required to save lives, limit destruction, and meet basic human needs fall under the response phase. Mobilizing the American Red Cross, the state's militia, or the National Guard are examples of activities in the response phase of disaster. In some cases, emergency personnel, such as firefighters, paramedics, and police officers, need to be brought from other states to a disaster area to supplement the resources in the local community. This occurred in Florida after Hurricane Andrew. Sometimes satellite communication systems must be set up because the communication system of a community has been destroyed. All of these activities and many more occur in the reaction phase of a disaster.

EMS Role All the mitigation and preparedness activities should make the actual response to a disaster run efficiently and effectively. Disaster research indicates that there are three important elements of disaster management that fail most frequently in an actual disaster—command, communications, and interagency cooperation. Proper planning and practice for disaster operations helps to avoid the three main failure points when the EMS system is called upon to respond to a disaster.

EMS units are usually among the first operations units on the scene of a disaster. In some instances they are the only units on the scene for several minutes before other help arrives. There are numerous steps that first arriving units must take to ensure that the situation is properly managed. If they fail to do these things first and instead get directly involved in patient care, the situation can quickly worsen. EMS units that arrive on the scene first must:

* Access the situation
* Assess the situation
* Determine the magnitude of the incident

- Determine if there are additional dangers to themselves or to other responding personnel
- Assume temporary command
- Establish communications
- Declare a disaster
- Call for assistance
- Inform the communications center of the situation and its magnitude and identifiable dangers
- Request specific resources for deployment to the site
- Establish a temporary command post
- Establish a perimeter
- Choose a staging area
- Select a triage/treatment area
- Prioritize rescue and lifesaving functions
- Communicate with incoming units
- Assign incoming units to specific functions until higher level command personnel arrive and assume command
- Ensure that initial operations are as safe as possible
- After an initial report surrender command functions to appropriate command personnel upon their arrival and then turn attention to access, rescue, triage, treatment, transportation, logistics, or other functions as required

It is very hard for trained EMS people, who arrive first at a disaster site, to take the steps outlined above and not get directly involved in rescue, triage, and treatment functions. Jumping into the rescue and treatment aspects of a disaster may feel right at the time, but it is clearly the wrong thing to do. It will only add to the chaos and confusion of a disaster because incoming units will have to assume the neglected functions. Ultimately, jumping right into action delays the organization of the disaster situation and endangers oneself as well as other responders to the site.

Recovery

Recovery covers any activities designed to put the community back on its feet. During the recovery period, victim needs are assessed, cost estimates are established, and resources are coordinated and deployed for the long-term care of victims. The recovery period is also a time when lessons from the disaster can be learned and a new and improved disaster plan can then be drawn up, practiced, and refined in the mitigation and preparedness phases. Debris removal, loans to small businesses, and the reconstruction of highways and bridges are all recovery activities. So are activities such as postdisaster counseling and temporary housing for people who have lost their homes.

All four phases are essential in disaster management and all four are dependent on each other to ensure a comprehensive, coordinated, and systematic approach to handling the extraordinary demands of a community-wide crisis event. Disaster management programs start off with mitigation and preparedness and then move on to response and recovery. After recovery, a community reviews its performance in the disaster and attempts to draw whatever lessons it can from the experience. The community can then utilize what it has learned to further mitigate the potential for future problems and to prepare for the next potential disaster. The mitigation—preparedness—response—recovery cycle continues indefinitely in a community. There are always improvements that can be made to a community's disaster program. Furthermore, to properly manage a disaster, local, state, federal, and private organizations must be willing to work together for the common good in each of the four phases. A great deal of effort must be put into gaining cooperation of the various segments of a community and into coordinating their efforts should a disaster occur.

Continuous programs for the prevention of disasters or for community preparation for disaster management is a challenging and time-consuming process that demands interagency cooperation and leadership. EMS systems should not only be a cooperating entity in disaster programs, but they should play an active leadership role in such programs.

EMS Role Once the disaster is concluded EMS systems may be requested to provide the community with medical education or information that might assist in the community's recovery. In situations in which the normal medical system has been badly disrupted, EMS systems may be asked to make field visits to assess medical needs or to provide limited medical care. These services are most needed by children and the elderly especially those living in poverty. There have been a few instances in history in which EMS systems were requested to temporarily supplement nursing staff in small hospitals where nurses were killed or injured during the disaster and insufficient staff members were available to keep the hospital running.

It is also common for one EMS system to assist another by providing direct EMS response services when that EMS system has encountered a severe loss such as a line-of-duty death or such severe impact of the disaster that the personnel are directly affected. A flood situation would be one in which personnel may need to attend to personal family issues before they can return to normal work shifts. Relief from other EMS agencies is greatly appreciated during the recovery phase of a disaster.

It would be irresponsible for EMS agencies to disregard the powerful psychological impact a disaster can have on their own personnel. A comprehensive, systematic, and multicomponent approach to support for personnel should be in place routinely. They are even more necessary in the aftermath of a disaster. Support programs for emergency personnel are called **critical incident stress management (CISM)** programs. The research in the CISM field strongly indicates that people who are able to discuss their experiences in a disaster or other distressing event recover faster and return to normal work functions with less disruption than people who tend to hold distressing events within their minds without the benefit of talking to others. When properly organized, CISM programs provide education and planning services before a disaster strikes. They also provide on-scene support services while an incident is ongoing. After a disaster has concluded, a wide range of support services are provided to assist personnel in recovering from the emotional effects of the incident. Most personnel, who receive the proper support, are able to return to normal work. Support services should include, but are not limited to:

- Stress education
- On-scene support services
- Demobilizations and group informational briefings
- Defusing
- Critical incident stress debriefings (CISD)
- Individual support services
- Family support
- Follow-up services and referrals

It is also during the recovery phase that EMS systems can review their procedures, write after-action reports, and decide what alterations to the disaster plan should be addressed in the mitigation and preparedness phases of disaster management.

HAZARDS

A **hazard** is a dangerous event or circumstance that can lead to an emergency or possibly even a disaster. Hazards are all around us in our daily lives. Small objects are a hazard to a baby who might put them in his mouth and choke. Smoking in bed is a hazard that might cause a fire and possibly a death. Failing to stop at a red light is a hazard that endangers us as well as others. A hazard can turn into an emergency. For example, failing to stop at a red light may cause an accident between two vehicles. The driver of one vehicle and a passenger in another are seriously injured. Local fire and EMS resources respond to this emergency and treat and transport the injured to a hospital.

The same hazard can also turn into a disaster. Suppose the vehicle that failed to stop at the red light hits a truck carrying volatile chemicals. There is a massive explosion that flattens an entire city block and kills 62 people and injures over 100. Fires rage throughout the area and threaten other areas of town. Local emergency resources are inadequate to manage the situation without outside help. Other communities have to be called in to assist with the situation. That community would then be dealing with a mass casualty incident and a type of technological disaster.

Mitigation is the best method of dealing with hazards to prevent them from becoming emergencies or turning into disasters. It is important to identify hazards, locate them, and do whatever is possible to eliminate them entirely or to make them less dangerous. If hazards cannot be eliminated or made less dangerous, then efforts need to be made to shield the community so that if the emergency or disaster occurred, it would do the least amount of damage. Mitigation is all about lowering the risks associated with a hazard.

A **risk** is the degree of susceptibility of individuals or an entire community to the hazard becoming an emergency or a disaster that can lead to death, injury, or destruction. Another way to describe risk is to use the word "chance." People often use the phrase, "I'll take my chances" when they are warned not to do something. For example, when told that the ice on a pond is thin and they should not be walking on it, people who deny the presence of the hazard will often increase the risk of an emergency occurring by continuing to expose themselves to the hazard. Not using seat belts in a car and continuing to smoke when the scientific evidence is stacked against such behaviors are other examples of people who are "taking their chances."

There are four important ingredients that create risk. They are:

1. Hazards
2. Exposure
3. Location
4. Vulnerability

Hazards are the dangerous conditions that could generate an emergency or a disaster. **Exposure** refers to the lack of protection of a community from the hazard. For example, not having properly installed lead shields to protect people from x-rays in a hospital setting exposes both patients and hospital workers to significant health threats. Exposure also refers to the hazard being unprotected from conditions such as weather that might cause the hazard to produce an emergency or a disaster. **Location** refers to the placement of a hazardous condition. The storage of explosives in a warehouse within a city is far more dangerous than the storage of the same materials in a remote area. **Vulnerability** is associated with the potential that a hazard could be attacked, stolen, impacted, and/or manipulated so as to become more dangerous and increase the chance that a disaster could occur. For example, not providing fences or other security devices around hazardous materials makes them more vulnerable to contact by people who do not know how to handle them or who might deliberately use those materials to harm others.

Hazard Analysis

Hazard analysis is the methods by which hazards are to be identified, located, assessed for risks, and mapped on the community map. Maximum threat areas need to be identified and secondary hazards must also be identified. A hazards analysis has three segments. First, hazards are identified and listed. Second, information on the hazards is collected. The information includes geographical information as well as demographic information. Detailed information on the specific hazards must be carefully reviewed. This would include the types of hazards, the primary and secondary effects of each, the historical occurrences, the vulnerable populations, and the possible mitigation programs. Third, a report must be developed that clearly outlines the potential hazards, their exposures, location, and their vulnerability to conditions that might cause a problem. Specific recommendations should advise community leaders and emergency personnel on how to limit the risks of having a disaster and what to do should a problem arise.

A well-executed hazard analysis can then be used to justify resource allocation. It can help to motivate the community to mitigate the hazards and prepare for a potential disaster. A hazard analysis sets the stage for the development of a disaster plan. A good hazard analysis can also serve as a platform for public education and information that might avert a tragedy.

Many years ago, in a large eastern city, an industrial area was developed in a remote area. Few people had cars at that time and public transportation to the area was inadequate. The workers built homes in nearby areas within walking distance of the factories. Over time the industrial facilities bought up land around the housing areas and expanded their chemical and manufacturing plants. The housing areas were therefore surrounded by industrial facilities. After a series of fires, explosions, and toxic leaks, people living in the community became concerned for their health and safety. A community hazard analysis was performed. First, every hazardous material or condition within any of the factories or chemical plants was identified and listed. Second, information was collected on a wide range of topics. Information on streams in the area, access and egress routes, location of emergency services stations, the types, amounts, and danger levels of each chemical or condition, and the history of dangerous events was collected. Third, a detailed report was developed and presented to plant owners and the city managers. This report included detailed information on the hazards and the potential for those hazards to turn into a disaster. Specific recommendations were provided to mitigate or eliminate the potential problems.

Emergency plans were improved based on the report's recommendations. The chemical and manufacturing facilities and the city, however, went further. The general consensus was that the people living in the area were being exposed to considerable health and safety risks and needed to be moved out of the area. The city condemned the buildings in the residential area. By means of a combination of federal, state, city, and private funds, the residents were bought out and assisted in moving to another area. In this way, a potential disaster was averted.

INCIDENT COMMAND SYSTEM (ICS)

The **incident command system (ICS)** is an organized method of managing a large-scale incident such as a search for a missing child, a major wild fire or a disaster. It was developed in California in 1972 after a series of large, uncontrolled fires destroyed vast areas of forest, homes, businesses, and other structures and killed numerous people and countless numbers of animals. At the time of those fires, thousands of firefighters worked independently of each other in separate departments in a totally uncoordinated manner. There was no unified command structure, no standardized procedures or equipment, no interagency communications, no common terminology, and no standardized training. The losses encountered in those fires motivated emergency organizations to formulate an integrated and coordinated system to manage large fires and other major incidents. The ICS has been formulated, tested, refined, and retested since 1972. Today, it has become a standard operating procedure in most emergency services organizations. Communities throughout the world are utilizing the system. Lives have been saved, injuries have been lessened, and destruction has been mitigated by the coordinated and standardized procedures of the ICS. Without the ICS, disaster management today would be chaotic, inefficient, and ineffective.

The ICS was designed to address the eight primary components of a good emergency management system. They are:

- Common terminology
- Modular organization
- Integrated communications
- A unified command structure
- Consolidated action plans
- Manageable span of control
- Designated incident facilities
- Comprehensive resource management

The ICS is a management tool characterized by a unified command structure in which the leaders of all of the agencies participating in a disaster come together under one key leader (unified command structure). They develop a strategic plan and then follow the primary leader who orchestrates the overall response strategy. The word, **strategy**, means the big plan of the disaster. A strategy is directed toward a large goal. For example a strategy in a typical disaster is to extinguish the fire, control the situation, and rescue the wounded without causing additional deaths or injuries. To carry out the strategy, a number of smaller tasks must be achieved by a series of steps or specific procedures. These steps or procedures are called **tactics**. In other words, tactics are the steps that need to be taken to increase the likelihood that the overall strategy can be accomplished.

The ICS utilizes commonly accepted, standardized terminology, procedures, training, communications, and equipment to perform the tactics and accomplish the strategy. One key characteristic of ICS is the use of **sections** (modular structure). A section (sometimes called a **sector**) is an area of responsibility. Examples of sections would be operations, logistics, command, administration, and plans. Section leaders have the responsibility to help develop the overall strategy and to manage the major areas of responsibility at the disaster.

The ICS utilizes a **manageable span of control** concept. This means that a command officer has responsibility for only between three and seven people. This helps to avoid overwhelming the commanders with too much input from too many people or too much responsibility for too many people. The **incident commander** (IC), the person in charge of all the personnel working at a disaster, only receives information and feedback from five or six key commanders in charge of sections.

The personnel who are in charge of sections receive input from and have the responsibility for a limited number of commanders under their area of responsibility. The person in charge of all fire-related activities, for instance, would be considered a "branch" officer. That person would report to operations (a section officer). So would the individuals in charge of law enforcement activities, EMS, and communications. Each of them would be a branch. All of them would report to the operations section officer.

The branch officer in charge of all fire-related activities would then have five or six people who would provide input and feedback. These people would be called division officers. The division officers for fire suppression, extrication, and search would report to the person in charge of the fire branch. Likewise, division officers for triage, treatment, and transportation would report to the branch officer in charge of all EMS activities. Similar arrangements exist for the law enforcement or other main areas of responsibility. Division officers are the people who develop the actual tactics in a disaster. They usually direct single resources, task forces, or strike teams that carry out the specific tactics assigned to them.

In summary, the typical response of an EMS system in a disaster might follow the description in the following paragraphs. EMS units would be deployed to the scene. The first arriving unit would access the situation, assess it, communicate with its dispatch center, and advise them of the nature of the incident and request a multiagency disaster response. The first arriving unit would assume temporary command until higher-ranking personnel arrived on the scene. Staging areas would then be chosen and a temporary command post would be established. Other responding units would be directed to assume certain tasks or to report to specific areas to begin their work. Early tasks would include the establishment of a perimeter and a patient collection/triage area. As soon as additional EMS personnel arrived they would be assigned to triage, treatment, and transportation functions. These assignments would only be made if scene security and safety could be ensured. If not, personnel and equipment would be staged until specialized resources could secure the scene and ensure the safety of the response personnel.

Once higher-ranking personnel arrived, they would be briefed on the incident and command would be surrendered to them. The ICS system would then be established and the first arriving EMS units would be assigned as required by the situation. The highest ranking EMS officer (branch officer) would report to the operations chief and ensure cooperation and communication with the other branch officers. Division commanders in the EMS field would most likely include the personnel in charge of medical staging, supplies, triage, treatment, transportation, and communications with the hospitals. Each of those command personnel would have under their control individual resources, strike forces, or task forces to carry out the tactics. **Individual resources** mean one unit such as one ambulance, one fire engine, or one police car. A **strike team** means a combination of same-type single resources assigned to a specific function. For example, four ambulances might be assigned to serve one function of the overall operation. A **task force** is a combination of resources that are assigned to deal with one problem in a disaster.

EMS field operations would continue in a disaster until the situation was managed. If a disaster is prolonged, the number of EMS units assigned to the scene may be downgraded once most of the wounded have been removed from the scene. In many cases

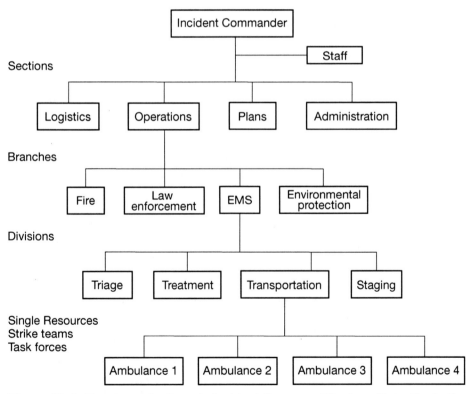

Figure 12-1 Structure of a Generic Incident Command System. *Note:* Illustration focuses on EMS functions.

of a prolonged search after a disaster, one or two EMS units are held at the scene in case another survivor is located. The EMS personnel are also held near the scene in case one of the other operations personnel is injured during the operation.

Figure 12-1 illustrates a typical incident command structure. It focuses on EMS aspects of incident command. Note carefully the primary segments of the incident command system with its sections, branches, divisions, and resource leaders. The objective of this illustration is not completeness, but simply to illustrate the main points of the incident command system.

FEDERAL ROLE IN DISASTERS

Most disasters are the responsibility of local and state jurisdictions. The federal government's role is relatively small in situations that have not been declared disasters by the president. It does, however, provide disaster management education and training to local and state disaster managers and emergency services personnel. It also provides additional assistance with hazard assessment and mitigation to most communities on a regular basis. In addition, the federal government provides other types of services in disaster mitigation, response, and recovery. The Army Corps of Engineers conducts an extensive flood control program in the U.S. The Centers for Disease Control and Prevention monitors and responds aggressively to communicable diseases that threaten the overall health of the nation.

Even without a presidential declaration of a major disaster, the federal government provides assistance to local communities for search and rescue operations. The National Park Service has assisted communities in large-scale search operations. The U.S. Air Force coordinates land-based aerial search and rescue support and the U.S. Coast Guard takes responsibility for search and rescue operations on the seas, rivers, bays, and tributaries of U.S. waters. In major wild fires, the Bureau of Land Management and the U.S. Forest service provide fire suppression assistance.

There are many other ways in which the federal government provides direct and indirect support in local disasters that do not receive a presidential declaration. But, the magnitude and the sources of assistance are significantly magnified once a presidential declaration is made.

Presidential Declaration of a Disaster

The federal government provides assistance in disasters in accordance with the Robert T. Stafford Disaster Relief and Emergency Assistance Act. Congress passed the latest version of this act in 1994. Periodically the act is amended by Congress to better meet the needs of disaster victims. Formal declarations of federal disasters are only provided in major disasters. A major disaster is any fire, flood, explosion, or natural disaster regardless of cause in the United States, which, in the determination of the president, causes damage of sufficient severity and magnitude to warrant major disaster assistance to supplement the resources of states, local governments, and disaster relief organizations.

To begin the process of requesting a federally declared or presidential disaster, the local and state resources must be overwhelmed. Only a governor of a state or an acting governor can request a presidential declaration in a disaster situation. The governor contacts the regional office of the Federal Emergency Management Agency (FEMA). Local, state, and FEMA representatives survey the affected area. Disaster specialists determine the extent of the private and public damage and estimate the extent of federal disaster assistance that will be required. Further consultations with the FEMA regional office to determine eligibility for federal disaster assistance are conducted. FEMA officials are then notified that the governor intends to request federal aid.

The governor's staff prepares the formal request and indicates clearly in the document that an effective response is beyond the capabilities of the state and that the state's resources have already been deployed and are overwhelmed. The governor's office must certify that the state will assume any costs not covered under the federal disaster assistance laws. Detailed estimates of the types and amount of federal assistance must be included in the document. The governor signs the request and it is then forwarded to the FEMA regional office. The regional office evaluates the request and makes recommendations to the director of FEMA. The director of FEMA makes the final recommendations to the president. The president reviews the documents and decides whether or not a formal declaration will be signed. The governor's office is notified if the declaration is approved and then Congress and the participating Federal agencies are notified. A coordinating officer is appointed by FEMA and lists of the types of assistance are developed and forwarded to the governor's office. Available resources are then matched with the types of assistance required. From that point on, the resources of the federal government are brought together to assist the community in managing and recovering from the disaster.

SUMMARY

Disasters are the most significant operational challenge for EMS systems. Although somewhat rare in most communities, they are so demanding that EMS agencies and other emergency response organizations must spend a considerable amount of time preparing for them. A lack of preparation leaves a community vulnerable to a disorganized response that can be costly in terms of life loss, injuries intensified, and destruction to the community. The energy and expense put forward now to prepare for a disaster will pay great dividends in an efficient and effective response when one is necessary.

A community does not have to wait for a big disaster, however, in order to reap some benefit from disaster preparations. Immediate benefits are available. They include better working relationships between the various emergency response organizations.

They also include enhanced leadership and decision making on more routine events. Practice for the major event enhances performance on the everyday emergencies. Up-to-date resource lists are frequently useful in unusual or complicated emergency responses that are clearly not disasters.

If EMS organizations can see that disaster preparations make their communities safer and their emergency services more efficient, they will be more willing to expend the resources that are necessary to make a real difference when a disaster strikes in their jurisdiction.

STUDY QUESTIONS

1. Define disaster.
2. List three examples each of natural disasters and technological disasters.
3. Discuss the relationship of the four key phases of disaster management.
4. Compare and contrast hazard assessment and hazard analysis.
5. Using a bulleted list, state the key points associated with EMS involvement in all phases of a disaster.
6. Diagram the incident command system structure for a natural disaster involving a flood in your local area.
7. Describe the procedure to obtain federal assistance in a disaster.

BIBLIOGRAPHY

Auf der Heide, E. (1989). *Disaster Response: Principles of Preparation and Coordination*. St. Louis, MO: C.V. Mosby Company.

Comfort, L. K. (1988). *Managing Disaster: Strategies and Policy Perspectives*. Durham, NC: Duke University Press.

FEMA Staff, Emergency Management Institute. (1986). *Emergency Management U.S.A.* Washington, DC: US Government Printing Office.

FEMA Staff, Emergency Management Institute. (1990). *Integrated Emergency Management Course: Hazardous Materials*. Washington, DC: US Government Printing Office.

FEMA Staff, Emergency Management Institute. (1994a). *Federal Response Plan for Public Law 93-288, As amended*. Washington, DC: US Government Printing Office.

FEMA Staff, Emergency Management Institute (1994b). *Integrated Emergency Management Course: All Hazards*. Washington, DC: US Government Printing Office.

FEMA Staff, Emergency Management Institute. (1995a). *ICS/EOC Interface Workshop: Participant Handbook*. Washington, DC: US Government Printing Office.

FEMA Staff, Emergency Management Institute. (1995b). *Consequences of Terrorism: Integrated Emergency Management Course: Student Manual.* Washington, DC: US Government Printing Office.

Grant, H. D. et al., Rescue Training Associates, Ltd. (1985). *Action Guide for Emergency Service Personnel.* Bowie, MD: Brady Communications Company, Inc.

Hildebrand, M. S. and Noll, G. G. (1999). *Propane Emergencies.* Washington, DC: Propane Education and Research Council.

Mitchell, J. T., & Everly, G. S. (1996). *Critical Incident Stress Debriefing (CISD): An operations manual for the prevention of traumatic stress among emergency services and disaster workers.* Ellicott City, MD: Chevron Publishing.

Ursano, R. J., McCaughey, B. G., & Fullerton, C. S. (Eds.). (1994). *Individual and Community Responses to Trauma and Disaster: The Structure of human chaos.* Cambridge, UK: Cambridge University Press.

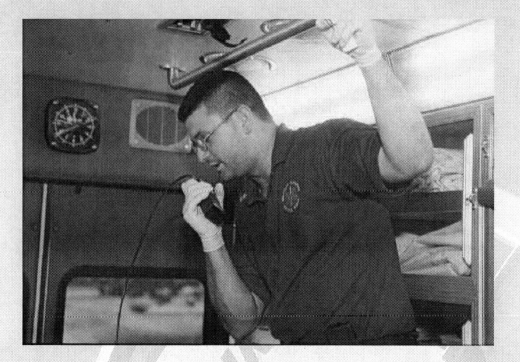

Case Study

The scene is a serious automobile crash involving two college freshmen who had been out partying and ran off the road into a utility pole. The advanced life support crew has assessed and stabilized the patients. They are now consulting to determine transport destination.

"Paramedic 56 to Base"

"Paramedic 56," responds the dispatch center.

"Request County General and Mercy Regional Trauma online for a transport consultation."

"Paramedic 56 switch to talk group Alpha and standby." The dispatch center now contacts the local hospital, County General, and the nearest trauma center and brings both facilities online.

"Paramedic 56 go ahead with County General and Mercy Trauma."

"Paramedic 56 to County and Trauma, we are on scene, auto crash into utility pole involving two males, both 19 years old. Subjects were belted front seat passengers with air bag deployment, no entrapment. Both subjects are conscious and oriented times four with patent airways. Chief complaint of the driver is chest wall pain with decreased motor and sen-

(continues)

CHAPTER 13

Clinical Care

Outline

Objectives

Upon completion of this chapter, the reader should be able to:

*   State the importance of the receiving hospital as part of an EMS system.

*   Identify historical trends that have led to an increased utilization of the emergency department by the general population.

*   Identify recognition of emergency medicine as a medical specialty as a positive factor in the improvement of emergency department care.

*   Describe the basic organization of an emergency department.

Case Study (continued)

sory response from about the nipple line down. Full spinal immobilization. Stable vital signs. Passenger has possible tib-fib fracture and possible shoulder injury. No other significant complaint. Also immobilized and has stable vital signs. We'd like to send the driver to Trauma given indications of possible spinal cord injury. As for the passenger, he can go to County, unless you advise otherwise. We have a land ETA to Trauma of about 35 minutes. Paramedic 56 to County and Trauma over."

"Paramedic 56, this is Dr. Karr at the Trauma Center. We will definitely accept the driver due to the possible spinal injury. Can you advise as to the speed of the crash or extent of deformity to the vehicle, over."

"Paramedic 56 to Trauma, we have about a foot of deformity to the front of the car. The pole was struck pretty much head on. The passenger compartment is basically intact. Driver states he was going around 55–60 when he hit the pole. Over."

"OK Paramedics 56, given the mechanism of injury, why don't you go ahead and send us both patients, especially since you are going to come here anyway. Is that OK with you County General?"

"This is County General, we concur. County clear."

"OK Paramedic 56 will see you shortly. Please advise of any change in the status of your patients and follow your spinal injury protocol en route. Mercy Trauma clear."

"Paramedic 56 direct. Switching back to talk group Charlie."

"Base direct Paramedic 56, I'll show you en route to Mercy Trauma."

- List common management positions within the emergency department.
- State the advantage of special emergency department areas such as fast track and chest pain ERs.
- Differentiate between categorization and designation of medical facilities.
- Identify the clinical components of a trauma system.
- List the components of a trauma center.
- Identify the three levels of trauma center designation.
- Cite an example of a specialty referral center.

- Discuss development of freestanding emergency departments or clinics.

- List the major requirements of the Emergency Medical Treatment and Active Labor Law.

- Discuss the role of critical care transport.

- Discuss expanded scope of practice for paramedics.

- State the role of a trauma registry.

Key Terms

American Board of
  Emergency Medicine
  (ABEM)
American College of
  Emergency Physicians
  (ACEP)
Categorization
Coding
Consolidated Omnibus
  Reconciliation Act
  (COBRA)

Critical care transport
Designation
Emergency department
Emergency Medical
  Treatment and Active
  Labor Law (EMTALA)
Emergency room
Fast track
Fellows of the American
  College of Emergency
  Physicians (FACEP)

Patient dumping
Shock-trauma centers
Society for Academic
  Emergency Medicine
  (SAEM)
Trauma care system
Trauma center
Trauma registry

CLINICAL CARE

A community could be served by the best EMS system in the world, responding in the latest vehicles, and with the highest trained personnel. However, the system would be essentially worthless if it could not transport patients to definitive care. For the average patient transported by EMS, definitive care is provided at the local hospital's emergency department (ED). The public in general sees the role of EMS as a means of transportation to the ED. Although modern EMS involves more than just simple transportation, it is still a temporizing solution to a medical or trauma problem that most often requires resolution in a hospital.

Because EMS is a system of attributes that work together, the hospital is an integral component of a total community EMS system. The importance of clinical care was recognized both by Boyd in the original 15 components of an EMS system and as one of the 14 system attributes in the *EMS Agenda for the Future*. In addition to serving as the terminus for prehospital EMS, the ED is also a major supplier of medical care for the general public. In 1998, it was estimated that 19.7% of all adults and 20.2% of all children were seen in EDs across the country (NCHS, 2000). For patients unable or unwilling to utilize private or group physicians, the ED is seen as a community "doctor's office."

The current structure and function of the modern ED has evolved from a simple "accident" ward for charity or accident victims to a sophisticated medical care unit capable of handling the entire spectrum of medical and trauma emergencies. As a result of this evolution, the practice of emergency medicine has developed into a recognized medical specialty with four subspecialties.

History of Emergency Medicine

In 1979, the **American Board of Emergency Medicine (ABEM)** was recognized by the American Board of Medical Specialties and the American Medical Association. This made emergency medicine the twenty-third recognized medical specialty. This approval led to the development of residency programs in EM and certification of physicians as **Fellows of the American College of Emergency Physicians (FACEP)**. Prior to this time, emergency room physicians were trained in a number of specialties such as surgery, internal medicine, general practice, anesthesiology, and cardiology. Some hospitals required house staff to cover shifts in the emergency room as part of their overall hospital duties, regardless of the physician's expertise or interest. Emergency rooms were occasionally staffed only by interns.

The demand for hospital emergency care grew rapidly after World War II. A number of socioeconomic factors caused a significant shift in the way Americans sought medical care. A major force behind this change was the demise of the "house call" by private physicians. It was common practice for the local general practice physician to visit the sick at their home. Likewise, if someone was injured, they were either rushed to the physician's office or the physician was summoned to the scene. Only in the more populated urban areas where people lived close to a hospital, were patients taken directly to the hospital for care. The second factor that changed the practice of medicine was the increased mobility of the general public. The availability of affordable transportation meant that more people were able to travel. The development of the "suburbs" required that people commute to work on a daily basis. This mobility resulted in increased auto crashes and demographic changes. People were less connected with the family physician as they had been in the past. The hospital **emergency room** replaced the local physician as the source of emergency and after-hours medical care.

In addition to the social changes of the postwar period, the practice of medicine was also changing. The experiences of physicians during World War II coupled with advances in battle field medical evacuation during the Korean War was leading to the investigation and development of new approaches to emergency and trauma medicine. The advantages of rapid transport of the trauma victim, ideally by helicopter, were now being recognized.

As a result of increased national attention to EMS, emergency medicine began to develop along two parallel routes. The quality of medical care in emergency rooms was improved as the importance and value of the ED was recognized by hospitals and medical staffs. At the same time, research into shock and trauma was leading to the development of a systems approach to the treatment of the severe trauma victim. The concept of a trauma system centered around a **trauma center** was emerging. As the two paths continued to develop and, in some circumstances intersect, the specialty of emergency medicine and the concept of the modern **emergency department** emerged.

Scope of Emergency Medicine

Patients present to EDs with a wide and varied spectrum of medical and trauma conditions. This variety requires a medical staff with a broad preparation in all areas of medicine. The organizations representing emergency medicine, **American College of Emergency Physicians (ACEP)**, American Board of Emergency Medicine (ABEM), and the **Society for Academic Emergency Medicine (SAEM)**, have jointly developed a Core Content for Emergency Medicine (see Table 13-1). As stated in the Core Content's preamble:

> The Core Content's purpose and function are threefold: It represents the breadth of emergency medicine practice. For the American Board of Emergency Medicine, it outlines the content at risk for examination in emergency medicine. Finally, it serves as a guide in the development of graduate and continuing medical education programs for those involved in the practice of emergency medicine. Because emergency medicine is changing rapidly, the Core Content requires periodic revision.

The Emergency Department

Hospital emergency departments serve as a direct point of contact with the public. They have been called the "front door" of the hospital. Nationally, approximately 40%–50% of hospital admissions occur through the ED. Additionally, the ED serves as the primary care center for a significant portion of the population.

Hospitals have provided some form of emergency room or accident room almost since their inception. In the mid seventeenth century, physicians from the Hotel Dieu of Paris, France, held sessions on Wednesdays and Saturdays to assist the poor. Early emergency rooms were simply rooms in which a private physician would greet patients presenting with urgent conditions. In larger teaching hospitals, interns or residents were assigned to see patients in the emergency room. These early endeavors have given way to the modern emergency department which is staffed 24 hours a day, seven days a week by trained emergency medicine specialists.

In addition to tradition, hospitals that are accredited by the Joint Commission on Accreditation of Healthcare Organizations (JCAHO) are required to provide at least one of four levels of emergency care (Table 13-2). The most basic, Level IV, provides only assessment and immediate stabilization. The typical ED is categorized as Level II (JCAHO, 1991).

Table 13-1   Core Content for Emergency Medicine

- Abdominal and Gastrointestinal Disorders
- Cardiovascular Disorders
- Cutaneous Disorders
- Endocrine, Metabolic, and Nutritional Disorders
- Environmental Disorders
- Head, Ear, Eye, Nose, and Throat Disorders
- Hematologic Disorders
- Immune System Disorders
- Systemic Infectious Disorders
- Musculoskeletal Disorders (Nontraumatic)
- Nervous System Disorders
- Obstetrics and Disorders of Pregnancy
- Pediatric Disorders
- Psychobehavioral Disorders
- Renal Disorders
- Thoracic-Respiratory Disorders
- Toxicologic Disorders
- Traumatic Disorders
- Urogenital/Gynecologic Disorders
- Administrative Aspects of Emergency Medicine
- Emergency Medical Services/Disaster Medicine
- Drug Classes
- Procedures/Skills

Source: American Board of Emergency Medicine. (1997). *Core Content for Emergency Medicine* [On-line]. Available: http://www.abem.org/corecnt.html

As a true department within the hospital, the ED is most often a stand-alone service or division within the administrative structure of the hospital. In some hospitals however, the ED is part of the department of surgery. Most EDs are managed by an emergency department director or manager. Traditionally this has been a physician who also served as the ED medical director. More recently, administrators with special training in emergency services management have either assumed the position of director or serve as the department's administrative officer reporting to the ED director or ED medical director. The director usually reports to the hospital's chief operating officer.

Table 13-2   Levels of Emergency Services

Level I

A Level I emergency department/service offers comprehensive emergency care 24 hours a day, with at least one physician experienced in emergency care on duty in the emergency care area. There shall be in-hospital physician coverage for medical, surgical, orthopedic, obstetrical/gynecological, pediatric, and anesthesiology services by members of the medical staff or by senior level residents. Other specialty consultation shall be available within approximately 30 minutes. Initial consultation through two-way voice communication is acceptable. The hospital's scope of services shall include in-house capabilities for managing physical and related emotional problems on a definitive basis. The above requirements also apply to a comprehensive level emergency department/service provided by a hospital offering care only to a limited group of patients, such as pediatric, obstetrical, ophthalmological, and orthopedic.

Level II

A Level II emergency department/service offers emergency care 24 hours a day, with at least one physician experienced in emergency care on duty in the emergency care area, and with specialty consultation available within approximately 30 minutes by members of the medical staff or by senior level residents. Initial consultation through two-way voice communication is acceptable. The hospital's scope of services includes in-house capabilities for managing physical and related emotional problems, with provision for patient transfer to another organization when needed.

Level III

A Level III emergency department/service offers emergency care 24 hours a day, with a least one physician available to the emergency care area within approximately 30 minutes through a medical staff call roster. Initial consultation through two-way voice communication is acceptable. Specialty consultation shall be available by request of the attending medical staff member or by transfer to a designated hospital where definitive care can be provided.

Level IV

A Level IV emergency service offers reasonable care in determining whether an emergency exists, renders lifesaving first aid, and makes appropriate referral to the nearest organizations that are capable of providing needed services. The mechanism for providing physician coverage at all times shall be defined by the medical staff.

Source: Emergency Services Standards. Oakbrook Terrace, IL: Joint Commission on Accreditation of Healthcare Organizations, 1991.

The ED medical director is responsible for overseeing the clinical operation of the ED and the management of the medical staff. Hospitals, especially those that are not teaching hospitals, routinely contract out for ED medical staff services. Physician groups bid for contracts to provide physician coverage. Groups may include physician's assistants and nurse practitioners as well as physicians. This practice reduces the administrative demand on the hospital as such routine matters as staffing, hiring, and compensation are handled by the group.

In the early years of the ER, many administrative and clinical duties were performed by the head nurse. This was especially true in ERs that did not have in-house or dedicated physician staffing. In the modern ED, the role of the head nurse has expanded into the nurse manager. Nurse managers now have operational, personnel, and financial responsibilities. They oversee not only the nursing staff, but ED technicians, unit secretaries, and in some EDs registration personnel. They report to the ED director as well as the hospital's director or vice president of nursing. Unlike the ED physicians, the nursing and clerical staff are hospital employees.

Some EDs have created the position of EMS coordinator or liaison. The coordinator serves as the bridge between the hospital and the ED and the prehospital EMS community. This may be a full-time position or assigned to a member of the nursing staff. The coordinator may also be responsible for providing training in prehospital EMS-related topics to the ED staff and prehospital providers. In addition to a training function, the coordinator ensures effective communication between EMS services and the hospital, assists with patient feedback information, quality assurance issues, medical direction and command, and ambulance restocking. The EMS coordinator may also be responsible for arranging ambulance transports and transfers to and from the ED or hospital at large.

Functions within the ED vary but can be categorized into the following basic activities:

- Triage
- Registration
- Nursing evaluation
- Physician evaluation
- Laboratory/radiology ordering
- Consultation
- Discharge from ED

As the demand for ED services increases, some hospitals have sought creative ways to meet the demand. One common approach is the **fast track** ED. Walk-in patients arriving at the ED are quickly triaged. If their complaint is minor and not an emergency, they are sent to fast track where they are evaluated and treated. Fast tracks have their own dedicated staff and facilities. They often utilize physician extenders which lessens the burden on the ED medical staff. By having a separate facility, patients with minor conditions do not have to wait for a regular ED bed or tie up resources that may be needed for more urgent cases.

Occasionally, patients seen in the ED require a period of observation before being discharged. It is not practical to admit such patients to the regular hospital, so they remain in the ED. If an ED does not have a dedicated observation area, such patients continue to tie up an ED bed and resources. As a result, some EDs have designated specific beds or even an area of the ED for observation patients. This makes it possible to keep patients in the hospital for up to 23 hours without having to admit them to a floor bed. Observation areas are also used for direct admission patients. A private physician can admit a patient to the hospital when a regular bed is not available. Such patients routinely enter the hospital through the ED and thus must remain in the ED area until a bed is available. During peak times, the presence of these patients may place a strain on the ED and limit its ability to deal with emergency patients. The observation area can also be used as a "staging area" for patients who are being admitted through the ED, but for whom a bed is not yet available in the hospital.

Hospital EDs that serve a large number of patients presenting with specific conditions or comprise a particular patient population, may open specialty EDs. Some hospitals open such units to increase their catchment area and thus increase revenue. Examples of specialty EDs include chest pain ERs, pediatric ERs, and psychiatric ERs. These specialty ERs are often similar to fast tracks for a specific patient group. Staffing includes medical specialists and nursing staff with special or advanced training as well as special resources and equipment.

Freestanding EDs As hospital emergency departments become more crowded and the business of private physician services changes due to managed care, the availability of traditional primary care has also changed. Faced with an unexpected or non-emergency medical condition, the patient has the choice of either waiting for an extended time in the hospital ED or seeing a private physician. As more and more physicians join HMOs and practice groups, the availability of the private physician is limited. To address this unmet need, freestanding urgent care clinics have come into being, some of which are sponsored by hospitals as a means to reduce demand on the ED.

The urgent care clinic is often open 24 hours, seven days a week, or at least with early morning and late evening hours, to meet the needs of working clients. The centers are staffed with a physician(s) and often a physician extender and nurses. Basic services such as a clinical laboratory and radiology may be available. Patients are usually seen on a walk-in basis although some centers do make appointments for routine medical procedures and follow up. Typical services include:

- Acute, non-life threatening medical conditions
- Asthma
- Colds and flu

- Pediatric ear infections
- Wound care and suturing
- Minor fractures, sprains, and strains
- Crisis intervention
- Obstetrical evaluation and testing
- STD testing and treatment
- Allergy treatment

Although not recognized as a transport destination by most EMS systems, some systems allow prehospital providers to transport patients with minor complaints to free-standing clinics, thus lessening the burden on hospital EDs. This is especially true in rural areas with limited hospital services or long transport times. Urgent care clinics may also be found in remote or isolated areas such as in an island or mountain community that cannot support a community hospital. Clinics also serve resort areas that have increased populations during peak times. Examples include clinics at ski and seashore resorts. Some major ski resorts operate clinics that are essentially hospitals without wards, having ED, radiology, laboratory, and out-patient surgical services.

CATEGORIZATION AND DESIGNATION

The Emergency Medical Services Systems Act of 1973 called for the regionalization of EMS and trauma care. The idea was to maximize the resources available in an area and to pool resources and patients to support centers to serve specific patient groups such as spinal cord injury and burn patients. In order to bring about regionalization, it is necessary to first determine what resources exist in an area. This involves the process of categorization. Once all the facilities have been categorized, certain facilities can be designated for specific purposes. This is the process of designation.

Categorization is often thought of as being "horizontal" in its approach. For example, all of the EDs in a region would be asked to categorize their ability and resources related to emergency care, trauma care, and care of special patient groups. Only the capabilities of the ED would be assessed, not the total resources of the hospital. Although a set criteria can be used, categorization is voluntary and based on the facility's own assessment. There is no independent verification. Also, categorization can change over time as well as the EDs ability to meet a previously assessed level. Categorization is nonbinding on prehospital providers. Just because a hospital may categorize itself as providing pediatric ED services, prehospital providers are not required to transport all pediatric patients to that particular hospital. Although the basic reason for categorization is to regionalize services, categorization does not limit the number of hospitals in an area that can provide the same or similar services.

Designation, on the other hand, is a more formal process than categorization. The process is usually codified in local or state law. Designation is vertical in that it involves the resources and capabilities of the entire hospital, not just the ED.

Approval for designation involves independent verification against established standards and criteria. Once designated, a hospital must continue to meet the designation standards and reapply for designation on a regular basis. Because designation is legally binding and designed to regionalize EMS and trauma resources, prehospital providers are required to follow transport protocols designed to deliver patients to the facility that will provide the best possible care for a given injury or illness. The most common example of a designated facility is the regional Level I trauma center.

TRAUMA CARE

One of the driving forces in the development of modern EMS was the recognition of automobile crash injuries as a significant source of death and disability. But most significantly was the realization that a significant portion of automobile trauma deaths could be prevented if proper emergency care was provided. Trauma victims were arriving alive at local hospitals, only to die a few minutes or hours later. Interestingly, research showed that similar victims transported to large urban academic medical centers often survived (Cowley, 1976). This fact, coupled with the military's experience with battlefield casualties, led to the concept of a dedicated hospital service for trauma victims. These early **shock-trauma centers** developed into the modern day trauma center which is at the hub of a trauma system. Such centers are necessary because trauma is a surgical disease. The only definitive intervention for the trauma patient is rapid surgical intervention. The efforts of prehospital providers and EDs are only temporizing. If a trauma patient is to survive the "golden hour" they must receive rapid surgical intervention.

Trauma research has shown that there are three periods in which trauma patients are likely to die. The first is at the time of insult. Death results immediately from severe injury such as brain stem injury, spinal cord laceration, aortic rupture, and heart rupture. The next grouping consists of those patients who live through the traumatizing event but die within one to two hours. This time frame was called the "golden hour" by R Adams Cowley, one of the pioneering researchers in shock and trauma. It is these patients that the EMS and trauma system are designed to save. The final group of patients are those who die weeks later due to sepsis or multiple organ failure.

The EMS Systems Act of 1973 called for the availability of critical care units within each EMS region or in an adjacent region. Trauma care centers were identified as one of the critical care units that should be available to an EMS region.

Trauma Care System

The **trauma care system** is really a subsystem of the total EMS system. A trauma care system cannot exist alone without support from the many other attributes of an EMS system. In its simplest form, a trauma system consists of a designated trauma center at the hub which receives serious trauma patients either directly from the field or from other hospitals within the region. Protocols exist for the transfer of patients to the trauma center by prehospital personnel. A system also exists for the transfer of critical patients from other facilities to the trauma center. Such systems are usually supported by an established communications system.

At the most sophisticated level, the trauma system consists of a number of interrelated components. The trauma victim is evaluated by prehospital providers and through medical direction, they decide on the appropriate receiving facility. The patient may go to a local trauma center, a specialty referral center, or the central Level I trauma center. A series of local or regional trauma centers, often designated Level II centers, serve the needs of the trauma patient with severe single-system injury or moderate multisystem trauma. Severe trauma patients are sent to the area-wide Level I trauma center most often associated with an academic medical institution. Admission to the Level I center may be directly from the incident site, via a local trauma center, or as a referral from a community hospital ED.

Cales and Heilig (1986) have identified twelve clinical components of a trauma system. These include:

1. Medical direction
2. Prevention
3. Communications
4. Training
5. Triage
6. Prehospital care
7. Transportation
8. Hospital care
9. Psychosocial rehabilitation
10. Public participation
11. Medical evaluation
12. Specialty care

As can be seen, these twelve components encompass many of the attributes common to an overall EMS system. In the case of a trauma system, the attributes have been "fine tuned" to provide optimal response and care for the trauma victim. A trauma system's main operational areas are prevention, clinical care, and research.

The Trauma Center

A typical trauma center consists of the following components:

- Trauma resuscitation area (may be dedicated space in the ED)
- Dedicated operating room(s)
- Intensive care unit(s)

- Surgical ward
- Rehabilitation services

Depending on the center's level, these components may be dedicated solely to the needs of the trauma center or shared on a priority basis with the hospital.

The Committee on Trauma of the American College of Surgeons has established three levels of trauma center designation. All of these levels involve formal designation of facilities by the authority having jurisdiction. These levels of trauma center designation should not be confused with the four levels of emergency care recognized by JCAHO and discussed earlier in the chapter.

Level I. This is the highest level of trauma care. Level I centers are usually associated with major, urban academic centers that admit over 700 trauma patients a year. Facilities, staff, specialists, and intensive care beds are available 24 hours per day on site. In addition to trauma care, the Level I center engages in trauma medical education, trauma research, and trauma prevention.

Level II. This level of trauma center is often found in major suburban community hospitals or associated teaching hospitals. The clinical level of trauma care should be the same as found in the Level I center. However, the dedicated facilities and availability of 24 hour per day on-site specialty services of the Level I center is not required or possible. However, specially trained trauma surgeons and associated medical staff are available on site or on call.

Level III. The Level III trauma center or facility is found in the neighborhood or community hospital. The primary role of the Level III center is to stabilize the trauma victim for transfer to a higher-level center. In rural areas, the Level III center may be the only available trauma service. In this case, a means is provided for the local surgeon or emergency physician to consult with specialists at a Level I or II center. Depending on the availability of transport services, especially air medical transport, the extent of stabilization and treatment may vary. It is also possible that a team from a higher-level center may be transported to the Level III center to provide ongoing stabilization and transfer.

In addition to facilities, the Committee on Trauma has also established guidelines for the training of trauma care personnel. These include surgeons, ED physicians, allied health personnel, and prehospital providers.

Specialty Referral Centers

Not all trauma patients experience severe multisystem trauma. Some patients suffer severe trauma to one particular body system, for instance, the auto crash victim who suffers blunt trauma to the spinal cord with loss of neurologic function. Such individuals may be transported to a trauma center, but would be better served by being transported to a facility that specializes in spinal cord injury. The same would hold true for burn patients or amputation victims with potential for reimplantation. Similarly, certain patient populations, most notably pediatrics, are better served in a facility with equipment and personnel geared to their needs. Examples of specialty referral centers include:

- Spinal cord
- Head injury
- Burns
- Eye trauma
- Replantation
- Pediatric
- Hyperbaric

Trauma Registry

As trauma care systems developed, questions about their efficiency and efficacy were raised given the high cost of such systems. Additionally, information about the patients seen in trauma centers and their injuries were of interest to public health and prevention researchers. What was needed was a means to uniformly collect patient data from all of the nation's trauma centers. This collection of data is known as a **trauma registry**. A trauma registry contains detailed information about moderate to severely injured patients admitted to a trauma center. It is cost prohibitive to include information on all trauma patients. A trauma registry will include information on all trauma deaths, trauma patients transferred to another facility, patients cared for by a trauma system, and those patients hospitalized for more than 48 hours and with specified discharge diagnoses.

Information entered into the trauma registry includes demographics, time intervals, type and severity of injury, physiological response to injury, treatment modalities, patient disposition, and discharge diagnosis. The process of reviewing a patient's medical record and entering them into the registry is called **coding**.

The purpose of a trauma registry is to provide a comprehensive database of trauma patients that can be queried by researchers and system administrators to assist with analysis and problem solving. It also provides baseline information for injury control and epidemiologic research. Additionally, the registry can assist with continuous quality improvement and resource utilization and cost containment. By knowing the types of patients seen by a trauma system, local resources can be better managed and education can be tailored to the local case mix.

State and federal agencies may require participation in a trauma registry as a requirement for facility designation and/or reimbursement. There are various commercial trauma registry programs available, including the American College of Surgeons (www.facs.org) NATIONAL TRACS®, a trauma registry software package.

Because of the various trauma registries existing nationwide, the American College of Surgeons has also developed the National Trauma Data Bank (NTDB). This subscription service is designed to collect data nationwide from the various commercial trauma registry programs. By combining data, a national repository of trauma data can be maintained. This will improve the scope of trauma and injury prevention research by providing data from a larger base population.

COBRA LEGISLATION

In the 1980s the U.S. Congress passed legislation to bring deficit spending by the government under control. As a result of these actions, changes were made to Medicare including adoption of a prospective payment plan. Hospitals now saw an increasing number of uninsured or underinsured patients. To reduce their losses, private hospitals would immediately transfer patients to public or charity hospitals. The practice of transferring patients for economic as opposed to medical reasons became known as **patient dumping**. In extreme cases, ambulances found themselves driving from hospital to hospital with a patient nobody wanted. Other patients were transferred without initial stabilization and treatment, resulting in complications and even death. To put an end to patient dumping, Congress passed the **Emergency Medical Treatment and Active Labor Law (EMTALA)** of 1986 as part of the **Consolidated Omnibus Budget Reconciliation Act (COBRA)** (Public Law 99-272). The EMTALA has subsequently become known in EMS as simply COBRA.

The purpose of COBRA was to require hospitals receiving Medicare funding to provide initial assessment and stabilization to any individual presenting to an ED or to any woman in active labor. COBRA also enacted strict guidelines for patient transfers. As the result of COBRA, some hospitals have closed their EDs and/or obstetrical departments due to the economic loss from uncompensated care.

The primary provisions of EMTALA are:

- Hospital must provide an appropriate medical screening examination to determine if an emergency exists. This examination is the responsibility of the ED physician. The screening may include laboratory tests, radiological studies, and consultation as medically necessary.

- If a true emergency condition is found, the patient must be appropriately stabilized prior to discharge or transfer.

- A woman with contractions is considered unstable until delivery of the child and placenta. Complicated deliveries may be transferred if necessary.

- A patient may be transferred after evaluation if the physician feels such a transfer is medically necessary and the patient's condition is properly documented.

- Hospitals must maintain a list of on-call specialists who are available to evaluate the patient. If an on-call specialist is not available or fails to show "in a reasonable period of time," the patient may be transferred.

- The hospital receiving the patient must agree to accept the patient, have a bed available for the patient, and have qualified staff and resources to care for the patient.

- An appropriate level of care must be maintained during the transfer. Requirements for transport must be specified by the referring physician.

- Hospitals not in compliance with the COBRA regulations are subject to a fine and loss of Medicare benefits. Physicians can also have sanctions imposed upon them that are not covered by malpractice insurance.

Of specific concern to EMS providers is the requirement for maintenance of care during transfer. It is required that the patient be transported by personnel with the proper training and equipment. It would not be appropriate, for instance, for a patient with chest pains to be removed from a cardiac monitor and transferred by a basic life support (BLS) crew. It is not uncommon for a nurse to accompany some patients during transfer.

CRITICAL CARE TRANSPORT

There was a time when a person could go to just about any hospital and receive all the medical care needed. The attending physician and the hospital would just bill the person's insurance company. Today, that is not the case. With new developments in medical equipment and procedures, as well as new approaches to managing health care costs, patients may not be able to receive "full service" at a single hospital. To contain costs, not all hospitals are able to afford every piece of major medical equipment and the staff to utilize it. Hospitals now specialize in certain areas of care such as cardiac care, cancer treatment, etc. Likewise, managed care organizations contract with specific hospitals for the most economic delivery of services. It is to the managed care organization's benefit for a member to go to a hospital or facility that offers a pre-arranged competitive rate. Because of all these changes and advances in medicine, it is not uncommon for patients to be moved from one hospital to another. In most cases, this movement occurs by ambulance.

The transfer of patients by ambulance can be as simple as a BLS crew moving a patient with a casted leg fracture to the sophisticated transfer of a patient from one intensive care unit to another intensive care unit. Transfers may require ambulances equipped with special medical devices and a specially trained staff of nurses and technicians. A typical interfacility transfer crew consists of a critical care nurse and a paramedic. Stable patients without mechanical support such as respirators or balloon pumps may be transported by ALS units depending on local medical protocols.

As the demand for interfacility transports increases, there is a need to properly train paramedics and nurses to work in the **critical care transport** environment. For both the nurse and the paramedic, providing critical care life support in the back of an ambulance can be challenging at times. Because of this, and the desire to increase the ability of paramedics to handle a wider scope of transports without the assistance of a nurse, special critical care transport training programs were developed. The programs are offered either by the in-house nursing and medical staff of a medical institution that has, or contracts for, a critical care transport team, or are offered through an established EMS educational program such as the critical care transport course offered by the University of Maryland, Baltimore County (www.ehs.umbc.edu) and available nationwide. The critical care transport program is an intense 80 plus hour program that introduces the paramedic or nurse to all aspects of critical care transport both by land and air. Topics covered in a typical critical care transport course include:

- Critical care environment
- Breathing management
- Surgical airway management
- Hemodynamic monitoring and management
- Cardiac management
- Pharmacological management
- GI, GU, and renal management
- Neurological management
- Transport considerations

As the role of the paramedic in critical care transport becomes more defined, state and regional EMS systems are developing protocols and amending the scope of practice to allow paramedics to assume an increasing level of responsibility during interfacility transports. Given this trend, future paramedics will either be trained to provide 911 scene response and care or specialize in critical care interfacility transport.

EXPANDED SCOPE OF PRACTICE

Changes in health care delivery have also given rise to the idea that paramedics could do more for patients than just scene assessment, stabilization, and transport. It has been suggested that paramedics could be involved in wellness programs and basic primary care. By adding additional knowledge and skills, the paramedic could help reduce health care costs by helping to prevent illness and injury as well as by providing care for minor medical and trauma conditions. Patients with such complaints as a sprained finger or minor laceration would be evaluated on scene. Through physician consultation, the paramedic could transport the patient or provide initial treatment without transport. Paramedics could also provide routine health monitoring and inoculations.

Initial programs to expand the scope of practice for paramedics have met with mixed results. Successful programs, such as the training of paramedics to be community health providers in Red River, New Mexico, seem to be those that address a specific skill or set of skills or are designed to meet the needs of a defined population. Attempts to have paramedics provide services that have traditionally been within the scope of other health care providers, such as wound care and home health visits, have met with the most resistance. Concerns related to the ability of EMS services to be compensated for expanded care have had a chilling effect on acceptance of the idea. Expanded scope continues to be discussed and investigated but remains an area of controversy.

THE FUTURE

The future of clinical EMS care looks promising. However, it is closely tied to medical advances and operational issues, most notably reimbursement. Advances in telemedicine and miniaturizations of diagnostic devices hold the potential for more definitive assessment and triage of patients in the field. Legislation is pending at the federal and state level to more fully recognize what services EMS provide and to establish a fair and equitable reimbursement schedule. The evolution of managed care will continue to redefine the role of EMS and provide opportunity for new and integrated relationships among patient care providers.

SUMMARY

The development of modern clinical care has come a long way from unstaffed emergency wards to modern trauma centers supported by an established EMS system. The importance of time in the survival of the most critical trauma patients remains a prime reason for the establishment of trauma systems. In addition to trauma centers, emergency departments continue to provide the majority of clinical care to sick and injured patients whether or not they are transported by EMS.

STUDY QUESTIONS

1. Discuss the development of the Emergency Department.
2. Describe how categorization and designation allow regionalization of EMS system hospital resources.
3. Identify the role(s) of a trauma registry.
4. Discuss how COBRA regulations effect local EMS operations.
5. Discuss the role of Critical Care Transport in interfacility patient transfers.

BIBLIOGRAPHY

American Board of Emergency Medicine. (1997). *Core Content for Emergency Medicine* [On-line]. Available: http://www.abem.org/corecnt.html

Cales, R. H. and Heilig, Jr., R. W. (1986). *Trauma Care Systems.* Aspen Publishers: Rockville, MD.

Cowley, R A. (1976). The resuscitation and stabilization of major multiple trauma patients in a trauma center environment. *Clinical Medicine. 83*(14).

Joint Commission on Accreditation of Healthcare Organizations (1991). *Emergency Service Standards.* JCAHCO: Oakbrook Terrace, IL.

National Center for Health Statistics. (October, 2000). [On-line]. Available: http://www.cdc.gov/nchs/products/pubs/pubd/hus/00tables.htm#Ambulatory Care.

Public Law 99-272, §9121, 100 Stat. 82, 164. (1986). (Codified as amended 42 USCA §§1395cc, 1395dd).

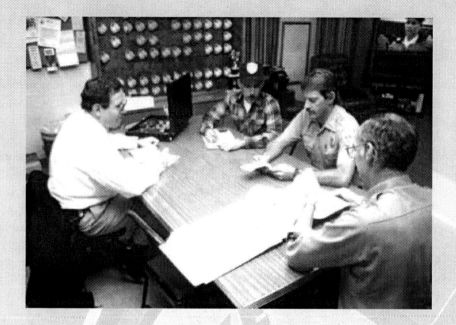

Case Study

The scene is a meeting of the regional managers of a private ambulance company with a public relations consultant.

Consultant: "I have been going through your annual reports and your monthly productivity reports. There is a lot of data here, but I'm afraid it is not in the form the public can understand."

A regional manager: "Well, that's how the corporate office wants us to report things. We have never thought of sharing our system information with the public. You'll just have to work with the data you have I guess."

Consultant: "I see, well that will make my job harder, but I'll see what I can do."

CHAPTER 14

Information Systems

Outline

Objectives

Upon completion of this chapter, the reader should be able to:

- State the importance of information in EMS.
- Recognize the role of a strategic information plan in EMS system management.
- Defend the need for information system integration.
- List barriers to information system integration.
- Differentiate between data and information.
- State the importance of the National Standard EMS Data Set.
- List the three general types of data collected in EMS.

- Discuss the various EMS data collection tools.
- State the role of analysis in producing useful EMS system information.

Key Terms

Analysis	HL7 standards	Optical mark recognition
Clinical data	Hybrid paper forms	Paper forms
Data	Information	Patient care record
Data elements	National Standard EMS	Performance and process
Data formats	Data Set	measures
Data validation	Operational data	Real-time checks
Encryption	Optical character	Strategic information plan
Firewall	recognition	Support data
Formatting standard	Optical imaging	Voice recognition

INFORMATION SYSTEMS

Contemporary EMS systems have access to large volumes of **data** from many different sources such as 911 systems, patient care reports, computerized dispatch systems, physiological monitoring devices, and billing systems. The challenge for EMS is to take this raw data and transform it into **information** that can be used to manage and improve the system by adding intelligence to the data. Data is just a record of an event in time. By itself, it is useless. But when data is placed in a framework or context, it has meaning and becomes information. Senior managers of EMS systems play a crucial role in transforming data into information and using information by:

- Creating and fostering an organizational culture that makes decisions based on facts instead of opinions
- Encouraging the sharing of information
- Establishing a clear information strategy

This chapter covers some of the issues to consider in developing and maintaining an information system for a contemporary EMS organization.

STRATEGIC INFORMATION PLANNING

Developing a sound information strategy begins with a clear mission and vision that state why the organization exists and what the organization wants to become. Overall strategic planning is used to decide how the organization is going to get there. A **strategic information plan** is a plan of the information needs of an organization so that it can meet its mission and vision by determining:

- How will we develop the information system's capabilities needed to support the overall organizational strategy and goals? What types of hardware, software, and staff are needed to collect the data and transform it into information that will be useful to the organization? This is an important step and is more than just buying a computer and a commercial software package. It involves determining the information needs of the entire organization and then working backward to determine what hardware and software can provide this information. A common mistake made by organizations is to purchase hardware and software and then try to "fit" the organization's needs into the information provided by the system.

- How will we provide our people with the skills and tools they need to support our information strategy? Data and information are only as good as the data captured by an information system. If the end users are not trained and motivated to properly collect data, the system will be inaccurate at best and most likely useless. It is important that organizations plan for training personnel to use the information system as well as how to use the information the system provides. By valuing the purpose of an information system, users are more inclined to input correct information and use the system in a positive way.

- How will we monitor our progress toward implementation of our information strategy? Planning alone does not equal success. Evaluation is an integral part of the implementation process. Therefore it is necessary for milestones or critical events to be identified during the planning process that will provide an indication of implementation status. For example, a milestone might be completion of the initial phase of training for field personnel in data entry using a palm computer.

- How will we measure the effectiveness of our information strategy? In the early days of computing, the saying "garbage in, garbage out" was commonly used to stress the importance of entering proper data into a computer. A computer is not capable of improving the data entered into it, just manipulating it in some way. Therefore, it is important for an organization to have a strategy for determining if the strategic information plan is working. This can be assessed by reviewing how information is used by the organization to increase efficiency and make better decisions.

One of the most significant influences on EMS information strategy is the explosion of Internet-based services and technologies. Wireless access is being integrated into devices such as personal digital assistants and cellular phones. High-speed data connections are rapidly becoming available at relatively low cost in more and more areas, making it economical to assemble and maintain the infrastructure components for a robust information system. EMS managers need to think through the implications and possibilities of having suppliers, institutional customers, and the entire workforce equipped with Internet-connected devices.

INFORMATION SYSTEM INTEGRATION

An EMS system is one component of a community's overall health care system. The various components of these health care systems are becoming increasingly reliant upon information systems to guide decisions and extract greater efficiencies and efficacy from health care processes. Most of these gains in efficiency and efficacy are found by looking at health care from a systems perspective rather than just looking at individual service components. Consequently, this is creating a growing demand for integration of information from all components of the health care system, including EMS, in order to reap those rewards (Figure 14-1).

Contrary to these incentives for integration, EMS faces significant social, political, legal, and technical barriers. Of these, the social and political barriers can be the most formidable. There are often very strong competitive factors wedging themselves between entities in health care systems. Legal barriers to integration stem from issues of privacy and confidentiality. Technical barriers come from both software and hardware compatibility issues. In the long run, the incentives are more than likely to prevail against the barriers, but it will be a struggle that EMS should be prepared for. The speed at which the integration occurs will likely be directly related to the magnitude of the mutual economic incentives to do so.

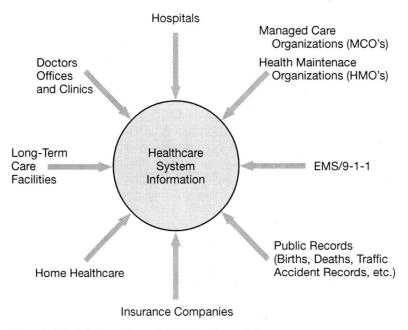

Figure 14-1 Integration of EMS system data

INFORMATION SYSTEM DESIGN CONSIDERATIONS

EMS must consider the wide variety of information needs in the organizations they interact with. These needs must be kept in mind when developing specifications or making actual selections of hardware and software components for information systems. EMS must work through the issues in facilitating data exchange with:

- *Other internal functions.* For example, if EMS is part of a larger organization, how would a central billing office integrate payment from a third-party payer if all other organization functions are direct billed.

- *Institutional customers and other types of customers.* Institutions such as hospitals and nursing facilities may be able to be linked electronically to an organization's computer network.

- *Billing systems.* Most third-party payers have a mechanism to receive billing information electronically as well as provide claim-processing data to the claimant.

- *Regulatory agencies.* Agencies such as the Health Care Finance Administration require regular reporting that can be done electronically as well as be incorporated into report-generating software.

- *Other entities involved in patient care to maintain clinical continuity.* This is an especially important requirement and one that continues to plague health care information systems. In most cases, there is no universal identifier to link a prehospital patient care report with hospital medical records and rehabilitation facility records.

- *Quality management activities.* To ensure quality care, it is necessary to review reports and information for correctness and proper patient care. Software is available that can review reports for accuracy and completeness and provide exception reports that identify questionable reports and inconsistent information.

- *Research activities.* These activities depend heavily on data. The ability to exchange raw field data with statistical software packages will greatly facilitate research.

The information system will need hardware and software components for data input, transfer, storage, analysis, and output. The overall information system design should also consider costs for daily operation, maintenance, repair, and upgrades. Upgrade costs are a particularly important consideration in the face of rapidly changing information technologies.

An often overlooked aspect of information system design considerations are the challenges and costs associated with initial, advanced, and refresher training for the organization's staff. Ideally, some general concepts on the needs and benefits of information systems are covered in the EMS curricula used for training clinical staff. At some point in the evolution of information system utilization in an EMS organization, some level of computer literacy may be appropriate to consider as a prerequisite or a corequisite for employment. If an organization's strategic plans are heavily dependent upon capturing data from the field, keyboard skills and basic computer literacy may be needed before voice recognition and other software advances are able to eliminate the need for those skills. More specific training on the hardware and commonly used software applications might be included in the new employee orientation process. Continuing education might include in-depth software and data entry training.

Data analysis and reporting is one of the last steps in most information system processes, but it should be one of the very first steps in designing an information system. Analyses and reports are the main reasons that organizations have information systems in the first place. If the mission and vision for the organization are known, a strategy can be developed to achieve these goals. With a chosen strategy, the information needed to build, implement, and manage it can be identified. That information is most always in the form of reports that are used by managers and staff working inside the processes to manage, support, operate, maintain, and continuously improve their processes. Starting with the larger processes and working down to the smaller component processes, managers and staff can design the reports they need to accomplish their tasks and meet their goals. From those report designs, the **data elements** (specific items of data recorded) and calculations needed to generate those reports can be identified. All too commonly, the exact opposite approach is taken. Managers and staff make an itemized list of data they can collect, have collected in the past, or think that might be helpful at some point in the future. Just because it is possible to collect a piece of data doesn't mean you should. While adding an individual data element can seem a trivial matter in the design phase, consider the time it takes to collect it, enter it, quality check it, correct it (if needed), transfer it, and store it— multiplied by the number of times that data element is collected in a given time frame. If it is a data element on a **patient care record** (a report completed by the EMS provider for each patient contact) in a busy system, the cost and hassle associated with superfluous data elements can be huge. Therefore, it is wise to limit data collection to items that are needed for a specific purpose for a specific internal or external customer.

Once it has been decided what data to collect (based on the design of reports to be used as the end-products of a data system) managers can now move forward confidently in the design process to:

- Identify a source for each of the pieces of data needed
- Determine what format the data is needed in
- Decide how to collect the data
- Decide how to validate the data

- Decide how to move the data from the point of collection to the point of storage
- Decide how to move the data from the point of storage to the point of analysis
- Decide how to move the information (*Note:* We no longer have just data—we have Information—after the analysis step.) from the point of analysis to a point of storage
- Decide how to move the information from the points of storage to the internal and external customers who need the information

DATA FORMATS

Data formats precisely define each piece of information and in what form the information is obtained and stored. There are several data formatting standards related to EMS, but the most notable is the **National Standard EMS Data Set** developed by the EMS Office of the National Highway Traffic Safety Administration. The standards list the information to be collected and the format in which the data is recorded for a typical prehospital EMS event. Another widely recognized set of health care data set standards are the so-called **HL7 standards**. The HL7 is a standard for the collection, integration, and exchange of clinical patient care data among health care data systems (www.HL7.org). Both the National EMS Data Set and the HL7 attempt to provide a national standard that facilitates the movement and sharing of information among the various producers and users of health care information. The types of data collected by theses standards are discussed below under data collection. Regardless of the external standards an EMS organization might adopt, none of these standards are likely to include all the pieces of data an EMS organization needs to monitor, manage, and improve its key processes.

Another strong factor in EMS data format standards is the variety of commercial EMS software packages available, such as EMScan/Keydata®, Fire Programs 2000™, Firehouse Software®, or SweetSoft®. When an EMS system chooses to use a particular EMS data collection software package, the software usually comes with a very comprehensive complete data set and **formatting standard**. These software packages often include the National Standard EMS Data Set and have the ability for some customization to allow collection of unique data elements needed by a particular EMS system.

DATA COLLECTION TOOLS

There are many ways to collect data in the field during an EMS response, but the most preferable are those that allow crews to maintain their focus on their patients.

Paper Forms

Paper forms are the most commonly used tool for field data collection. Their main advantages are portability, ease of use, ability to generate multiple copies (with special papers), flexibility, legal acceptance, ease of filing, and moderate costs. The costs for printing forms on paper that can generate multiple copies can be quite substantial, but the value of having instantly available copies to provide to receiving facilities usually justifies the expense. The main disadvantages are potential legibility problems with handwritten entries, limited ability to provide real-time data validation, large forms or multiple forms necessary to collect large data sets, and the expense of labor and cycle time delays when typing in data from the paper reports for billing and other reporting purposes. The design of paper forms is almost an art form. A great form is easy to read and understand, easy to fill out, and uses space very efficiently. Trade-offs are made between clear complete labels for each field on a form and using as little space as possible in an effort to collect the desired information on a single page.

Hybrid paper forms utilize electronic processes to reduce the need for manual keyboarding into a computer system. **Optical mark recognition** forms use one or more small circles filled in by pen or pencil to return a value for a particular data element. These can work well when crews are careful to neatly darken the circles. These types of forms tend to take up a lot of space. Paper forms can also use **optical character recognition** technology making spaces for individual characters. These are read by a computer scanning device and converted to computer text, numbers, and symbols. These forms require reasonable handwriting by the field crews. Another paper/computer hybrid is provided by **optical imaging**. The entire form is scanned with a fax or similar device. A more robust type of handwriting recognition software is used that does not have the same strict spacing requirements as standard optical character recognition methods. Some blocks of text that do not need to be electronically processed may be simply saved in an image and kept available in the database record for that particular patient care report. Other hybrid technologies may incorporate handheld barcode readers that allow crews to input certain types of information.

Paper strips with text and physiological waveforms (i.e., ECG, pulse oximetry, capnography) are often generated by medical devices. Paper patient care report designs often include spaces for attaching these strips of information with tape or adhesive strips added to the form in the printing process.

Stationary Computer Workstations

Another paper/computer hybrid strategy utilizes paper forms in the field. The information from the forms is typed by the crews into computer workstations at their crew quarters or in the receiving hospital. This option can work well for systems in which crews have sufficient time to enter their own data into the workstations between calls. The big advantage here is using computers in an environment less susceptible to the dirt, moisture, temperature changes, and mechanical forces that a field computer is subjected to.

Field Computers

Light and durable computers used directly in the field can offer many benefits. One of the most common reasons they are used is to streamline the billing and payment process by collecting information in a computerized format at the point of care. These efficiencies alone can often provide a sufficient return on investment to pay for the hardware and software. These systems can then be used for the many other administrative and quality management benefits that field computers have to offer. Other advantages of field computers include the real-time quality and validation checks that can be performed on the data. This can lead to even further reductions in data collection costs. The disadvantages include high initial costs, loss of data in the event of system failures, susceptibility to damage or malfunction in the field environment, short service lives due to rapid technical obsolescence, and the bulk and weight of many of the hardware platforms. The good news is that computers suitable for the field are getting smaller, faster, lighter, less expensive, and more durable. Newer-generation field-capable computers and medical devices are being equipped with wireless data transfer capabilities that allow the information previously transferred on paper strips to be moved electronically and added to the electronic patient care report.

Data entry into field computers typically requires a keyboard or touch screen/stylus technology. The technology for **voice recognition**, which allows a provider to speak and have his words recognized by the software, is rapidly advancing and may soon be a practical and affordable way for crews to enter their data into their field computers. When combined with smaller hardware components configured into wearable devices, this technology will allow crews to enter data with both hands free to provide patient care.

DATA COLLECTION

There are three general types of data collected in EMS: clinical, operational, and support process data.

- **Clinical data.** Data directly related to the assessment, treatment, and clinical outcomes of injuries and illnesses (e.g., cardiac care)
- **Operational data.** Data related to the nonclinical activities taking place in direct support of field operations (e.g., fleet management and dispatch)
- **Support data.** Nonclinical and nonoperational data that comes from processes used to lead, manage, and support the overall organization (e.g., administration, payroll, human resources, training)

Data from operations and support activities are generally easier to obtain because the processes usually take place in fixed locations in controlled environments. Well-tested generic computerization and data collection systems are widely available for these processes from a wide range of business hardware and software providers. Data from the field EMS setting is far more challenging because of the highly variable and relatively uncontrolled settings in which field EMS crews perform their duties.

One of the biggest problems in EMS data systems has been making sure the data entered into a paper or electronic system is complete and correct. This is where strong leadership, management, and training must come together to make sure that:

- The processes of field care are designed to include data collection. Protocols should integrate documentation into the process steps for assessment and care.

- Training processes for field care include data collection. ACLS, BTLS, PHTLS, and other commonly utilized EMS scenario training programs all but ignore data collection in their processes. Therefore, it should not come as a surprise that EMS data collection suffers because the design of clinical processes and training fail to incorporate data collection. As a result, field crews are often inadequately trained to collect data during their care and assessment processes.

DATA VALIDATION

After all the time, effort, and expense to collect data, it is of no value if the data is not valid. Invalid data can actually have a negative value because it can lead staff and managers to costly mistakes. Fortunately, **data validation** can be addressed at several levels. Data collection tools can often be designed in a way that increases the likelihood that data collected is valid. Paper forms can limit the range of inputs to valid choices with checkboxes and lists or specific number of digits or characters. Reminders can be included on a data collection tool to help define valid entries.

Computer-based data collection tools can be designed to perform **real-time checks** on data for proper format and validity, and advise how to correct the entry in many cases. For example, 360 is entered for an adult pulse rate, the computer could give back an error message that states what range of values it will accept as valid.

DATA TRANSFER, STORAGE, AND ANALYSIS

Once the data related to a prehospital EMS event or out-of-hospital transport is collected in the field, it must be transferred to a central data storage point where it can be aggregated with other patient care records for analysis and centralized billing, accounting, and reporting activities. How the transfer occurs will depend on the type of data collection used. This could include paper reports, computer media, or dial-in modem transfer. The widespread availability of Internet technologies is making it possible to use cables and wireless Internet connections to move data from the field or crew station to the EMS organization's headquarters directly without having to physically transfer a data source. Because these records contain sensitive and confidential information, any such data sent across the Internet must be adequately safeguarded with **encryption**, a **firewall** (a protective measure that limits direct access to a computer or program), and other appropriate security measures to protect patient privacy and ensure data integrity. Federal regulations establish certain standards that EMS systems must abide by when moving patient information across the Internet.

EMS leaders must also consider needs for data security from threats of many different types. For these reasons, organizations are well served to make electronic backups of their data files and store those backups in another physical location that offers security against manmade threats and natural disasters.

Analysis is necessary to transform simple data into actionable information that can be used for different processes and to improve the overall system. Most of the types of analyses performed should be traceable from the mission, to the vision, to the strategic plan, to **performance and process measures** associated with the strategy, to top level reports, to the data sets and the individual data elements collected in the field and elsewhere in the system. The use of data and information to monitor and measure performance is discussed in more detail in Chapter 16.

DATA USAGE

One of the most common problems with EMS data systems is that they collect vast quantities of data that are not used by managers for any specific purpose or benefit to the system. EMS managers need to make sure that there is a legitimate and valuable purpose for each piece of data being collected. When field personnel don't feel this is the case, their efforts to ensure that all data is completely and correctly collected rapidly diminishes, and justifiably so.

In addition to using data to monitor performance and process measures, data and information are useful tools for all levels of an organization. For example:

- Management uses information to make better decisions. Anytime a decision is made, there is some risk involved unless the manager knows for certain what the outcome of the decision will be. To reduce risk, the manager needs information that will help him or her decide the best alternative with the most acceptable amount of risk.

- Internal customers are customers within an organization. Internal customers have various other internal customers and function both as consumers and producers of services. Information is important in both roles. For example, the supply manager for a large commercial ambulance service has the organization's fleet of vehicles field crews as customers. In order to provide a constant and consistent supply of equipment and expendables to the units, the supply manager needs information. He needs to know, for example, the number of units on the road and the number and types of responses handled by the units. By linking the supply operation with data collected in the field, the supply manager can better anticipate the restocking needs of the fleet and prevent supply shortages without having to resort to having costly volumes of inventory sitting on warehouse shelves.

- External customers receive the services provided by the organization. As an example, a nursing care facility may have a contract with a commercial ambulance company to transport all of its residents to physician offices and other health care facilities. By linking the unit availability status of the ambulance company to the scheduling database of the nursing facility, delays and reschedules can be reduced or avoided. And conversely, providing the ambulance company with the needs of the nursing facility allows the company to better schedule and utilize units for more efficient and reliable service.

SUMMARY

EMS systems collect data related to patient care, operations, and support processes. In order for this data to be useful, it must be collected in the proper format, validated, and analyzed. Only then will the data become useful information. Information is an important tool for EMS system managers in that it helps managers make informed decisions. For system information to be truly useful, it must be integrated into the total health care information network. Technological advances have the prospect of making integration easier as well as improving the capture and validation of EMS system data.

STUDY QUESTIONS

1. Differentiate between data and information.
2. Support the need for a strategic information plan in an EMS system.
3. Identify current factors that inhibit integration of health care system information.
4. List at least five entities that EMS systems need to share information with.
5. What are data elements and how are they standardized nationally?
6. List the three types of data used by EMS systems.
7. Compare and contrast the various methods of collecting EMS data elements in the field.
8. Describe the role of analysis in the utilization of EMS data.

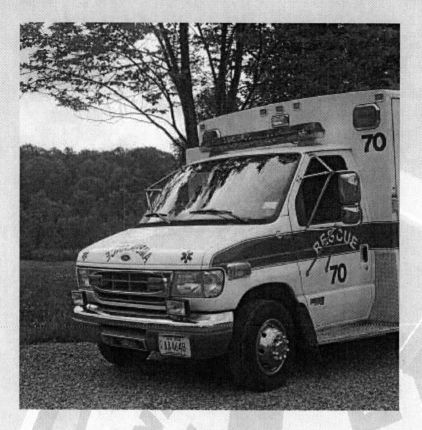

Case Study

The following announcement appeared in the local newspaper.

The Sunshine and Community Volunteer Ambulance Corps announces the initiation of ambulance billing. As of July 1, all patients transported by the SCVAC will be billed for ambulance service. The cost for a transport will be $250. Direct third-party billing will be available. However, any person needing emergency ambulance service should call 911 regardless of ability to pay. *No one will be refused ambulance service based on ability to pay.*

The necessity to bill for ambulance service has been brought about by rising operational costs and reduced response by volunteer personnel. All funds generated through ambulance billing will be used to support part-time paid personnel on duty during weekdays and direct operational costs.

An open meeting will be held at the ambulance corps' headquarters on Tuesday, June 20 at 8:00 PM. Any resident who has questions or concerns about ambulance billing is urged to attend.

Remember, the Sunshine and Community Volunteer Ambulance Corps will continue to provide quality ambulance service to all in need regardless of ability to pay.

CHAPTER **15**

System Finances

Outline

Objectives

Upon completion of this chapter, the reader should be able to:

- Identify the three types of organizations providing EMS.
- Describe the cost-income relationship for each of the three organizational types.
- Identify sources of income for each of the three organizational types.
- Describe basic accounting approaches used by each of the three organizational types.
- State the financial effects of managed care on each of the three organizational types.
- Discuss the role of government in financially supporting EMS.
- Identify future trends in EMS funding.

Key Terms

Balance sheet
Billing for service
Charitable giving
Contracts
Fail-safe public utility
  model

Fee-for-service
For-profit company
Government services
Grants
Income statement
Medicaid

Not-for-profit company
Rates of reimbursement
Start-up money
Subsidy
Third-party payers

SYSTEM FINANCE

Health care costs in the United States now exceed one trillion dollars every year and represent approximately one-seventh of all money spent for goods and services in the U.S. (see Figure 15-1). Despite efforts by the government and industry to control these costs, health care cost increases continue to substantially exceed the yearly rate of inflation as measured by the U.S. Consumer Price Index. Future projections of the demand and cost of health care show a significant increase based on two major factors; the aging of our population and the development of new and expensive medical technologies.

EMS services, though they make up only a relatively small part of the total health care expenditure, nevertheless face the same dilemma; increasing cost for personnel and equipment coupled with an increasing demand for services in an environment where government and industry are trying to control the costs. Because EMS services are a

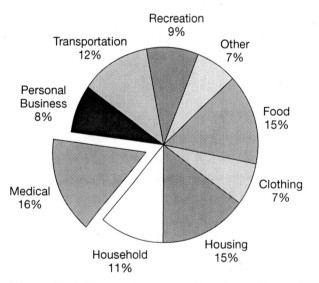

Figure 15-1 Personal Consumption Expenditures 1997

major entry point into the health care system, how these systems operate has taken on additional importance in attempts to control costs. EMS managers today must not only be concerned with the services they provide, but also understand the financial structure and constraints under which EMS systems operate.

SYSTEM ORGANIZATION

Underlying any discussion of the financing of prehospital care and transportation is the business structure of the company providing the service. The type of business will, in large part, determine both the source of funds as well as how these funds are managed. Three major business organizations provide services: for-profit companies, government agencies, and not-for-profit companies.

For-Profit Companies

For-profit companies might be as small as a single unit "mom and pop" company or as large as the international companies that have developed in the last several years. For-profit businesses are organized by investors who expect to earn money on their investment in the company. Therefore, there is an incentive in the company to operate so that revenues exceed expenses and a portion of the resulting profit is shared with the investors. A company that cannot generate a profit will not stay in business for very long because investors will seek other opportunities for their investments.

In a for-profit company, revenues are dependent upon the volume and type of services provided. Prices charged for these services are constrained by competition from other companies as well as government reimbursement policies. Besides increasing revenue, a for-profit company will strive to reduce its costs, however, it is constrained in its cost cutting by the necessity to maintain an acceptable quality or risk losing its market.

Government Services

Government services, or agencies, are exempt from taxes and do not have investors to share in the profits. They are authorized by legislatures and operated by the executive branch of federal, state, and local governments, and are dependent on their legislatures to provide a yearly operating budget from tax revenues which may be augmented by fees and grants. The financial focus tends to be on accountability rather than efficiency, ensuring the legislature that the funds provided were spent properly in accordance with policies set by the government. Funds received in excess of need are usually returned to the government's general fund and may even result in action to reduce future appropriations by the legislature. This practice tends to encourage government agencies to expend all of their allocated funds each year and shifts the incentive for cost containment to the legislature.

Not-for-Profit Companies

Volunteer companies are organized as independent **not-for-profit companies**. Such businesses do not have investors and are organized under special provisions within the federal tax code to encourage the provision of services for social welfare. Such organizations are exempt from taxes and donations made to the organization are tax deductible for the donors. Because they do not have to return money to investors, there typically is less incentive to increase revenue over costs. Any excess funds (profits) are retained within the company for future use. In order to ensure their future viability and maintain the confidence of lenders and donors, including the government, not-for-profit organizations must be concerned with providing services efficiently and handling their funds in a responsible manner.

Nothing in the general descriptions of the three types of organizations should be interpreted to imply that one form is better suited to provide services than another. Examples of the best and the worst can be found in each of the organizational types.

SOURCES OF FUNDS

In order to understand the funding of EMS, imagine yourself as the owner of a private ambulance service, the chief officer of a government service, or chief of a newly formed volunteer service. You have two major financial concerns. First you must find the money to meet the start-up costs of housing and equipping the service and then you need to be able to meet the ongoing operational costs.

For-Profit Company

If you're a for-profit business you will need to raise your **start-up money** in the private sector. You may invest your own savings in the business or bring in partners or other investors by selling shares of the company. In addition, you may turn to commercial banks to lend you a portion of the start-up cost. Once you are in operation you will need to generate revenue through patient billing and contracts to meet your operational costs, compensate your investors, pay the interest on the bank loans, and generate funds for future development.

Because of the number of payment mechanisms and their complexity, **billing for services** has become a major component in the successful operation of EMS service. In some cases you will bill the patient directly in what is termed **fee-for-service**. This is a simple business transaction where you provide the service and the patient pays you directly out-of-pocket for the services provided. Your only problem is ensuring that the patient pays the bill.

It is far more likely that the patient will have some sort of health insurance through a commercial firm or federally run medical program that insures the elderly and totally disabled. These insurance programs, termed **third-party payers**, pay all or a portion of the billed charges depending on the program. While the patient remains responsible for the bill, you will need to assist in filing the paperwork necessary to support the insurance claim. Under some programs you will be paid directly by the insurance company, while in others they will pay the patient and you must collect from the patient. In the case of Medicare your allowable charges will have been established in advance by the government based on a formula of "usual and customary" rates in your area of operation. Under most insurance programs, including Medicare, the patient is still directly responsible for a portion of the bill so you will still need to bill the patient directly or consider offering your own form of insurance through a subscription program. Under such a program, the member pays a modest fee in advance that guarantees that he will not be responsible for any charges beyond those covered by his insurance.

Instead of billing the patient for services, you may enter into **contracts** with health care facilities and managed care insurance programs to provide services to the patient in their program or you may agree to accept a reduced fee-for-service charge based on the expected volume of service.

In order to ensure that necessary services are provided to all their constituents, states and local governments have established several programs to assist patients who cannot pay for services. The best known of these programs is the state run **Medicaid** program which uses federal and state funds to compensate health care providers for services to program enrollees who otherwise would be unable to pay for services. Under guidelines established by the federal government, states determine who will be covered and what services will be provided. The states also determine the **rates of reimbursement** that will be paid to providers. These rates are usually significantly less than what would otherwise be billed, but cannot be so low that health care providers would be unwilling to provide services. If a company bills Medicaid they agree to accept the state reimbursement in full satisfaction of the claim and cannot bill the patient for the difference. Another mechanism that is used by local governments to ensure service is to provide a yearly **subsidy** (grant) to compensate a for-profit company for providing service to an area that would otherwise not be financially attractive to a business.

Several local governments have decided to privatize their EMS systems. This method, popularly known as the "public utility model" (see Chapter 5), relies on a performance based, competitive bid contract with a for-profit ambulance service to provide EMS services in lieu of the more traditional government service. There are a few variations on this method, but the most popular is termed the **fail- safe public utility model**. Under this model the local government establishes a public corporation that owns all the assets of the EMS service including the vehicles, equipment, and facilities. The public corporation does the billing and in most cases receives a subsidy from the local government to reduce the billing amount. The corporation in turn contracts with a private ambulance service to provide the staffing and run the day to day operations of the service.

Government Services

As the director of a government EMS service most of your start-up funding will come from the legislative body of your local jurisdiction. In addition, some grants from the state and federal government as well as from private foundations may be available for the purchase of equipment and to assist in training. **Grants** are made by these organizations in order to encourage development and assist in improving services. Unlike business contracts, there is no specific product or service returned directly to the organization making the grant. Grants are usually made for a limited time period and are not meant to pay for ongoing operational costs.

As with start-up costs, most of the operational cost of the service will be provided by the legislature through an annual or biannual budget process. Some charitable giving may occur by grateful patients and their families. These funds are kept separate and used for specific charitable projects that improve the service.

Increasingly, government services have turned to patient billing as a way of reducing the pressure on tax revenue. Usually the local government does the billing and payments are returned to the general fund of the government. While some jurisdictions have handled the process well, in many cases there have been problems because taxpayers feel they are paying twice for the same service and government service employees resent being required to collect patient billing information. The process has also been hindered by the complexities of billing patients for health care services.

Not-for-Profit Companies

To meet the start up costs of a volunteer company you will need to depend upon charitable giving, grants and business loans. **Charitable giving** can take many forms from responses to direct solicitations to participation in fundraising events. Volunteer members can sponsor fundraising activities such as bingo or fireman's fairs and use the proceeds tax free under the special provisions of the tax code for charitable organizations.

As a private business, volunteer units may also borrow money from commercial banks as long as they can show that their assets and expectations of future revenue will allow them to repay the debts. In order to meet ongoing operational costs, the volunteer company will rely on several methods including charitable giving, government subsidies, and increasingly patient billing, contracts, and subscription programs similar to those offered to for-profit businesses.

Charitable giving, the traditional method of fundraising for volunteers, remains the most important source of funds, but these funds are proving inadequate to meet the costs associated with modern EMS systems. Consequently, volunteer units have had to rely more heavily on government funding in order to meet their obligations. Most local governments subsidize volunteer companies to some degree, but there are wide disparities in the amounts. In some areas, local governments will pay all, or almost all of the unit's operational costs and consider it a bargain in that they don't have to provide a government service or contract with a for-profit provider. In other areas, local governments have been unwilling or unable to make more than a token contribution to the volunteers. State governments also assist in meeting the operational costs of volunteer units through grants to replace and upgrade equipment and programs to train personnel.

If a volunteer unit decides to bill patients for services, it faces all the complexities of the for-profit ambulance provider. Because of the time and the experience required to do the billing effectively, many volunteer units contract with private firms to take on this task. Volunteer units are very concerned with maintaining the goodwill of their donors and therefore tend not to pursue payments from individuals too aggressively and in many cases will sponsor subscription programs to lessen the burden on individuals.

Table 15-1 is a recompilation of the various funding sources used by the different types of EMS organizations. No matter what type of EMS organization is providing the service, all must follow some form of accounting practice, but as you will see in the

Table 15-1   Funding Sources for EMS Organizations

| Funding Source | EMS Organization Type | | |
	Government Services	Not-for-Profit Services	For-Profit Services
Donations and Charitable Fundraising Events	O	M	O
Grants	F	F	
Government Subsidies		M	F
Contracts	O	O	M
Fee-for-Service	O	F	M
Medicare	O	F	M
Medicaid	O	F	M
Subscription Programs		O	O
Business Loans		F	M
Stock Investment			M
Direct Governmental Operational Funding	M		

Major Funding Source
Frequent Funding Source
Occasional Funding Source

next section, these practices will vary sharply, largely because of the varying sources of funds described in this section.

ACCOUNTING AND BUDGETING

Over the years attempts have been made to compare the different types of prehospital EMS service providers based on their financial records. Such attempts have immediately run into problems because accounting and budgeting practices logically differ according to the form of the organization. For comparison, the following is a brief description of the accounting and budgeting practices of each of the major prehospital care provider types.

For-Profit Company

For-profit ambulance services keep their accounting records like other for-profit businesses, using the traditional report forms. The **balance sheet** records the assets, liabilities, and owner's equity at a point in time and the **income statement** reports the revenue and expenses for a given period. The business may be organized as a corporation, partnership, or sole proprietorship based on such factors as size, need for capital, and liability. Most larger firms will be organized as corporations but they can differ from the large corporation that offers ownership shares to the public to the closely held corporation with limited shareholders. Regardless of the type of the for-profit organization, the goal is the same: increase revenue, reduce costs (including taxes where possible), and return a profit to the owners.

The particular form of the business determines how reports are made to the Internal Revenue Service and how profits and losses are apportioned for tax purposes. Firms that offer shares of ownership to the public are required to have a yearly audit by an outside accounting firm that attests to the company's compliance in following accepted accounting procedures.

In accordance with Internal Revenue Service guidelines, costs associated with the capitalization of assets, such as depreciation, are allowed as expenses before taxes are computed for for-profit businesses. Because taxes are not a concern for government and not-for-profit providers, the same expenses may be disregarded by these organizations.

Budgeting in a for-profit business usually involves managers setting goals regarding the type and volume of services to be provided in terms of the expected return on investment. Each item on the balance sheet and income statement is projected forward based on past experience and anticipated cost and revenue. Progress is monitored during the budget year for variances and corrections and adjustments made to the projections.

Government Services

In contrast, government agencies rarely use the financial reports used by for-profit businesses because they don't apply. Because government services don't pay taxes they don't report to the Internal Revenue Service except to report salaries paid to their employees. Liabilities are usually limited to current purchases and there is no owner's equity to be considered. Instead, the most important financial activities are focused on developing and justifying the budget and measuring variances against approved appropriations. Rather than profit, the emphasis is on accountability, i.e., that funds were spent appropriately following established guidelines.

As stated earlier, the tendency is to ensure that all appropriated funds are spent because the "reward" for saving money may be a reduced budget in the future. It is the legislature that normally acts to limit expenditures through the budgeting process although the state governor or local chief executive officer may intercede and curtail spending in an emergency. During normal times, agency budgets tend to grow incrementally as agency requests for additional funds are only partially pared down by the legislature. This usually provides a mechanism for auditing how the agency expended their funds.

Not-For-Profit Companies

Not-for-profit organizations usually follow accounting practices somewhere between those followed by for-profit businesses and government agencies. The larger the organization, the more likely it is to follow for-profit procedures. Profit is not a primary goal, but the organization needs to track its revenue and expenses to ensure its ability to meet current and future needs. Consequently an income statement is frequently prepared. Although the organization is exempt from taxes, it is required to file a yearly report with the Internal Revenue service concerning its activities and financial transactions so it must maintain records for this purpose. Not-for-profit organizations do not have investors to report to, or to share profits with from the operation. However, they frequently incur long-term liabilities through loans and therefore may be required to keep financial records to demonstrate to lenders their ability to meet future payments on the debt.

Not-for-profit organizations usually budget in a manner similar to for-profits except there is less emphasis on profits and more concern with meeting the future demands for the services the organization provides.

Not-for-profit organizations are established with a voluntary board of directors that is responsible for the conduct and procedures of the organization. This can be problematic if someone on the board cannot assume knowledgeable leadership for the safeguarding of funds.

Not-for-profit organizations are dependent on the continued goodwill of donors and supporters so that any evidence of fraud by employees or members can be devastating. Unfortunately, this is not an unusual occurrence and many well-known organizations have had to deal with the consequences of lack of financial oversight.

In accounting, as in other endeavors, form follows function and each of the provider types discussed follows the procedures that are important for their operation. The result is that comparisons are difficult and often flawed or biased by individuals and groups with a particular agenda. The story is often told in accounting about the CEO who hired his accountant based on the question "How much is two plus two?" The obvious answer was four, but the person hired responded "How much do you want it to be?"

ISSUES AND TENSION

There are several issues within EMS that, depending on whom you discuss them with, either offer the best hope for EMS in the future or mean the end of effective EMS. The ideas have created tensions and all have implications for the future financing of EMS. Two of the most important are the role of government and managed health care. Perhaps the most basic issue is the proper role of government in EMS. Is prehospital care and transportation a government responsibility in whole or in part, and should the government provide the service directly or only be responsible for ensuring that a system is in place? There isn't yet a uniform response to these questions and there may never be. We have the full spectrum of responses in place from local governments that disclaim any responsibility to governments that provide services in the same manner as police and fire protection, or those that contract with private providers to supply the service. It is probably safe to assume that we will continue to see this variation in accordance with local custom unless state and local budgets are forced to make cuts in the future. Then we could see a more vigorous adoption of the privatization of services.

One of the most significant trends in the last decade has been the growth of private managed health care organizations (HMOs). It is estimated that over 185 million Americans now receive their health care through such organizations.

In the past, health care providers received their revenue from patients and third-party payers based on the type and frequency of the care provided. The more care provided, the more revenue generated. The incentive clearly was to provide as much care as could be reasonably justified, erring on the side of excess.

Managed care systems seek to change the financial incentives by prepaying the provider. This in effect rewards the provider who limits services because the provider has already received payment and any medical costs subsequently generated reduce the provider's profit. Ideally, the goal is to keep the patient as healthy as possible to avoid medical care and to eliminate excess care when medical intervention is required. This change of incentives has affected prehospital care and transportation in several ways.

Everyone with experience in EMS knows that there is a percentage of emergency calls that are unnecessary. Yet, traditionally government and volunteer ambulance services have operated on the basis that all patients requesting emergency care will be transported and that they will be taken to the nearest hospital that can provide appropriate care. Predictably, in order to reduce costs, managed care companies have sought to control access to emergency care by screening calls and routing ambulances to hospital facilities within the HMO's system so that they can control costs. This process is known as pathways management (see Chapter 5). Constrained by public opinion and in some cases state legislation, managed care companies have only been marginally successful in controlling access to emergency care. Where they have been most successful is in those situations where they have been able to contractually provide ambulance service to their members through a private provider. It is fair to assume that managed care firms will continue in their efforts to control emergency access to care through more contractual arrangements with ambulance services even, conceivably, with governmental and volunteer organizations.

SUMMARY

The financing of EMS will continue to be an issue for EMS managers. At the present we have a variety of providers pursuing a number of funding sources. To manage successfully will require that the manager understand the financial functioning of her organization as well as the health care financing environment.

STUDY QUESTIONS

1. Briefly describe the history of EMS funding.
2. Compare and contrast the three types of organizational groups providing EMS services.
3. Discuss the role of accountability in government EMS operations.
4. Identify ways that managed care has affected EMS funding.

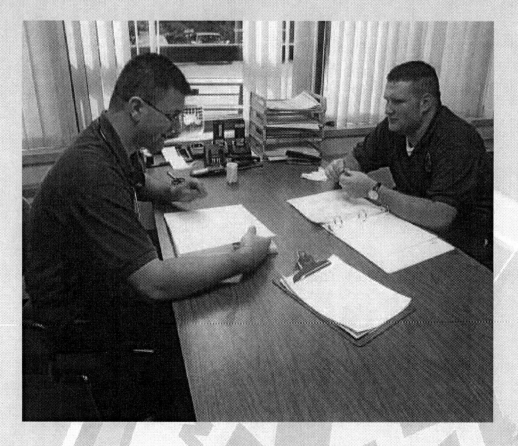

Case Study

The scene is a conference room at a commercial ambulance company.

Group Leader: "Let's get started by looking at the process indicators we identified in our last meeting related to interfacility transport of cardiac patients. Russ, I believe you have developed the indicators?"

Russ: "That's correct. I looked at all aspects of how we transport cardiac patients from community hospitals to tertiary care facilities. I broke the transport down into a series of processes. I grouped the processes into categories. Now we need to take each process and determine the criteria for assessing quality and then relate that to cost."

Leader: "Thanks, Russ. I have distributed to each of you the processes identified by Russ. Now let's get started on determining quality indicators for each process."

CHAPTER 16

Evaluation

Objectives

Upon completion of this chapter, the reader should be able to:

- Relate quality, cost, and value to system performance.

- Define a high performance EMS system using the series of equations presented in this chapter.

- State the value of the Baldrige Criteria as a measure of overall performance.

- Identify the role of planning in quality management.

- Defend the need for key performance indicators in process measurement.

- State the needs of a data system to support measurement of key performance indicators.

- Describe process assurance.

- Describe process improvement

- Identify personnel to be included on a cross-functional team.

Key Terms

Baldrige Criteria for
    Performance
    Excellence
Component processes
Cost
Cost indicator
Cross-functional team
Deming Cycle
High performance EMS
    system

Key performance
    indicators
Mission
Organizational
    assessment
Performance
Performance indicator
Plan-Do-Check-Act
    (PDCA) Cycle
Process

Process assurance
Process improvement
Quality
Quality indicator
Shewhart Cycle
Utstein Guidelines
Value
Value indicator
Vision

QUALITY AND PERFORMANCE EVALUATION

One of the most fundamental responsibilities of an EMS management team is monitoring and improving the quality and performance of its organization's services. Yet most EMS systems have relatively primitive quality and performance management systems. The most common reason is that the agencies that oversee or regulate EMS activities have similarly primitive systems for assessing quality and performance. Most people involved want to improve quality and performance, but have difficulty making measurable progress. This chapter is intended to provide insights and exposure to some strategies and tools that can make real improvements in the quality and performance of EMS systems.

Quality, Cost, and Performance

To place the information within this chapter into proper context, the relationship between quality, cost, and performance should be clearly understood. In the context of this discussion, **quality** is a measure of how well a given process is working. It might be expressed in measures such as response time intervals, survival rates, customer satisfaction ratings, or employee turn-over rates. **Cost** is a purely financial expression, usually in terms of dollars (or other currencies), of how efficiently a process is working. It might be expressed in terms of cost per fleet mile, cost per ALS unit hour, average cost per resuscitation attempt, cost per bill, or cost per new employee recruitment and orientation. **Performance**, in the context of this chapter, is synonymous with **value**. It reflects the combined effects of quality and cost, as expressed in the equation below:

$$\text{value or performance} = \text{quality/cost} \qquad \text{(Equation 1)}$$

MEASURING OVERALL PERFORMANCE

One of the first issues managers confront when trying to take an organized and logical approach to quality and performance management is determining their current level of quality and performance. One of the best ways to measure overall quality and performance is the **Baldrige Criteria for Performance Excellence**. These criteria were developed as part of the National Quality Improvement Act of 1987 (Public Law 100-107) which established the Malcolm Baldrige National Quality Award. Despite the award, the real focus is on the use of the Baldrige Criteria as a framework for organizations to improve overall performance. These criteria are widely recognized for their validity and utility. The criteria and a host of related information and resources are available online at no cost from the NIST website at http:/www.quality.nist.gov.

The EMS Office of the National Highway Traffic Safety Administration (NHTSA) undertook a project in the mid-1990s to develop a model for EMS system quality improvement. The result was not a new program, but a discovery and strong endorsement of the Baldrige Criteria as the best available model. A special information package on the Baldrige Criteria and EMS quality management, called the Leadership Guide to Quality Improvement of EMS Systems, is available at no charge from the NHTSA EMS Office website at http://www.nhtsa.gov/people/injury/ems/leaderguide. html. The Leadership Guide provides EMS managers with an excellent primer to quality management concepts and tools. It also has en excellent bibliography on EMS-specific quality management literature.

Examining organizational performance with the Baldrige Criteria is not a pass/fail process. It's more like measuring your organization's performance with a very long tape measure. These same criteria can be used over and over again to measure EMS system progress from year to year. The overall results are expressed on a scale of 0 to 1000. The Baldrige Criteria results are divided into seven broad areas:

1. Leadership system
2. Strategic planning
3. Information and analysis
4. Customer systems
5. Human resources
6. Process management
7. Results

The feedback report from a properly performed **organizational assessment** using the Baldrige Criteria provides an objective and detailed analysis of the organization's overall performance. The feedback is not prescriptive, but gives insights on how well things are going in terms of an organization's approach to performance improvement, how well those efforts are deployed throughout the organization, and how effective those efforts have been in yielding meaningful results.

Conducting a complete Baldrige assessment is a significant task in itself. Many organizations begin the assessment portion of their quality and performance management journey by using one of several less elaborate assessment tools that are based on the Criteria. A survey-style tool developed by Mark Graham-Brown (Graham-Brown, 1994), based on the 1995 edition of the Baldrige Criteria, is a very useful example of this type of tool. Many states have their own versions of the Baldrige Criteria and corresponding sets of abbreviated assessment tools, such as the State of Florida's Sterling Challenge (http://www.floridasterling.com/assessment/challeng.html).

Regardless of which version or which type of Baldrige assessment an EMS organization uses, the feedback provides an excellent starting point for the strategic planning process. In many successful organizations, the Baldrige assessment process is conducted on an annual basis and the feedback is used to start a new annual cycle of strategic planning, budgeting, implementation, and reassessment.

HIGH PERFORMANCE EMS SYSTEMS

Stout is well known in the field of EMS systems for the concepts of designing **high performance EMS systems** (Stout, 1996, 1983) (see Chapter 5). He effectively makes the case that it is relatively easy to have high costs and high quality, but that does not make for a high performance system. For example, a system can easily lower response times and thereby improve survival from cardiac arrest by putting many more ambulances or rescue units with defibrillators on the street. Plugging numbers into the value equation, you can see how spending more money might get a higher level of quality, but the corresponding level of performance may not change because the numerator and denominator are both increasing in that scenario. Similarly, it is not difficult to build a system with a few units and low survival from cardiac arrest for low costs and low quality. Lower costs and lower quality also do not make a change in performance by the equation.

The challenge is to build a high performance EMS system in which costs are held constant or lowered while simultaneously increasing quality. In our example, that translates into making improvements in survival without increasing costs. Preferably, survival (quality) increases while costs simultaneously decrease. It's all about spending money smarter on the processes that really matter. A good starting point for improving quality in an organization is with an examination of its mission. The **mission** states why the organization exists. For many EMS organizations, it may be to simply provide out-of-hospital care and medical transportation services to a specified community. The **vision** of an organization describes what it aspires to be while fulfilling its mission. Lofty words such as the best, finest, and excellence are often used in statements of an organization's vision. If an EMS organization has a vision to provide the highest level of quality in out-of-hospital care and medical transportation services, the strategy of the organization needs to identify how the organization plans to achieve that vision.

Most organizations with successful long-term efforts have discovered that quality is far more than a program or function. It is something that cannot be delegated to the "quality manager." It is a philosophy of management that gets woven into the very culture of the organization. It is something that every person in the organization should participate in. This philosophy is based on several fundamental premises, including the following:

- All organizations (or systems) are composed of interrelated **processes** that collectively fulfill its mission and serve the needs of its customers.

- The performance (or value) of a process is the result of the combined effects of quality and cost. The goal is to be a high performance organization, one that provides a high level of quality at a low level of cost (a point that deserves frequent repetition).

- You cannot effectively manage what you cannot effectively measure.

- The performance of most every process can be directly or indirectly measured.

- The performance of most every process can be improved (by improving its quality and/or reducing its cost).

- Every process in an organization should contribute toward fulfilling its mission.

- The people who best understand how a process really works and how it can be improved are those who work inside that process and those who directly use the products or services that come from the process.

Leadership System

The role of the senior leader and the senior management team is essential to the success of a quality and performance management system. The leaders must focus the organization on the mission, create and communicate a vision, and take clear steps in their policies, procedures, and processes to steer the organization toward achieving their vision. Too commonly, leaders talk about lofty quality themes and values when their actions are inconsistent with their words. This is one of the quickest ways for leaders to undermine such efforts and diminish their own credibility within their organization. High performance leaders in high performance organizations not only "talk the talk," they "walk the talk" of continuously improving quality, performance, and value.

Improving quality and performance in an organization must also be recognized as a never-ending process. Many liken it to a never-ending journey in which the organization reaches many exciting milestones along the way, but there are always higher levels of quality and performance to aspire to. In a business like emergency medical services, with the lives and well-being of the community at stake, there should never be a point at which an EMS organization is content and no longer seeks to make further improvements in decreasing the morbidity, mortality, and suffering of the citizens it serves.

Strategic Quality Planning

Most organizations use strict financial performance measures and budgetary planning as a routine part of their business activities. The senior managers of the organization are held accountable for meeting specific budgetary targets related to expenses, revenues, and other financial measures of performance. This same type of planning, measurement, and accountability can be applied to meeting quality-related performance targets.

The overall strategy of the organization identifies how it plans to achieve its vision. The strategic planning process should provide sufficient detail to enable plans to be made on how to attain goals that reflect attainment of that vision. Many of those goals will relate to issues of quality, cost, and returns on investment (in both public and private sector EMS organizations).

Strategic quality planning starts by articulating all of the quality-related goals that stem from the organization's vision. From those goals, the next step is to break them down into specific quality objectives. Each of those objectives can be broken down even further into specific milestones with associated timelines, budgets, and measures that will indicate how well the goals and objectives are being met. Some of these goals might be attainable sooner than others. Because the overall strategic planning and budgeting process in most organizations works on an annual cycle, the strategic quality plan should also be organized into one-year increments.

For example, a component of an EMS system's vision is to have the highest rate of survival from cardiac arrest. That might be articulated in even more specific terms— the highest rates of survival from cardiac arrest per the **Utstein Guidelines** on reporting survival from cardiac arrest (Cummins et al., 1991). The Utstein Guidelines are an international set of standards and templates for the recording of prehospital cardiac arrest resuscitation outcomes. Assuming that the organization is early in its quality journey, the main objectives for the first year might be to establish a reliable data collection and analysis process that will enable the system to measure its current rate of survival as a baseline. For most EMS systems, this is no small task. Working through all of the initial process design problems and then refining the process to a high level of reliability could easily take a year or more. Meeting this objective will require planning, budgeting, and establishing managerial accountabilities, just like organizations have for financial planning and performance. Assuming this objective is met in year one, the goal for the next year might be to improve survival to a higher level, based on lessons learned in the first year. Experience gained in those first two years will be extraordinarily helpful in identifying opportunities for further improvement and setting realistic goals for the following years. This same approach can be taken to all functions of the organization from fleet management, human resources, billing and collections, supply and dispatch, to administration.

Information and Analysis

The performance measures for key processes in an EMS organization, whether clinical, operational, or administrative, are referred to in quality management terminology as **key performance indicators**. These key processes may be broken down into smaller and smaller levels of **component processes** and corresponding **performance indicators**. Regardless if they are "key" performance indicators or components thereof, they should all ideally be developed to include both the quality and cost aspects of performance. When developing a **quality indicator**, it is helpful to ask, "What changes would I expect to see if this process was working very well or very poorly." Measuring these changes may be the basis for a quality indicator. Try to choose indicators that are influenced only by the process under examination, or as close to this ideal as possible. Vehicle emissions from your EMS fleet might reflect on the performance for your engines and exhaust system, but using the city-wide pollution index is not specific enough to your EMS vehicles to be a useful indicator. A direct measurement of emissions from the tailpipes of your EMS vehicles would be a more specific, and therefore more useful, performance indicator.

Careful judgment is necessary in choosing indicators because in some cases, the less direct indicators may be more useful. For example, the time spent on-scene could be used as a quality indicator for the EMS processes used in the care of acute coronary syndrome patients. But with deeper consideration, a better process might have slightly longer EMS scene time to obtain a prehospital 12-lead ECG, but have a lower total time from the onset of symptoms until a decision is made for providing thrombolytic therapy or other definitive treatment. The time interval from the onset of symptoms to the time a decision is made regarding definitive treatment may be a better indicator, although it is not as specific as we might like it to be.

When developing a **cost indicator**, it is helpful to ask, "What costs do I have from this process?" Some of those costs may be direct and others may be indirect. Like the quality indicators, careful consideration is necessary to choose good cost indicators. Using the acute coronary care example again, the cost of all equipment and supplies used in the field on a suspected acute myocardial infarction might be a good direct cost indicator for that clinical process. A lower cost process might suggest a better performing process. On deeper consideration, a better process in some systems with longer transport times might include prehospital administration of thrombolytic and/or antiplatelet drugs. This early timing of drug administration might increase the EMS costs but decrease the total costs of care.

A quality indicator can be combined with a cost indicator to derive a **value indicator**, as referred to in Equation 1. For example, an EMS fleet might use the number of breakdowns per 100,000 fleet miles in each month as a quality indicator. A cost indicator might be the monthly average cost per fleet mile. If the fleet ran 334,562 miles this past month and had 17 breakdowns, that would equate to 17/334562 or approximately 5.1 breakdowns per 100,000 fleet miles. That same fleet had an average cost per fleet mile of $34.18.

To use the value equation mentioned earlier, we would have to express the quality numbers in the numerator in such a way that better results have higher values and worse results have lower numbers. A lower number of breakdowns is better than a higher number of breakdowns. To flip the direction of the breakdown numbers to be usable in our value equation, we would simply use its reciprocal (1/number of breakdowns per 100,000 fleet miles). In the cost values for the denominator, the opposite needs to be true. A higher number needs to reflect a higher cost. The use of dollars in the denominator will work fine as is for this purpose. The resulting fleet value indicator is shown in equation 2:

(1/5.1 breakdowns per 100,000 fleet miles) /
($34.18 average cost per fleet mile) = 0.196/34.18 = 0.00573   (Equation 2)

If that fleet was able to reduce how often it had breakdowns over the next month to 4.5 per 100,000 while keeping its average cost per fleet mile steady at $34.18, the fleet value indicator would go up to 0.00650, as shown in equation 3:

(1/4.5 breakdowns per 100,000 fleet miles) /
($34.18 average cost per fleet mile) = 0.222 / 34.18 = 0.00650   (Equation 3)

If the breakdowns stayed at 5.1 per 100,000 fleet miles but the average cost per fleet mile went down to $30.50, the fleet value indicator would go up to 0.00643 as shown in equation 4:

(1/5.1 breakdowns per 100,000 fleet miles) /
($30.50 average cost per fleet mile) = 0.196/30.50 = 0.00643   (Equation 4)

We could also see a smaller improvement in the number of breakdowns per 100,000 fleet miles to 4.7 and a smaller decrease in the average cost per fleet mile to $32.25. But the value equation would reflect their combined effects as shown in equation 5:

(1/4.7 breakdowns per 100,000 fleet miles) /
($32.25 average cost per fleet mile) = 0.212/32.25 = 0.00660   (Equation 5)

It is interesting to consider other commonly used EMS quality indicators such as survival rates from cardiac arrest or response times in combination with appropriate cost indicators to derive value indicators. These types of value indicators can be far more useful to EMS system managers than quality or cost indicators alone. In order to calculate any of these quality or cost indicators, it is necessary to carefully design, implement, and manage data processes that address:

- What specific pieces of data are needed?
- Where does each piece of data come from?
- How will each piece of data be collected?

- How will each piece of data be moved from where it collected to where it needs to be stored and used in calculations?

- How will the accuracy for each piece of data be ensured?

- How can it be ensured that all pertinent data has been collected?

Putting the infrastructure in place for a data management system that addresses these issues is another significant challenge (see Chapter 14). It is an absolutely vital step for building a robust quality and performance management system.

PROCESS ASSURANCE AND IMPROVEMENT

Having data collection and analysis processes are great steps forward, but the journey to high performance is just beginning. The next step is to make sure that the processes under evaluation are being followed consistently. Consider a situation in which an EMS system is studying the performance of its clinical process (protocol) for the management of chest pain of suspected cardiac origin. On the quality side, they are looking at changes in the patient's level of pain on a scale of 0 to 10. The protocol (or clinical process), calls for the administration of a 0.4 mg nitroglycerin spray sublingually every 5 minutes as long as the patient reports continuing pain or discomfort and their systolic blood pressure remains above 100 mm Hg. The data from the first month of study might show that for patients starting with a pain level of 7 and having transport time intervals of 10–12 minutes, the pain level only goes down to an average of 6 by the time they arrive at the hospital ED doors. For the patients whose systolic BP remained above 100, there should be at least 3 doses of nitroglycerin in that time frame (at minutes 0, 5, and 10). Closer study of the data revealed that these patients were only getting an average of 1.4 doses. Discussion of the process by the cross-functional team (to be described later in this section), which included field crews, suggested that some of the problems may be related to difficulties in keeping track of the elapsed time between nitroglycerin doses. With many tasks to accomplish, it can be difficult for crews to keep track of the five-minute intervals. The team came up with the idea of putting timers in the drug kits that could be set to beep every five minutes once they were activated. Crews were asked to turn the timers on when they gave their first dose of nitroglycerin. The following month after the timers were put into place, the cases starting at a level of 7 went on average down to a level of 3. The average number of doses was now 2.8 out of 3 available doses.

This example illustrates **process assurance**. Initially, the protocol was not being followed consistently. Over the next couple of months, these and other problems in process assurance were discovered and corrected to the point that the results from month to month were consistent and the cross-functional team felt that they now had a good idea of what their clinical process was capable of accomplishing in terms of pain relief. Until the process was being followed as written by all crews, the results did not reflect how well the process was capable of performing. In an unknown number of cases the results were clouded by noncompliance to the stated nitroglycerin dosage protocols.

Once an organization has completed the first big steps of putting processes in place to collect and analyze data that reliably measures its levels of performance, it will be ready to begin the next phase—**process improvement**. In this phase, processes are examined to find ways to make them perform with higher quality and ways to make them perform at lower cost. The goal is to bring the processes to a higher level of overall performance.

Many organizations use cross-functional teams to oversee and improve processes. **Cross-functional teams** are typically composed of people who supply a process (suppliers), those who work inside a process (processors), and those who use the outputs of a process (customers). The cross-functional teams are often charged with developing the performance indicators, designing the processes for data collection and analysis, evaluating the results, and coming up with ideas for improvements to the processes.

For example, a cross-functional cardiac team might take stewardship of the protocols for acute coronary syndromes, cardiopulmonary resuscitation, stroke, and congestive heart failure. The team members might consist of a field EMT, field paramedic, field supervisor, ED physician, CCU nurse, cardiologist, and a representative from a cardiac patient support group. To come up with ideas for protocol changes, the group might use brainstorming, literature reviews, surveys, polls, or get ideas from other EMS systems that have good results in their cardiac processes (benchmarking).

Referring back to the chest pain example, a cross-functional cardiac care team might have come to recognize that the current protocol for pain relief in suspected acute coronary syndrome cases, with near 100% compliance, was not capable of providing complete relief of pain in cases where the pain level started at a 7 or higher. In those cases, a quality improvement project might try to "test" a change in the protocol to see if a better level of performance can be obtained. The "test" should be conducted using the scientific method (see Chapter 17). A change in a process (protocol) represents a hypothesis that the new process will perform better than the current one. Therefore, quality improvement teams should develop strong skills in the design and analysis of experimental data.

The cardiac team, after reviewing the literature and their own data, came to the conclusion that if the patient's chest discomfort was not completely relieved by three EMS nitroglycerin sprays, it was unlikely to make additional improvements. Therefore, the protocol (process) was modified to add 2 mg doses of morphine sulfate at three-minute intervals if three EMS doses of nitroglycerin failed to completely relieve the chest pain. The results of the new protocol can be compared to the prior protocol to determine if there was a statistically significant improvement under the new protocol. If the data from the new protocol (process), with reliable and consistent data, showed better performance, the new protocol (process) change could be permanent. If it failed to show better results, another idea for improvement could be developed and tested. This continuous cycle of planning a change, implementing it, checking the results, and acting on results is referred to by several names in the literature, the **Plan-Do-Check-Act (PDCA) Cycle**, the **Shewhart Cycle**, or the **Deming Cycle**.

SCOPE OF PERFORMANCE IMPROVEMENT EFFORTS

There are many administrative, operational, and clinical key processes in an EMS system. It is impossible for a designated quality improvement officer and the medical director to study, collect data, measure performance, analyze trends, maintain consistency, and generate improvement ideas, and then implement and test them all by themselves. Despite this fact, that is the way in which many EMS quality programs are currently designed. As a result, most EMS quality programs only look at a couple of performance indicators. Most of the available man hours for quality efforts are spent on quality assurance activities and externally mandated data collection and reporting requirements. This leaves little to no time available for legitimate quality improvement efforts.

The organizations that are most successful in their performance improvement efforts have overcome this issue (in EMS, healthcare and non-health care industries) with a very broad scope of participation from a large portion of the workforce. The activities associated with performance improvement are designed into the employee selection criteria, job descriptions, orientation, training, education, schedules, and budgets for *all* departments, divisions, workgroups, and work processes in the organization. For example, those working in fleet management participate on teams that address fleet processes and participate on cross-functional teams for other processes. The managers serve as coaches and road block/hassle removers for the teams they work with. The performance improvement staff trains the staff in the use of performance improvement strategies and use of analytical tools. They may also serve as facilitators and internal consultants for specific problems that the teams might need additional assistance with. Performance improvement staff might also consolidate reports between multiple teams and conduct global performance audits such as an annual self-assessment with the Baldrige Criteria.

SUMMARY

It is up to the senior leaders of an EMS system to make sure that all job descriptions, budgets, managerial accountabilities, reward and recognition programs, policies and procedures have performance (quality and cost) improvement components deeply integrated into them and are at the very core of what each person is expected to do in the organization. It has to be more than talk—it has to be measured and held to the same level of accountability and get as much (or more) time as the budget or other primary responsibilities of the management team.

STUDY QUESTIONS

1. Define a high performance system in terms of this equation:

   performance = quality/cost.

2. Differentiate between an organizational mission and vision.

3. Describe the role of quality within an organization.

4. Discuss the Baldrige Criteria for Performance Excellence.

5. Defend the need for strategic quality planning.

6. Identify and describe key performance indicators within an EMS organization.

7. List members to include on a cross-functional team to study transport of fall patients from nursing facilities.

BIBLIOGRAPHY

Cummins, R. O., Chamberlain, D. A., Abramson, N. S., Allen, M., Baskett, P. J., Becker, L., Bossaert, L., Delooz, H. H., Dick, W. F., Eisenberg, M. S. et al. (1991). Recommended guidelines for uniform reporting of data from out-of-hospital cardiac arrest: The Utstein style. A statement for health professionals from a task force of the American Heart Association, the European Resuscitation Council, the Heart and Stroke Foundation of Canada, and the Australian Resuscitation Council. *Circulation, 84*(2), 960–75.

Graham-Brown, M. (1994, December). Measuring up against the 1995 Baldrige Criteria. *Journal for Quality and Participation.* 66–72.

Stout J., (1983). Measuring your system. *Journal of Emergency Medical Services, 8*(1):84–91.

Stout J. (1996, June). High performance mobile healthcare services. Sponsored by the 4th Party and the University of Maryland, Baltimore County. St. Petersburg Beach, FL.

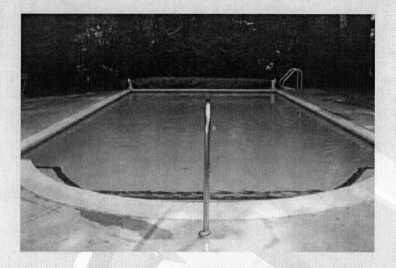

Case Study

One year, in Pinnellas County, Florida, the paramedics began to notice a disturbing trend (Harrawood et al., 1994). There appeared to be an increase in the number of pediatric drowning cases. In the past, if such a trend were noticed, it is likely that the EMS community would have looked for ways to decrease the response times for these emergencies. Or, they might have instituted a program to teach parents about CPR. But in this case, something truly remarkable occurred. First, a coalition was formed. It included not only EMS personnel, but also physicians, nurses, firefighters, public health officials, and local elected officials. The first thing the group did was to document the extent of the problem. They found that the trend had indeed been rising over the previous few years. Then they asked a historic question. Instead of asking how they could speed ambulances to the scene faster, or do CPR better, they asked "What can we do to prevent these drownings?" The coalition then worked together to develop guidelines and implement interventions. As a result of their efforts, the pediatric drowning rate in that county was cut by 50%.

CHAPTER 17

Research

Outline

Objectives

Upon completion of this chapter, the reader should be able to:

- Define research.
- List reasons why research is necessary in EMS.

- List the steps of the scientific method.
- Define various research designs.
- Identify the components of a research study.
- Differentiate between a null and an alternate hypothesis.
- Define reliability, validity, and bias.
- List reasons why research should be published.

Key Terms

Alternate hypothesis
Bias
Double-blind,
   randomized control
   study

Institutional review board
   (IRB)
Interventional study
Literature review
Null hypothesis

Observational study
Reliability
Standard deviation
Validity

WHAT IS RESEARCH?

One way to define research is organized curiosity. It is a way to ask questions and develop answers. It is a way for us to examine the world. Perhaps most importantly, it is a method we use to understand the world around us. Researchers use this understanding to predict a patient's response to medication, the effect of a procedure used for trauma patients, and the changes that can be expected from new policies or procedures.

WHY DO RESEARCH?

EMS personnel have been extraordinarily good at coming up with innovative solutions to problems, but not as good at sharing accomplishments. Perhaps it is because problem solving means that a problem exists and some managers refuse to admit that their agency has a problem. Perhaps it is because there are few role models or mentors to help EMS personnel work their way through the research process. Whatever the reasons, it is now recognized that research is a crucial component of future EMS development. Other reasons to do research include:

- Improve patient care
- Improve the system
- Reduce hazards
- Provide legal protection
- Improve the profession

Improve Patient Care

One of the most crucial reasons for health care professionals to conduct research is to improve patient care. An organized research project allows researchers to consider a number of interventions for a particular type of patient complaint or condition. As an example, consider the use of the MAST (Military Anti-Shock Trousers). For many years, the MAST suit was considered the prehospital intervention of choice for hypotensive trauma patients. During those years much anecdotal evidence was accumulated that seemed to demonstrate the efficacy of the trousers. Then Dr. Paul Pepe and a team of researchers conducted a number of scientific research studies (Bickell et al., 1985; Mattox et al., 1986; Pepe, Bass, & Mattox, 1986; Bickell et al., 1987; Mattox et al., 1989). As a result of those studies, it was determined that the MAST does not improve patient outcomes and, in some cases may even increase mortality. As a result of this research, MAST protocols have changed dramatically.

Improve the System

Research can also be used to make improvements within an existing EMS system. In one study (Joyce, Dutkowski, & Hynes, 1997) a QI program was evaluated for its impact on the EMS system. Using criteria such as appropriate treatment, adequate documentation, call time intervals, and protocol compliance, the authors found that the new QI program resulted in significant improvement in 13 of 19 parameters evaluated.

Reduce Hazards

There are many hazards involved in EMS and research can be used to identify hazards and implement plans for reducing those hazards. In another study (Maguire & Porco, 1997), the authors reported on a research experiment aimed at reducing ambulance collisions. In this case the study was prompted by a number of dramatic ambulance collisions. Using a pre- and postintervention evaluation model, the collision rate was calculated prior to and after the implementation of two interventions. The combined use of a mandatory driver training program and a change in the departmental driving policies was associated with a 50% reduction in collisions following the interventions.

Provide Legal Protection

Research projects can both identify the legal risks associated with EMS (Goldberg et al., 1990; Soler et al., 1985) and can help protect practitioners who follow guidelines based on scientifically verified procedures. For example, researchers in Brooklyn, NY, conducted an eight-year retrospective review of all legal cases related to one hospital-based EMS agency (Maguire and Porco, 1997). They found that 100% of the litigation was associated with motor vehicle collisions. They also discovered that the lack of seat belt use was a recurring factor in much of the litigation.

Improve the Profession

For the medical and health care communities, research is the language of professionals. It is the way professionals communicate with one another and it helps separate the professions from the trades. It is the method professionals use to improve their professions.

INTRODUCTION TO THE SCIENTIFIC METHOD

As described above in the MAST example, the lack of an organized, objective examination of the facts can lead to erroneous assumptions and beliefs. Therefore, researchers have developed a systematic inquiry approach called the scientific method. This approach includes:

- Formulating a testable hypothesis from which verifiable predictions can be confirmed or deduced as true or false based on brute facts (facts not subject to controversy, interpretation, or dispute)

- The use of neutral and repeatable experimental procedures to test a hypothesis to screen out biases and preconceptions about the validity of the hypothesis being tested

- Submitting findings to the review of peers, and,

- Organizing knowledge into a system of general laws that reveal causal connections existing in the world.

The scientific method has allowed the natural sciences to have the following characteristics:

- Self-correcting methods that provide an increasingly accurate picture of nature

- Consensus generated, that is, practitioners come to agreement on which hypotheses are to be accepted and rejected (this differs from philosophy and religion where disagreements do not necessarily diminish over time).

Statistics

Although a formal review of statistical methods is beyond the scope of this text, it is now essential for EMS professionals to be familiar with at least the basic tenets of statistics. One of the most important statistical concepts is that of population distribution. We measure population distributions by calculating average scores and standard deviations. For example, if we measure the height of a randomly selected group of men from the population, we will find an average height and a distribution of heights that will be mostly near the average. So, if the average height is 5'8", most men will be about 5'8", fewer will be 6' and even fewer will be 6'5". If we graph the results using height as the x axis (the base) starting at under 4' on the left and going to over 7' all the way to the right, and if we put the number of subjects as the y axis, we will gen-

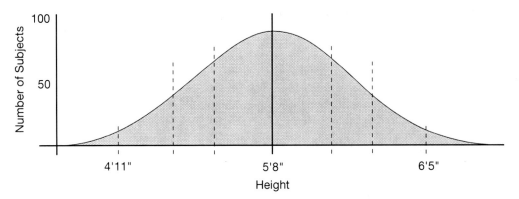

Figure 17-1 Standard Distribution Curve

erate a picture that looks like Figure 17-1. This is known as the standard distribution curve.

The **standard deviation** is a calculation that lets us predict, for example, how many men will be within certain ranges. In a normally distributed population, 68% of the subjects fall within one standard deviation of the mean. If, for example, the standard deviation for the subjects we tested was 3″, we would know that 68% of the group is between 5′5″ and 5′11″. Two standard deviations encompass 95% of the population. So, we would know that 95% of these men are between 5′2″ and 6′2″. Ninety nine percent of the population will be within three standard deviations of the mean. In this example, that means that 99% of the subjects will be between 4′11″ and 6′5″.

Consider the measurement of IQ. The IQ test is written to generate an average score of 100 and a standard deviation of 15. This means that 68% of the population has an IQ between 85 and 115, 95% between 70 and 130, and 99% between 55 and 145. Because the population is normally distributed, we can also calculate the percentage of people who have, for example, an IQ over 130. We know that 95% of the population has an IQ between 70 and 130. That leaves 5% of the population. We also know that there is the same number of subjects above and below the average. Therefore, we can calculate that 2.5% of the population has an IQ above 130.

Once we know the average and standard deviation, we can use those figures to determine if an intervention changes the average and standard deviation in our test population to a significant degree. Various statistical tests are used to measure that question under different circumstances.

RESEARCH DESIGN

Research projects can be divided into two broad categories: observational and interventional.

Observational Studies

In an **observational study** events are monitored and analyzed without an attempt to manipulate or alter the outcome. The causation is inferred based on the observed outcomes. The problem with observational studies is that they do not account for other variables. There is no way to control for the effects of outside influences. In fact, there is no way to know if you are even observing the proper variables. Observational studies are often done as a prelude to an interventional research project. They may define the problem or offer a baseline look at the prevalence of a condition or the incident rate of a factor to be studied.

Interventional Study

In an **interventional study**, the researcher influences the process and then analyzes the effects. The Maguire and Porco collision study (1997) is an example of an interventional project. In this case, the collision rate was calculated, an intervention was performed, and the collision rate was recalculated. It was found that there was a 50% reduction in collisions following the intervention.

Double-Blind, Randomized Control Study The gold standard in research is the **double-blind, randomized control study** (DBRCS) experimental design. This is a prospective (ongoing, not retrospective) research method. When using this approach the subjects are randomly assigned to the experimental and control groups (each subject has the same chance of being in the experimental group). When the experimenters and subjects are blind to the intervention being used on each subject, it is called double blinding. Let's use a hypothetical example.

A drug company has just released a new drug for experimentation. The hypothesis is that this drug will cause an increase in heart rate for any persons receiving the drug. If you are the experimenter, you might list the potential difficulties of performing such an experiment. For example, if you simply pick the next ten people that come into the emergency department and administer the drug to them, you might have some confounding effects. Maybe the ten people are all frightened of needles. Maybe they are all becoming hypotensive, or they are all becoming increasingly irate at being in the ED. Perhaps some (or all) of them just had coffee (or other stimulants) before coming to the ED. If the doctor administering the drug tells them that this will increase their heart rate, perhaps any noted increase was influenced by the doctor's suggestion.

In order to control for these types of variables we begin by randomly selecting a group of subjects from the population. There are rigorous standards for subject selection that will be covered later in the chapter. Once we have an adequate size group selected, we randomly assign each of the subjects to either the experimental (receives the intervention) or control (receives a placebo or no intervention) group. Next we prepare the drug. Syringes are prepared for each of the subjects. The subjects in the experimental group receive an injection of the drug. The subjects in the control group receive a placebo—in this case an injection of sterile water. The syringes all look identical except for an identification number.

In order for the study to meet the criteria of "double blind," the person administering the medication must not know the contents of the syringe. Therefore we select research assistants (perhaps medical students) to administer the drug. The research assistants are not told what the drug is supposed to do and they do not know the contents of the syringes.

Prior to the day of the experiment, the subjects are all given the same instructions as to diet, physical activity, and travel to the site of the experiment. They also completed a questionnaire that asked them about any factors that might affect the outcome of the experiment (although the questionnaire may not have indicated the nature of the experiment). On the day of the experiment, the subjects' vital signs are recorded, the drug or placebo is administered, and the subjects' vital signs are retaken at the appropriate time(s).

Using this step-by-step approach, we can be confident that if there is a significant increase in heart rate in the experimental group and, if there is a significant difference in heart rates among the experimental and control groups (that is, their distribution curves are significantly different), then the effects can be attributed to the drug.

Quasi-Experiment One of the problems with the gold standard is that some types of problems or environments do not lend themselves to randomization. If we were to do a study to test the effect of epinephrine on cardiac arrest in the field, we could not randomly assign subjects to the condition of cardiac arrest. Nor would many paramedics, or medical directors, feel comfortable with ambulances carrying syringes that might contain epinephrine or might contain water. In the MAST study, we could not randomly assign subjects to be hypotensive (or traumatized) and the rescuers could certainly not be blind to whether they were using the MAST. Under such circumstances, researchers use what is called the quasi-experimental model.

In the MAST study, patients who met the research criteria were assigned, on alternate days, to the MAST or no-MAST groups. After the study period the two groups were compared on the basis of age, sex, race, injury etiology, injury severity scores, and trauma scores. In a total population of 784 patients, the two groups were statistically identical for those indices. Therefore, the researchers felt comfortable with their findings that "the overall mortality of 31% in the MAST group, compared to 25% in the No-MAST group was statistically significant ($p = 0.05$)"(Bickell et al., 1987). The $p=0.05$ equation means that there was a 5% or less probability that the outcome could have occurred by chance.

THE RESEARCH STUDY

The components of a research study include a series of steps to formulate the research question or hypothesis, test the hypothesis, analyze the results, and make the findings known. The steps of a research study are:

- Identify the problem or question.
- Review the literature.
- Formulate a hypothesis.
- Define your team.
- Design the study.
- Perform the study.
- Analyze the data.
- Use the information.
- Share the findings.

Identify the Problem or Question

Problem identification occurs the moment someone says that something is wrong and must be fixed, or that something can be done better. In some studies, the researchers made statements such as: "There are too many ambulance collisions"; "There are too many pediatric drownings"; and "Do MAST really work?" These are the types of statements that promote thinking. They help researchers realize the opportunities for improvement. They may also inspire others (for example, funding agencies) to support the research project.

Review the Literature

The next step, the **literature review**, is to see if anyone has already answered the question or if anyone has done research that will assist in answering the question. There is a wealth of sources for this research. The sources available can be divided into a few different categories. The first is information available in scientific peer-reviewed journals. In the medical profession these papers are catalogued in a database called Medline. Other professions also have peer-reviewed papers catalogued in a variety of databases. EMS, nursing, and other health care professions have peer-reviewed and non–peer reviewed papers catalogued in a database called CINAHL.

A second resource for information and data is the Internet. Search engines can direct us to government databases, newspaper articles, and a variety of organizational and private web pages. Researchers must be cautious when using these sources. Peer-reviewed journal articles have been thoroughly critiqued by knowledgeable experts to ensure that the findings are valid and reliable. Information found on the Internet may not have had such a rigorous evaluation.

Finally, textbooks can also be a rich source of information. Libraries and commercial book retailers have searchable databases for textbooks.

Formulate a Hypothesis

This is the declaration to be proven or the outcome expected by the researcher. For example: "Drug *x* will cause an increase in heart rate" or "The prehospital use of MAST improves survival rates for trauma patients."

Researchers and statisticians use two terms when describing the hypothesis. The **null hypothesis** states that no significant difference will exist between the control (placebo) and experimental (intervention) groups. For example: "There is no difference in survival rates between prehospital trauma patients treated without MAST and those who were treated with MAST."

The **alternate hypothesis** states that a significant difference will be seen between the two groups (e.g., "Subjects in the experimental group will experience an increase in heart rate," or "Prehospital trauma patients treated with MAST will have improved survival rates").

Statisticians operate under the assumption that the alternate hypothesis can never be proven. That is, they are never 100% confident that drug *x*, for example, really does increase heart rate. Therefore, the statistical tests are designed to either prove the null hypothesis or disprove the alternate hypothesis.

Define Your Team

Determine who else is affected by the issue; who may benefit from the findings; and what expertise is required for the project (e.g., a statistician). Are there specific skills that team members will need? Who has those skills? What other perspectives may be useful to answer the research question?

In the Pinnellas County example, paramedics teamed up with physicians, nurses, firefighters, public health officials, and local elected officials. All lent valuable perspectives and resources to the process. Having such a team may also be valuable when attempting to implement changes based on the research findings. For example, if an EMS agency experiments with a new type of intervention, but does not include the medical community in the process, the agency may be blocked from implementing changes regardless of the research findings.

If human subjects are used, this is the point in the study to make contact with the appropriate **institutional review board (IRB)**. The IRB will, among other things, ensure that the following ethical guidelines are adhered to (Davis & Maio, 1993):

- Subjects give voluntary consent.
- All potential hazards are explained to the subjects.

- The research results may offer benefits to society.
- The research is based (when applicable) on animal models.
- Each subject can stop the experiment.

For some research, these guidelines may be untenable. Therefore, the U.S. Department of Health and Human Services (DHHS) has approved waiver regulations. To qualify for the waiver, four conditions must be met:

1. The research could not be practically carried out without a waiver.
2. Whenever appropriate, the subject would be provided with additional, pertinent information after participation.
3. The research involves no more than minimal risk to the subjects.
4. The waiver will not adversely affect the rights and welfare of the subjects.

The agency medical director will likely be the liaison to the IRB. It is important to meet with the IRB early in the research design phase and recognize that this person will be an integral part of the research team.

Design the Study

Experiments can be observational or interventional; retrospective or prospective; open, blinded, or double-blinded; quasi-experimental or experimental. Observational and interventional models were discussed previously. Retrospective and prospective refers to the time the observations are made. For example, a typical retrospective analysis is a chart review of all patients that were seen in the past three years. The observations are based on the past. A typical prospective study is the drug *x* example. A study is designed, a subject is selected, an intervention is made, and the results recorded. The observations are made in the present.

Open, blinded, and double blinded refer to the knowledge of the participants. For example, in the drug *x* example, an open model, the subject and the physician both know the contents of the syringe. In a blinded model, the subject would not know the contents of the syringe but the physician would. In a double-blinded model, neither the subject nor the physician knows the contents of the syringe. The quasi-experimental and experimental models were discussed previously.

Consider the data sources, what will be measured and how the measurement will be performed. When creating data collection instruments (e.g., data from questionnaires, observations, response to stimuli) begin by assessing the reliability and validity of the instrument.

Reliability means that repeated observations by different people at different times are in agreement. A straightforward example is the pulse check in the hypothetical drug test discussed above. Different people taking the same patient's pulse at the same time, should record the same rate. Furthermore, the results should be consistent every day of the experiment.

Validity means that the instrument is measuring what it is meant to measure. For example, using the MAST on healthy subjects may not be a valid means of determining the effect they will have on traumatized, hypotensive patients.

Controlling for Bias A **bias** is an influence that distorts the results of a test. The best defense against inadvertent bias is to be aware of its common causes. They include:

- *History.* This may include personnel changes. For example, if the hypotension study was begun using senior physicians to take the blood pressure and later nursing students performed that role, it may be possible that a change in blood pressure over time was, in some way, due to the change in the person performing the test.

- *Maturation.* Will subjects change over time (e.g., will their blood pressure improve even without treatment)?

- *Repeated measure.* Will subjects change their responses after being tested the same way repeated times?

- *Regression toward the mean.* This problem is most noticeable when subjects are chosen from the extremes of the distribution curve. In the hypotension study example, if only subjects with extremely high blood pressure were chosen in the beginning, subsequent measures will tend to be closer to the average, even without an intervention.

- *Instrument decay.* Will the equipment operate the same way at the end of the experiment as it did in the beginning of the experiment?

- *Subject selection.* Research will often be designed to predict the effects of an intervention on the general population. Therefore, subjects should be randomly selected from the general population and not from one particular group.

- *Loss of subjects.* Do the subjects lost to attrition differ in any way from the rest of the subjects?

- *Investigator bias.* The researcher, too, can unintentionally influence the outcome of an experiment. There is an old story of a horse that could count. People were amazed and came from miles away to see the horse. A person would shout out a number and the horse would tap his foot exactly the right number of times. A skeptical scientist put a sheet in front of the horse to block his view of the people. The horse suddenly lost his amazing ability. It turned out that the horse was simply reacting to the body language of the people in the room; he would tap his foot until they started smiling.

The same effect can be seen in medicine. A doctor believes a drug will work a certain way, the patient is told this is how it will work and, after administration, the patient begins to behave as if the drug worked in the described manner.

Sample Size The question of adequate sample size has perplexed many researchers. The competing objectives are:

1. To have enough subjects to ensure that any changes noted are the result of the intervention and not the result of chance. When researchers indicate "p<0.05" it indicates the results of a statistical test proving that there was less than a 5% probability that the results occurred by chance. In order to arrive at this conclusion, the study must have an adequate number of subjects.

2. To avoid having too many subjects. An overabundance of subjects may make the research unwieldy and/or very costly.

Employ a statistician to calculate the minimum number of subjects needed for your experiment.

Perform the Study

This is the moment to administer the drug, turn on the machine, teach the class, etc. Extensive planning in the design phase will ensure that this component of the study is implemented appropriately. This is also the time that data is collected. The 2000 presidential election is an excellent example of the problems researchers may face during data collection. Because it was not specified in advance, there was a great deal of debate about whether ballots that were not punched through entirely should be counted. Anticipating these problems in advance may save a researcher (or an election worker) countless hours of recounting.

Analyze the Data

The first issue to evaluate is whether the research answers the question. Also consider the demographic characteristics of the subjects: how do they relate to the population in terms of age, gender, race, and experience? What correlation exists between the interventions and the outcomes? What else was learned?

Use the Information

The information can be used in a variety of ways. The findings can help solve problems, reduce risks, and improve health. The findings are also used to constantly improve the process and outcomes. In many fields, there is usually no one "right" answer or "right" way to do something. Instead, managers, clinicians, and researchers use the "best" way based on information that is currently available. Ongoing research reevaluates this best way and seeks to find better ways.

Share the Findings

EMS professionals are typically very creative. Over the years a plethora of innovative practices have been implemented. Unfortunately, many of the experiences have not been shared. This has meant that EMS agencies must again and again "reinvent the

Table 17-1 Good Research Practices

- Be open-minded.
- Use your common sense.
- Think of yourself as the user as well as the supplier of information.
- Be creative.
- Self-confidence breeds success.
- Be consistent and care about the details.
- Develop your ability to communicate.
- Be honest.
- Have fun.

Finally, a quote from one of the most important philosophers of the late twentieth century, Gene Roddenberry: "In every revolution, there is one man with a vision." Be a visionary.

wheel." As a profession we all pay the cost when our limited resources are used on basic problems and not on creating new opportunities.

An early example of one paper that had a great influence on the profession is the research published by Pantridge and Geddes (1966). Their description of prehospital advanced life support inspired the world. There are other reasons to publish:

- That is what scientists (and professionals) do.
- It is a hallmark of a profession.
- It helps create a strong professional community.
- It's good for patient care.
- There may be some personal benefit in terms of professional, academic, or monetary recognition.
- It provides academic credibility for the profession.

Another way that professionals share their findings is through presentations at professional conferences. Such conferences are an ideal means of not only sharing research findings but also of meeting people with interests in either the findings or the research itself. Good research practices are outlined in Table 17-1.

FUTURE CHALLENGES

The scientific method works especially well with precise experiments conducted in controlled laboratories. In the drug example used earlier, to test the efficacy of a new drug designed to increase heart rate, an experimenter would bring a group of subjects to the lab, take their pulse, administer the drug, wait x minutes and retake the pulse.

When we combine this simple approach with an adequate sample size, random selection of subjects, placebos, and the double-blind method, we can be confident that our results are both reliable and valid. We will be confident that the drug does or does not increase heart rate.

If, on the other hand, our question is "Does CPR work?" the challenges include the following: we do not have controlled laboratories, we cannot randomly assign citizens (e.g., to the condition "cardiac arrest patient"), and we cannot randomly assign patients to the treatment (CPR) and placebo (no CPR) groups. In addition, many of the factors affecting outcome occur before the patient arrives in our laboratory (ambulance) and after they leave (i.e., their time in the hospital).

Furthermore, many EMS interventions cannot (or should not) be measured in isolation. That is, many EMS practices work, or do not work, largely because of influences from the entire system. For example, measuring cardiac arrest outcomes based on the quality of the field providers' CPR skills would obviously not account for the myriad of influences on cardiac arrest outcomes. These influences include the entire chain of survival from pre-event system design, through public education, 911 operations, EMS training, vehicles, and equipment and hospital designation, resources, and staffing.

SUMMARY

To meet the challenges of EMS-related research, EMS professionals must be resourceful, knowledgeable, and creative. There must be support for research projects and all EMS personnel must be familiarized with the importance of ongoing research into all aspects of EMS operations.

STUDY QUESTIONS

1. Using an EMS-related magazine or journal, identify a study that supports the null hypothesis.
2. Discuss the difference between reliability and validity.
3. Discuss the reasons for using a team approach when doing EMS research.
4. Write an example of a null hypothesis.

BIBLIOGRAPHY

Bickell, W. H., Pepe, P. E., Wyatt, C. H., Dedo, W. R., Applebaum, D. J., Black, C. T., & Mattox, K. L. (1985, March). Effect of antishock trousers on the trauma score: a prospective analysis in the urban setting. *Annals of Emergency Medicine, 14*(3): 218–222.

Bickell, W. H., Pepe, P. E. Bailey, M. L. Wyatt, C. H. Mattox, K. L. (1987, June). Randomized trial of pneumatic antishock garments in the prehospital management of penetrating abdominal injuries. *Annals of Emergency Medicine, 16*(6): 653–658.

Davis, E. A., & Maio, R. F. (1993, January–March). Ethical issues in prehospital research. *Prehospital and Disaster Medicine, 8*(1) Supplement S11–S14.

Goldberg, R. J., Zautcke, J. L., Koenigsberg, M. D., Lee, R. W., Nagorka, F. W., & Kling, M. W. (1990, May). A review of prehospital care litigation in a large metropolitan EMS system. *Annals of Emergency Medicine, 19*(5):557–561.

Harrawood, D., Gunderson, M. R., Fravel, S., Cartwright, K., & Ryan, J. L. (1994, June). Drowning prevention: a case study in EMS epidemiology. *Journal of Emergency Medical Services, 19*(6): 34–38, 40–41.

Joyce, S. M., Dutkowski, K. L., & Hynes, T. (1997, July–September) Efficacy of an EMS quality improvement program in improving documentation and performance. *Prehospital Emergency Care, 1*(3): 140–144.

Maguire, B. J., & Porco, F. V. (1997, June). An eight year review of legal cases related to an urban 911 paramedic service. *Prehospital and Disaster Medicine, 12*(2) 83–86.

Maguire, B. J., & Porco, F. V. (1997, November). Vehicle safety issues related to the provision of emergency medical services. *Emergency Medical Services, 26* (11): 39–78.

Mattox, K. L., Bickell, W. H., Pepe, P. E., & Mangelsdorff, A. D. (1986, September). Prospective randomized evaluation of antishock MAST in post-traumatic hypotension. *Journal of Trauma-Injury Infection & Critical Care, 26*(9): 779–786.

Mattox, K. L., Bickell, W., Pepe, P. E., Burch, J., & Feliciano, D. (1989, August). Prospective MAST study in 911 patients. *Journal of Trauma-Injury Infection & Critical Care, 29*(8): 1104–1111; discussion 1111–1112.

Pantridge, J. F., & Geddes, J. S. (1966). Cardiac arrest after myocardial infarction. *Lancet 1:* 808–808.

Pepe, P. E., Bass, R. R., & Mattox, K. L. (1986, December). Clinical trials of the pneumatic antishock garment in the urban prehospital setting. *Annals of Emergency Medicine, 15*(12): 1407–1410.

Soler, J. M., Montes, M. F., Egol, A. B., Nateman, H. R., Donaldson, E. A., & Greene, H. H. (1985, October). The ten-year malpractice experience of a large urban EMS system. *Annals of Emergency Medicine, 14*(10): 982–985.

Appendix A
EMS Systems Act
of 1973

Public Law 93-154
93rd Congress, S. 2410
November 16, 1973

An Act

To amend the Public Health Service Act to provide assistance and encouragement for the development of comprehensive area emergency medical services systems.

Be it enacted by the Senate and House of Representatives of the United States of America in Congress assembled,

SHORT TITLE

Section 1. This Act may be cited as the "Emergency Medical Services Systems Act of 1973".

EMERGENCY MEDICAL SERVICES SYSTEMS

Sec. 2 (a) The Public Health Service Act is amended by adding at the end thereof the following new title:

"TITLE XII—EMERGENCY MEDICAL SERVICES SYSTEMS

"DEFINITIONS

"SEC. 1201. For purposes of this title:

"(1) The term 'emergency medical services system' means a system which provides for the arrangement of personnel, facilities, and equipment for the effective and coordinated delivery in an appropriate geographical area of health care services under emergency conditions (occurring either as a result of the patient's condition or of natural disasters or similar situations) and which is administered by a public or nonprofit private entity which has the authority and the resources to provide effective administration of the system.

"(2) The term 'State' includes the District of Columbia, the Commonwealth of Puerto Rico, the Virgin Islands, Guam, American Samoa, and the Trust Territory of the Pacific Islands.

"(3) The term 'modernization' means the alteration, major repair (to the extent permitted by regulations), remodeling, and renovation of existing buildings (including initial equipment thereof), and replacement of obsolete, built-in (as determined in accordance with regulations) equipment of existing buildings.

"(4) The term 'section 314 (a) State health planning agency' means the agency of a State which administers or supervises the administration of a State's health planning functions under a State plan approved under section 314 (a).

"(5) The term 'section 314 (b) areawide health planning agency' means a public or nonprofit private agency or organization which has developed a comprehensive regional, metropolitan, or other local area plan or plans referred to in section 314 (b), and the term 'section 314 (b) plan' means a comprehensive regional, metropolitan, or other local area plan or plans referred to in section 314 (b).

"GRANTS AND CONTRACTS FOR FEASIBILITY STUDIES AND PLANNING

"Sec. 1202. (a) The Secretary may make grants to and enter into contracts with eligible entities (as defined in section 1206(a)) for projects which include both (1) studying the feasibility of establishing (through expansion or improvement of existing services or otherwise) and operating an emergency medical services system, and (2) planning the establishment and operation of such a system.

"(b) If the Secretary makes a grant or enters into a contract under this section for a study and planning project respecting an emergency medical services system for a particular geographical area, the Secretary may not make any other grant or enter into any other contract under this section for such project, and he may not make a grant or enter into a contract under this section for any other study and planning project respecting an emergency medical services system for the same area or for an area which includes (in whole or substantial part) such area.

"(c) Reports of the results of any study and planning project assisted under this section shall be submitted to the Secretary and the Interagency Committee on Emergency. Medical Services at such intervals as the Secretary may prescribe, and a final report of such results shall be submitted to the Secretary and such Committee not later than one year from the date the grant was made or the contract entered into, as the case may be.

"(d) An application for a grant or contract under this section shall—

"(1) demonstrate to the satisfaction of the Secretary the need of the area for which the study and planning will be done for an emergency medical services system;

"(2) contain assurances satisfactory to the Secretary that the applicant is qualified to plan an emergency medical services system for such area; and

"(3) contain assurances satisfactory to the Secretary that the planning will be conducted in cooperation (A) with each section 314(b) areawide health planning agency whose section 314(b) plan covers (in whole or in part) such area, and (B) with any emergency medical services council or other entity responsible for review and evaluation of the provision of emergency medical services in such area.

"(e) The amount of any grant under this section shall be determined by the Secretary.

"GRANTS AND CONTRACTS FOR ESTABLISHING AND INITIAL OPERATION

"Sec. 1203. (a) The Secretary may make grants to and enter into contracts with eligible entities (as defined in section 1206(a)) for the establishment and initial operation of emergency medical services systems.

"(b) Special consideration shall be given to applications for grants and contracts for systems which will coordinate with statewide emergency medical services system.

"(c) (1) Grants and contracts under this section may be used for the modernization of facilities for emergency medical services systems and other costs of establishment and initial operation.

"(2) Each grant or contract under this section shall be made for costs of establishment and operation in the year for which the grant or contract is made. If a grant or contract is made under this section for a system, the Secretary may make one additional grant or contract for that system if he determines, after a review of the first nine months' activities of the applicant carried out under the first grant or contract, that the applicant is satisfactorily progressing in the establishment and operation of the system in accordance with the plan contained in his application (pursuant to section 1206(b) (4)) for the first grant or contract.

"(3) No grant or contract may be made under this section for the fiscal year ending June 30, 1976, to an entity which did not receive a grant or contract, under this section for the preceding fiscal year.

"(4) Subject to section 1206 (f)—

"(A) the amount of the first grant or contract under this section for an emergency medical services system may not exceed

(i) 50 per centum of the establishment and operation costs (as determined pursuant to regulations of the Secretary) of the system for the year for which the grant or contract is made, or

(ii) in the case of applications which demonstrate an exceptional need for financial assistance, 75 per centum of such costs for such year; and

"(B) the amount of the second grant or contract under this section for a system may not exceed (i) 25 per centum of the establishment and operation costs (as determined pursuant to regulations of the Secretary) of the system for the year for which the grant or contract is made, or (ii) in the case of applications which demonstrate an exceptional need for financial assistance, 50 per centum of such costs for such year.

"(5) In considering applications which demonstrate exceptional need for financial assistance, the Secretary shall give special consideration to applications submitted for emergency medical services systems for rural areas (as defined in regulations of the Secretary).

"GRANTS AND CONTRACTS FOR EXPANSION AND IMPROVEMENT

"Sec. 1204. (a) The Secretary may make grants to and enter into contracts with eligible entities (as defined in section 1206 (a)) for projects for the expansion and improvement of emergency medical services systems, including the acquisition of equipment and facilities, the modernization of facilities, and other projects to expand and improve such systems.

"(b) Subject to section 1206(f), the amount of any grant or contract under this section for a project shall not exceed (i) 50 per centum of the cost of that project (as determined pursuant to regulations of the Secretary), or (ii) in the case of applications which demonstrate an exceptional need for financial assistance, 75 per centum of such costs.

"GRANTS AND CONTRACTS FOR RESEARCH

"SEC.1205. (a) The Secretary may make grants to public or private nonprofit entities, and enter into contracts with private entities and individuals, for the support of research in emergency medical techniques, methods, devices, and delivery. The Secretary shall give special consideration to applications for grants or contracts for research relating to the delivery of emergency medical services in rural areas.

"(b) No grant may be made or contract entered into under this section for amounts in excess of $35,000 unless the application therefor has been recommended for approval by an appropriate peer review panel designated or established by the Secretary. Any application for a grant or contract under this section shall be submitted in such form and manner, and contain such information, as the Secretary shall prescribe in regulations.

"(c) The recipient of a grant or contract under this section shall make such reports to the Secretary as the Secretary may require.

"GENERAL PROVISIONS RESPECTING GRANTS AND CONTRACTS

"SEC. 1206. (a) For purposes of sections 1202, 1203, and 1204, the term 'eligible entity' means—

" (1) a State,

"(2) a unit of general local government,

"(3) a public entity administering a compact or other regional arrangement or consortium, or

"(4) any other public entity and any nonprofit private entity.

"(b) (1) No grant or contract may be made under this title unless an application therefor has been submitted to, and approved by, the Secretary.

"(2) In considering applications submitted under this title, the Secretary shall give priority to applications submitted by the entities described in clauses (1), (2), and (3) of subsection (a).

"(3) No application for a grant or contract under section 1202 may be approved unless-

"(A) the application meets the application requirements of such section;

"(B) in the case of an application submitted by a public entity administering a compact or other regional arrangement or consortium, the compact or other regional arrangement or consortium includes each unit of general local government of each standard metropolitan statistical area (as determined by the Office of Management and Budget) located (in whole or in part) in the service area of the emergency medical services system for which the application is submitted;

"(C) in the case of an application submitted by an entity described in clause (4) of subsection (a), such entity has provided a copy of its application to each entity described in clauses (1), (2), and (3) of such subsection which is located (in whole or in part) in the service area of the emergency medical services system for which the application is submitted and has provided each such entity a reasonable opportunity to submit to the Secretary comments on the application;

"(D) the—

"(i) section 314(a) State health planning agency of each State in which the service area of the emergency medical services system for which the application is submitted will be located, and

"(ii) section 314 (b) areawide health planning agency (if any) whose section 314(b) plan covers (in whole or in part) the service area of such system,

have had not less than thirty days (measured from the date a copy of the application was submitted to the agency by the applicant) in which to comment on the application;

"(E) the applicant agrees to maintain such records and make such reports to the Secretary as the Secretary determines are necessary to carry out the provisions of this title; and

"(F) the application is submitted in such form and such manner and contains such information (including specification of applicable provisions of law or regulations which restrict the full utilization of the training and skills of health professions and allied and other health personnel in the provision of health care services in such a system) as the Secretary shall prescribe in regulations.

"(4) (A) An application for a grant or contract under section 1203 or 1204 may not be approved by the Secretary unless (i) the application meets the requirements of subparagraphs (B) through (F) of paragraph (3), and (ii) except as provided in subparagraph (B) (ii), the applicant (I) demonstrates to the satisfaction of the Secretary that the emergency medical services system for which the application is submitted will, within the period specified in subparagraph (B) (i), meet each of the emergency medical services system requirements specified in subparagraph (C), and (II) provides in the application a plan satisfactory to the Secretary for the system to meet each such requirement within such period.

"(B) (i) The period within which an emergency medical services system must meet each of the requirements specified in subparagraph (A) is the period of the grant or contract for which application is made; except that if the applicant demonstrates to the satisfaction of the Secretary the inability of the applicant's emergency medical services system to meet one or more of such requirements within such period, the period (or periods) within which the system must meet such requirement (or requirements) is such period (or periods) as the Secretary may require.

"(ii) If an applicant submits an application for a grant or contract under section 1203 or 1204 and demonstrates to the satisfaction of the Secretary the inability of the system for which the application is submitted to meet one or more of the requirements specified in subparagraph (C) within any specific period of time. the demonstration and plan prerequisites prescribed by clause (ii) of subparagraph (A) shall not apply with respect to such requirement (or requirements) and the applicant shall provide in his application a plan, satisfactory to the Secretary, for achieving appropriate alternatives to such requirement (or requirements).

"(C) An emergency medical services system shall —

"(i) include an adequate number of health professions, allied health professions, and other health personnel with appropriate training and experience;

"(ii) provide for its personnel appropriate training (including clinical training) and continuing education programs which (I) are coordinated with other programs in the system's service area which provide similar training and education, and (II) emphasize recruitment and necessary training of veterans of the Armed Forces with military training and experience in health care fields and of appropriate public safety personnel in such area;

"(iii) join the personnel, facilities, and equipment of the system by a central communications system so that requests for emergency health care services will be handled by a communications facility which (I) utilizes emergency medical telephonic screening, (II) utilizes or, within such period as the Secretary prescribes will utilize, the universal emergency telephone number 911, and (III) will have direct communication connections and interconnections with the personnel, facilities, and equipment of the system and with other appropriate emergency medical services systems;

"(iv) include an adequate number of necessary ground, air, and water vehicles and other transportation facilities to meet the individual characteristics of the system's service area-

"(I) which vehicles and facilities meet appropriate standards relating to location, design, performance, and equipment, and

"(II) the operators and other personnel for which vehicles and facilities meet appropriate training and experience requirements;

"(v) include an adequate number of easily accessible emergency medical services facilities which are collectively capable of providing services on a continuous basis, which have appropriate nonduplicative and categorized capabilities, which meet appropriate standards relating to capacity, location, personnel, and equipment, and which are coordinated with other health care facilities of the system;

"(vi) provide access (including appropriate transportation) to specialized critical medical care units in the system's service area, or, if there are no such units or an inadequate number of them in such area, provide access to such units in neighboring areas if access to such units is feasible in terms of time and distance;

"(vii) provide for the effective utilization of the appropriate personnel, facilities, and equipment of each public safety agency providing emergency services in the system's service area;

"(viii) be organized in a manner that provides persons who reside in the system's service area and who have no professional training or financial interest in the provision of health care with an adequate opportunity to participate in the making of policy for the system;

"(ix) provide, without prior inquiry as to ability to pay, necessary emergency medical services to all patients requiring such services;

"(x) provide for transfer of patients to facilities and programs which offer such followup care and rehabilitation as is necessary to effect the maximum recovery of the patient;

"(xi) provide for a standardized patient recordkeeping system meeting appropriate standards established by the Secretary, which records shall cover the treatment of the patient from initial entry into the system through his discharge from it, and shall be consistent with ensuing patient records used in followup care and rehabilitation of the patient;

"(xii) provide programs of public education and information in the system's service area (taking into account the needs of visitors to, as well as residents of, that area to know or be able to learn immediately the means of obtaining emergency medical services) which programs stress the general dissemination of information regarding appropriate methods of medical self-help and first-aid and regarding the availability of first-aid training programs in the area;

"(xiii) provide for (I) periodic, comprehensive and independent review and evaluation of the extent and quality of the emergency health care services provided in the system's service area, and (II) submission to the Secretary of the reports of each such review and evaluation;

"(xiv) have a plan to assure that the system will be capable of providing emergency medical services in the system's service area during mass casualties, natural disasters, or national emergencies; and

"(xv) provide for the establishment of appropriate arrangements with emergency medical services systems or similar entities serving neighboring areas for the provision of emergency medical services on a reciprocal basis where access to such services would be more appropriate and effective in terms of the services available, time, and distance.

The Secretary shall by regulations prescribe standards and criteria for the requirements prescribed by this subparagraph. In prescribing such standards and criteria, the Secretary shall consider relevant standards and criteria prescribed by other public agencies and by private organizations.

"(5) The Secretary shall provide technical assistance, as appropriate, to eligible entities as necessary for the purpose of their preparing applications or otherwise qualifying for or carrying out grants or contracts under sections 1202, 1203, or 1204, with special consideration for applicants in rural areas.

"(c) Payments under grants and contracts under this title may be made in advance or by way of reimbursement and in such installments and on such conditions as the Secretary determines will most effectively carry out this title.

"(d) Contracts may be entered into under this title without regard to sections 3648 and 3709 of the Revised Statutes (31 U.S.C. 529; 41 U.S.C. 5).

"(e) No funds appropriated under any provision of this Act other than section 1207 or title VII may be used to make a new grant or contract in any fiscal year for a purpose for which a grant or contract is authorized by this title unless (1) all the funds authorized to be appropriated by section 1207 for such fiscal year have been appropriated and made available for obligation in such fiscal year, and (2) such new grant or contract is made in accordance with the requirements of this title that would be applicable to such grant or contract if it was made under this title. For purposes of this subsection, the term 'new grant or contract' means a grant or contract for a program or project for which an application was first submitted after the date of the enactment of the Act which makes the first appropriations under the authorizations contained in section 1207.

"(f)(1) In determining the amount of any grant or contract under section 1203 or 1204, the Secretary shall take into consideration the amount of funds available to the applicant from Federal grant or contract programs under laws other than this Act for any activity which the applicant proposes to undertake in connection with the establishment and operation or expansion and improvement of an emergency medical services system and for which the Secretary may authorize the use of funds under a grant or contract under sections 1203 and 1204.

"(2) The Secretary may not authorize the recipient of a grant or contract under section 1203 or 1204 to use funds under such grant or contract for any training program in connection with an emergency medical services system unless the applicant filed an application (as appropriate) under title VII or VIII for a grant or contract for such program and such application was not approved or was approved but for which no or inadequate funds were made available under such title.

"AUTHORIZATION OF APPROPRIATIONS

"SEC. 1207. (a) (1) For the purpose of making payments pursuant to grants and contracts under sections 1202, 1203, and 1204, there are authorized to be appropriated $30,000,000 for the fiscal year ending June 30, 1974, and $60,000,000 for the fiscal year ending June 30, 1975; and for the purpose of making payments pursuant to grants and contracts under sections 1203 and 1204 for the fiscal year ending June 30, 1976, there are authorized to be appropriated $70,000,000.

"(2) Of the sums appropriated under paragraph (1) for any fiscal year, not less than 20 per centum shall be made available for grants and contracts under this title for such fiscal year for emergency medical services systems which serve or will serve rural areas (as defined in regulations of the Secretary under section 1203 (c) (5)).

"(3) Of the sums appropriated under paragraph (1) for the fiscal year ending June 30, 1974, or the succeeding fiscal year—

"(A) 15 per centum of such sums for each such fiscal year shall be made available only for grants and contracts under section 1202 (relating to feasibility studies and planning) for such fiscal year;

"(B) 60 per centum of such sums for each such fiscal year shall be made available only for grants and contracts under section 1203 (relating to establishment and initial operation) for such fiscal year; and

"(C) 25 per centum of such sums for each such fiscal year shall be made available only for grants and contracts under section 1204 (relating to expansion and improvement) for such fiscal year.

"(4) Of the sums appropriated under paragraph (1) for the fiscal year ending June 30, 1976-

"(A) 75 per centum of such sums shall be made available only for grants and contracts under section 1203 for such fiscal year, and

"(B) 25 per centum of such sums shall be made available only for grants and contracts under section 1204 for such fiscal year.

"(b) For the purpose of making payments pursuant to grants and contracts under section 1205 (relating to research), there are authorized to be appropriated $5,000,000 for the fiscal year ending June 30, 1974, and for each of the next two fiscal years.

"ADMINISTRATION

"SEC. 1208. The Secretary shall administer the program of grants and contracts authorized by this title through an identifiable administrative unit within the Department of Health, Education, and Welfare. Such unit shall also be responsible for collecting, analyzing, cataloging, and disseminating all data useful in the development and operation of emergency medical services systems, including data derived from reviews and evaluations of emergency medical services systems assisted under section 1203 or 1204.

"INTERAGENCY COMMITTEE ON EMERGENCY MEDICAL SERVICES

"SEC. 1209. (a) The Secretary shall establish an Interagency Committee on Emergency Medical Services. The Committee shall evaluate the adequacy and technical soundness of all Federal programs and activities which relate to emergency medical services and provide for the communication and exchange of information necessary to maintain the coordination and effectiveness of such programs and activities, and shall make recommendations to the Secretary respecting the administration of the program of grants and contracts under this title (including the making of regulations for such program).

"(b) The Secretary or his designee shall serve as Chairman of the Committee, the membership of which shall include (1) appropriate scientific, medical, or technical representation from the Department of Transportation, the Department of Justice, the Department of Defense, the Veterans' Administration, the National Science Foundation, the Federal Communications Commission, the National Academy of Sciences, and such other Federal Agencies and offices (including appropriate agencies and offices of the Department of Health, Education, and Welfare), as the Secretary determines administer programs directly affecting the functions or responsibilities of emergency medical services systems, and (2) five individuals from the general public appointed by the President from individuals who by virtue of their training or experience are particularly qualified to participate in the performance of the Committee's functions. The Committee shall meet at the call of the Chairman, but not less often than four times a year.

"(c) Each appointed member of the Committee shall be appointed for a term of four years, except that-

"(1) any member appointed to fill a vacancy occurring prior to the expiration of

the term for which his predecessor was appointed shall be appointed for the remainder of such term; and

"(2) of the members first appointed, two shall be appointed for a term of four years, two shall be appointed for a term of three years, and one shall be appointed for a term of one year, as designated by the President at the time of appointment.

Appointed members may serve after the expiration of their terms until their successors have taken office.

"(d) Appointed members of the Committee shall receive for each day they are engaged in the performance of the functions of the Committee compensation at rates not to exceed the daily equivalent of the annual rate in effect for grade GS-18 of the General Schedule, including traveltime; and all members, while so serving away from their homes or regular places of business, may be allowed travel expenses, including per diem in lieu of subsistence, in the same manner as such expenses are authorized by section 5703 of title 5, United States Code, for persons in the Government service employed intermittently.

"(e) The Secretary shall make available to the Committee such staff, information (including copies of reports of reviews and evaluations of emergency medical services systems assisted under section 1203 or 1204), and other assistance as it may require to carry out its activities effectively.

"ANNUAL REPORT

"SEC. 1210. The Secretary shall prepare and submit annually to the Congress a report on the administration of this title. Each report shall include an evaluation of the adequacy of the provision of emergency medical services in the United States during the period covered by the report, and evaluation of the extent to which the needs for such services are being adequately met through assistance provided under this title, and his recommendations for such legislation as he determines is required to provide emergency medical services at a level adequate to meet such needs. The first report under this section shall be submitted not later than September 30, 1974, and shall cover the fiscal year ending June 30, 1974."

(b)(1) Section I of the Public Health Service Act is amended by striking out "titles I to XI" and inserting in lieu thereof "titles I to XII".

(2) The Act of July 1, 1944 (58 Stat. 682), as amended, is further amended by renumbering title XII (as in effect prior to the date of enactment of this Act) as title XIII, and by renumbering sections 1201 through 1214 (as in effect prior to such date), and references thereto, as sections 1301 through 1314, respectively.

"TRAINING ASSISTANCE

SEC. 3. (a) Part E of title VII of the Public Health Service Act is amended by inserting after section 775 the following new section:

"TRAINING IN EMERGENCY MEDICAL SERVICES

"SEC. 776. (a) The Secretary may make grants to and enter into contracts with schools of medicine, dentistry, osteopathy, and nursing, training centers for allied health professions, and other appropriate educational entities to assist in meeting the cost of training programs in the techniques and methods of providing emergency medical services (including the skills required in connection with the provision of ambulance service), especially training programs affording clinical experience in emergency medical services systems receiving assistance under title XII of this Act.

"(b) No grant or contract may be made or entered into under this section unless (1) the applicant is a public or nonprofit private entity, and (2) an application therefor has been submitted to, and approved by, the Secretary. Such application shall be in such form, submitted in such manner, and contain such information, as the Secretary shall by regulation prescribe.

"(c) The amount of any grant or contract under this section shall be determined by the Secretary. Payments under grants and contracts under this section may be made in advance or by way of reimbursement and at such intervals and on such conditions as the Secretary finds necessary. Grantees and contractees under this section shall make such reports at such intervals, and containing such information, as the Secretary may require.

"(d) Contracts may be entered into under this section without regard to sections 3648 and 3709 of the Revised Statutes (31 U.S.C. 529; 41 U.S.C. 5).

"(e) For the purpose of making payments pursuant to grants and contracts under this section, there are authorized to be appropriated $10,000,000 for the fiscal year ending June 30, 1974."

(b) Section 772 (a) of such Act (42 U.S.C. 295f-2 (a)) is amended-

(1) by striking out "or" at the end of paragraph (12),

(2) by striking out the period at the end of paragraph (13) and inserting in lieu thereof " ; or", and

(3) by inserting after paragraph (13) the following new paragraph:

"(14) establish and operate programs in the interdisciplinary training of health personnel for the provision of emergency medical services, with particular emphasis on the establishment and operation of training programs affording clinical experience in emergency medical services systems receiving assistance under title XII of this Act."

(e) Section 774(a)(1)(D) of such Act (42 U.S.C. 295f-4(a)(1)

(D) is amended by inserting "(including emergency medical services)" after "services" each time it appears.

STUDY

SEC. 4. The Secretary of Health, Education, and Welfare shall conduct a study to determine the legal barriers to the effective delivery of medical care under emergency conditions. The study shall include consideration of the need for a uniform conflict of laws rule prescribing the law applicable of the provision of emergency medical services to persons in the course of travels on interstate common carriers. Within twelve months of the date of the enactment of this Act, the Secretary shall report to the Congress the results of such study and recommendations for such legislation as may be necessary to overcome such barriers and provide such rule.

Approved November 16, 1973.

Appendix B
Resource List

Air and Surface Transport Nurses Association (ASTNA)
9101 E. Kenyon Avenue, Suite 3000
Denver, CO 80237
(800) 897-NFNA (6362)
www.astna.org

Air Medical Physician Association (AMPA)
383 F Street
Salt Lake City, UT 84103
(801) 408-3699
www.ampa.org

American Ambulance Association (AAA)
1255 Twenty-Third Street, NW, Suite 200
Washington, DC 20037-1174
(202) 452-8888
www.the-aaa.org

American Association of Critical-Care Nurses (AACN)
101 Columbia
Aliso Viejo, CA 92656-4109
(800) 899-2226 or (949) 362-2000
www.aacn.org

American College of Emergency Physicians (ACEP)
1125 Executive Circle
Irving, TX 75038-2522
(800) 798-1822
www.acep.org

American College of Surgeons (ACS)
633 North Saint Clair Street
Chicago, IL 60611-3211
(312) 202-5000
www.facs.org

Association of Public-Safety Communications Officials (APCO)
351 N. Williamson Blvd.
Daytona Beach, FL 32114-1112
(888) APCO-911
(888) 272-6911
www.apcointl.org

Emergency Nurses Association (ENA)
915 Lee Street
Des Plaines, IL 60016-6569
(800) 900-9659
www.ena.org

International Association of EMTs and Paramedics (IAEP)
159 Burgin Parkway
Quincy, MA
(617) 376-0020
www.iaep.org

International Association of Fire Fighters (IAFF)
1750 New York Ave., NW
Washington, DC 20006
(202) 737-8484
www.iaff.org

International Critical Incident Stress Foundation
10176 Baltimore National Pike, Unit 201
Ellicott City, MD 21042
(410) 750-9600
www.icisf.org

National Association of Air Medical Communication Specialists (NAAMCS)
P.O. Box 3804
Cary, NC 27519-3804
(877) 396-2227
www.naacs.org

National Association of EMS Educators (NAEMSE)
700 North Bell Avenue, Suite 260
Carnegie, PA 15106
(412) 429-9550
www.naemse.org

National Association of EMS Physicians (NAEMSP)
P.O. Box 15945-281
Lenexa, KS 66285-5945
(913) 492-5858
(800) 228-3677
www.naemsp.org

National Association of EMTs (NAEMT)
408 Monroe Street
Clinton, MS 39056-4210
(800) 34-NAEMT
www.naemt.org

National Flight Paramedics Association
383 F Street
Salt Lake City, UT 84103
(800) 381-NFPA
www.nfpa.rotor.com

National Registry of EMTs (NREMT)
Rocco V. Morando Building
6610 Busch Blvd.
P.O. Box 29233
Columbus, OH 43229
www.nremt.org

Professional EMTs and Paramedics (PEP)
(888) 919-4PEP
www.boilermakers.org/2-WhoWeAre/pephome.html

Society of Emergency Medicine Physician Assistants (SEMPA)
950 N. Washington Street
Alexandria, VA 22314-1552
(703) 519-7334
www.sempa.org

Appendix C
Physician Medical Direction in EMS

Hector Alonso-Serra, MD, MPH
Assistant Professor
Chief, Emergency Medical Services Division
Section of Emergency Medicine
University of Puerto Rico

Donald Blanton, MS, MD
Medical Director
Nashville Fire Department, EMS
Clinical Assistant Professor of Emergency Medicine
Vanderbilt University Medical Center
Attending Emergency Physician
Columbia-Summit Medical Center

Robert E. O'Connor, MD, MPH
Chair, NAEMSP Standards and Clinical Practice Committee
and
Medical Director
State of Delaware EMS
Research Director and Associate Clinical Professor
Department of Emergency Medicine
Medical Center of Delaware
Newark, DE

Correspondence: National Association of EMS Physicians, Attn: Executive Director, P.O. Box 15945-281, Lenexa, KS 66285-5945.

Approved by the NAEMSP Board of Directors on July 12, 1997

INTRODUCTION

Modern EMS systems are designed to bring sophisticated emergency medical care to the patient's side. While contemporary EMS systems do not routinely utilize physicians to deliver care, the public expects to receive equivalent care provided by EMS personnel. As such, EMS systems require knowledgeable physician participation and supervision at every level. Active physician involvement in many EMS systems has brought needed improvements but guidelines for a Medical Director's qualifications, responsibilities, and authority continue to be refined.

The out-of-hospital mission is accomplished through varied approaches. Some systems are inclusive,

COMMUNICATIONS

The Medical Director should be involved in establishing or modifying dispatch training and protocols, and should ultimately be responsible for development of:

An enhanced 911 system.

Level of medical training of call-takers and dispatchers based on recognized national standards and modified as appropriate for local circumstances and regulations.

Caller inquiry protocols

Pre-arrival patient care instructions and their criteria for utilization

Ranking of call priority and triage by the potential medical significance of the patient complaint.

Criteria for dispatch of first responders

Criteria for dispatch of BLS versus ALS personnel

Criteria for emergency versus non-emergency response

Criteria for implementation of Disaster or Multiple Casualty Response

Procedures for reviewing and updating dispatch protocols

Continuous Quality Improvement (CQI) program evaluating compliance with dispatch protocols and identifying opportunities for improvement

Access to relevant records to accomplish CQI

Continuing Medical Education for Emergency Medical Dispatch personnel and testing to an approved level of proficiency

Evaluation recommendations of communications technology

Qualified direct (on-line) medical direction and implement protocols for their use and evaluation

System for Critical Incident Stress Management

FIELD CLINICAL PRACTICE

The Medical Director should be involved in establishing:

Entry level of medical training and credentialing of out-of-hospital personnel based on recognized national standards

Periodic testing to verify skill proficiency for personnel involved in out-of-hospital care

Protocols for transport and non-transport, including patient initiated refusals and EMS system initiated refusals with specific guidelines considering appropriate access to care, cost efficiency, and ultimately patient safety

Protocol for interaction with other responders or agencies

Protocol for utilizing direct medical direction

Criteria for determining patient transport and destination

Procedures for reviewing and updating patient care protocols

Set or approve medical standards for promotion of individuals to higher levels of patient care responsibility

- Standards of care for out-of-hospital providers' clinical practice
- For all patient care providers, official authority to limit the medical activities of patient care providers for cause secondary to deviation from established clinical standards of practice or by not meeting training standards
- Continuous Quality Improvement program(s)
- Access to relevant records to accomplish CQI
- Standard specifications for equipment used during patient care
- Evaluate and make recommendations on whether or not to adopt new patient care technologies
- Mechanism for the evaluation and management of occupational injury and illness
- System for Critical Incident Stress Management

PHYSICIAN CLINICAL RESPONSIBILITIES

Maintain a presence in the field to provide on-scene medical direction, assess compliance to protocols and policy, observe the quality of patient care, and be a resource and teacher

Maintain current knowledge and skills appropriate for the clinical practice of out-of-hospital emergency medicine

Participate in training and Continuing Medical Education for base station and out-of-hospital personnel in the classroom and at the patient's side

Knowledge of the Incident Command system

PERSONNEL EDUCATION

The Medical Director should be involved in establishing or modifying educational objectives, and should review and approve:

Requirements for initial training and CME for out-of-hospital personnel

Educational curricula that reflect topics identified in local quality improvement analysis

Evaluation of medical competency of out-of-hospital providers to assure maintenance of an adequate knowledge base and skill proficiency

Promotion of opportunities for additional education and advancement within the organization by establishing collaborative relationships with academic institutions

SYSTEM EVALUATION

The Medical Director must be involved in this process of continuing quality improvement (CQI). The CQI process must be integrated into the day-to-day operations of each distinct component, with data shared between these various agencies and reported to a CQI office and the Medical Director.

The Continuous Quality Improvement (CQI) process is a dynamic continuum. Evaluation of any shortcoming in patient care involves first looking at the protocol to assure its appropriateness or need for updating. Secondly, the educational system must be responsive to the CQI office and keep personnel up to date through routine reviews and supplemental attention to identified problem areas. With this approach, feedback may go appropriately to the system as a whole or to individual personnel; frequent feedback of positive performance is essential.

The Medical Director, with or through the CQI, staff should:

Establish measurable standards that reflect the goals and expectations of the EMS system and local community

Establish a mechanism for data collection that captures information reflecting standards

Establish and ensure compliance with written patient care protocols and standard operating procedures for Emergency Medical Dispatch and clinical patient care

Operate closely with the educational system to relay appropriate feedback and stimulate necessary changes to accomplish common goals

Solicit and incorporate consumers and other health care providers input into the evaluation process

Provide positive reinforcement to individuals and the system as well as corrective instruction

Analyze system efficacy and cost effectiveness with respect to patient outcomes

Clinical Supervisors should contribute to the CQI process

EMS RESEARCH

Not all EMS systems will have the resources to participate in formal research. However, a solid CQI program will generate useful data that will be of benefit to the EMS system and may perhaps enlighten other EMS systems.

The Medical Director is encouraged to:

Participate in, support, and encourage the application of research methods to improve patient care, cost effectiveness, and system performance

Identify local health care and operational issues related to out-of-hospital care that are in need of scientific evaluation and provide leadership to develop research in that area

Identify potential sources of funding for EMS research in the community or at the state and federal level

Establish collaborative relationships with academic institutions and other health care providers involved in scientific research

Incorporate basic principles of conducting research in the objectives for the local EMS provider CME

Assist the development of reliable methods for data collection

Investigate the effectiveness of EMS interventions, treatments, and system design

ADMINISTRATION

Patient outcome and the quality of care depend on the care provided by EMS personnel at the scene of an emergency. The quality of this care is influenced by system-wide policies, daily administrative and operational decisions, and interaction with other public agencies and health care providers. Issues such as public access to EMS, qualifications and utilization of personnel, mode of communication, financial planning and system evaluation may have a profound effect in patient outcome. As an advocate for quality medical care, the Medical Director must have the right and authority to provide input at every level of the decision making process within the organization.

MEDICAL DIRECTOR LIAISON ACTIVITIES

The Medical Director should demonstrate leadership through:

The facilitation of information flow among the community of care givers, from out-of-hospital to emergency department to in-patient care with regard to goals, expectations, and priorities of clinical care, and information regarding clinical outcomes

The facilitation of information flow among all EMS personnel

Establishing standards and requirements for concurrent direct (on-line) medical direction regarding base station education and physician field experience

Establishing minimal qualifications and training for the delegation of authority for direct (on-line) medical direction to surrogates (RNs, etc.).

Resolution of disputes involving medical care occurring within the EMS system

Strategies for integration of out-of-hospital emergency care and the global health care delivery system

Interactions with national, regional, state, and local EMS authorities regarding standards, requirements, and resource utilization

Coordination of activities such as mutual aid, disaster planning and management, and hazardous materials response

Participation in National EMS organizations

Serving as educator and liaison to local government

Serving as educator and liaison to local medical community

Delegation of authority to other physician(s) as Assistant Medical Director(s)

Serving as educator and liaison to the media

FINANCE

The Medical Director should demonstrate leadership through:

Budgetary, planning, and management issues

Grant application process for system funding, expansion, and research

Reviewing and making recommendations regarding EMS equipment

Establish funding priorities regarding issues directly affecting patient care

PUBLIC ACCESS

The Medical Director should demonstrate leadership through:

Collaboration with other health care providers and networks in the community to guarantee public access to EMS for the treatment of perceived medical emergencies

Collaboration with local agencies to assure EMS access to all members of society regardless of socioeconomic status, age, language barriers, etc.

PUBLIC HEALTH

Because of frequent interactions in the community, out-of-hospital providers are able to evaluate many public health issues first hand; their observations and insights should be a source of valuable information to other agencies and the community. The Medical Director should be aware of the community's health care needs and promote full integration of the EMS system as a public health resource.

PUBLIC EDUCATION

The Medical Director should demonstrate leadership through:

Assisting in public education regarding appropriate utilization of the EMS system, health-promotion, and the prevention of emergencies

Assisting in public education regarding prevention, initial approach, and basic management of common medical emergencies

Collaboration with other community providers and local authorities to assist in community health assessment and surveillance to determine public education needs

Promotion of public recognition of EMS personnel and function

ILLNESS AND INJURY PREVENTION

The Medical Director should demonstrate leadership through:

Promulgation of injury and illness prevention programs among out-of-hospital providers

Education of out-of-hospital providers in the principles of prevention as part of routine CME

Collaboration with other local health care providers and authorities in the assessment of the community's specific needs for prevention activities

Collection and analysis of data identifying factors that contribute to injuries and illness

Promulgation of public education on prevention of injuries and illness

Development of programs for injury or illness prevention

LEGISLATION AND REGULATION

The Medical Director should demonstrate active leadership through:

Analysis of legislation affecting local and/or regional EMS practice

Participation in development of legislation related to EMS. Articulation of EMS positions and explain EMS issues to law makers and to solicit support

Participation in local and national EMS organizations

INTEGRATION OF HEALTH SERVICES

The Medical Director should demonstrate active leadership through:

Collaboration with other health care providers in the community to integrate EMS interventions as part of continued health care and to identify outcome of patients accessing the system

Collaboration with other health care and social resources in data collection and transmittal of information leading to community's health needs assessment and surveillance

Developing innovative roles for EMS providers to participate in public health care issues responding to specific needs and resources within the community served

INFORMATION SYSTEMS

The Medical Director should demonstrate active leadership through:

Advocating adoption of uniform data elements and definitions within the EMS system consistent with nationally recognized standards

Working with health care administrators, health care organizations, agencies and authorities to develop an integrated information system that would allow the exchange of vital information

Assuring of legal protection of all data related to CQI activities

OBLIGATIONS OF THE EMS SYSTEM

The EMS system has an obligation to provide the Medical Director with the resources and authority commensurate with the responsibilities outlined above, including:

Compensation for services

Necessary material and personnel resources

Liability insurance for duties and actions performed by the Medical Director

REFERENCES

American College of Emergency Physicians: Medical Direction of Prehospital Emergency Medical Services. *Ann Emerg Med* 1993;22:767–768.

Krentz MJ, Wainscott MP: Medical accountability. *Emerg Med Clin North Am* 1990;8:17–32.

Stewart C: Communication with emergency medical services providers. *Emerg Med Clin North Am* 1990;8:103–117.

National Highway Traffic Safety Administration: *Emergency Medical Services: Agenda for the Future*. U.S. Department of Transportation. National Highway Traffic Safety Administration. August 1996.

Fitch JJ: *Prehospital Care Administration*. Mosby-Yearbook, Inc., St. Louis, 1995.

Alexander KE (ed.): *Prehospital Systems and Medical Oversight (2nd Edition)* National Association of EMS Physicians,.; Mosby-Yearbook, Inc., St. Louis, 1994.

Swor RA (ed.): *Quality Management in Prehospital Care;* Mosby-Yearbook, Inc., St. Louis, 1993.

Polsky SS, Krohmer J, Maningas P, McDowell R, Benson N, Pons P: Guidelines for medical direction of prehospital EMS. *Ann Emerg Med* 1993;22:742–744.

Polsky SS (ed.): *Continuous Quality Improvement in EMS* American College of Emergency Physicians, Dallas, 1992.

Roush WR (ed.): *Principles of EMS Systems* American College of Emergency Physicians, Dallas, 1989.

American Society for Testing and Materials: *Standard Practice for Qualifications, Responsibilities, and Authority of Individuals and Institutions Providing Medical Direction of Emergency Medical Services* Annual Book of ASTM Standards; Philadelphia, September, 1988.

Stewart RD: Medical direction in emergency medical services: The role of the physician. *Emerg Med Clinics North America* 1987;5:119–132.

Pepe PE, Stewart, RD: Role of the physician in the prehospital setting. *Ann Emerg Med* 1986;15:1480–1483.

APPENDIX PHYSICIAN MEDICAL DIRECTION IN EMS SELF-ASSESSMENT

The following form should be used as a self-assessment form for EMS medical direction. Use of this form should help to identify areas in need of improvement, and to monitor existing programs.

Emergency Medical Dispatch

The Medical Director will establish or modify and subsequently approve:

Existing practice of high quality; ongoing activities are maintenance level

    Existing practice, but little experience or quality requires significant improvement

        Non-existing practice; creation, organization, and implementation required

            Adoption of an enhanced 911 system

Level of medical training of call-takers and dispatchers

Caller inquiry protocols

Prearrival patient care instructions

Ranking of call priority by potential medical significance

Criteria for dispatch of first responders

Criteria for dispatch of BLS versus ALS personnel

Criteria for emergency versus non-emergency response

Criteria for implementation of Disaster or Multiple Casualty Response

Procedures for reviewing and updating dispatch protocols

Continuous Quality Improvement program

Access to relevant records to accomplish CQI

Continuing Medical Education for dispatch personnel

Evaluation/recommendations of communications technology

Qualified direct (on-line) medical control and protocols for its use

System for Critical Stress Management

First Responder/Non-Transport System (Field Clinical Practice)

The following are areas essential to adequate functioning of a first responder or non-transporting section of an EMS system. The Medical Director will establish or modify and subsequently approve:

Existing practice of high quality; ongoing activities are maintenance level

Existing practice, but little experience or quality requires significant improvement

Non-existing practice; creation, organization, and implementation required

Level of medical training

Patient care protocols/standing orders

Protocols for transport and non-transport patient contacts

Protocol for interaction with ambulance responders/other agencies

Protocol for utilizing direct medical direction

Procedures for reviewing and updating patient care protocols

Standards for promotion to patient care supervisory positions

Standards for medical supervision

Authority to limit activities of providers for cause

Continuing Medical Education program

Continuous Quality Improvement program

Standards for equipment used in patient care (specifications)

Evaluation and management of occupational injury/illness

System for Critical Incident Stress Management

Evaluation/recommendations of communications technology

Qualified direct (on-line) medical control and protocols for its use

System for Critical Stress Management

Ambulance Transport System

The following are areas essential to adequate functioning of the ambulance transport section of an EMS system. The Medical Director will establish or modify and subsequently approve:

Existing practice of high quality; ongoing activities are maintenance level

Existing practice, but little experience or quality requires significant improvement

Non-existing practice; creation, organization, and implementation required

Level of medical training

Patient care protocols/standing orders

Protocols for transport and non-transport patient contacts

Protocol for interaction with ambulance responders/other agencies

Protocol for utilizing direct medical direction

Criteria for determining patient destination

Procedures for reviewing and updating patient care protocols

Standards for promotion to patient care supervisory positions

Standards for medical supervision

Authority to limit activities of providers for cause

Continuing Medical Education program

Continuous Quality Improvement program

Standards for equipment used in patient care

Evaluation and management of occupational injury/illness

System for Critical Incident Stress Management

Evaluation/recommendations of communications technology

Qualified direct (on-line) medical control and protocols for its use

System for Critical Stress Management

Physician Clinical Responsibilities

The Medical Director should demonstrate leadership through:

Existing practice of high quality; ongoing activities are maintenance level

Existing practice, but little experience or quality requires significant improvement

Non-existing practice; creation, organization, and implementation required

Maintaining a presence in the field to provide on-scene supervision, direct medical control, to assess compliance to protocols and policy, to observe the quality of patient care, and to be a resource and teacher

Maintaining current knowledge and skills appropriate for the clinical practice of out-of-hospital emergency medicine

Participating in training and Continuing Medical Education for out-of-hospital personnel in the classroom and at the patient's side

Establishing knowledge of the Incident Command system

Personnel Education

The following are areas essential to adequate functioning of the education section of an EMS system. The Medical Director will establish or modify and subsequently approve:

Existing practice of high quality; ongoing activities are maintenance level

Existing practice of high quality; ongoing activities are maintenance level

Existing practice, but little experience or quality requires significant improvement

Non-existing practice; creation, organization, and implementation required

CME requirements of out-of-hospital personnel

Educational curricula reflecting national core curricula

Educational curricula reflecting topics identified in local CQI analysis

Evaluation of medical competency of out-of-hospital providers to assure maintenance of an adequate knowledge base and advancement skill proficiency

Promotion of opportunities for further education within the organization by establishing collaborative relationships with academic institutions

System Evaluation

The Medical Director, with or through the CQI staff, should:

Existing practice of high quality; ongoing activities are maintenance level

Existing practice, but little experience or quality requires significant improvement

Non-existing practice; creation, organization, and implementation required

Establish measurable standards that reflect goals

Establish a mechanism for data collection that captures information reflecting standards

Establish and ensure compliance with written patient care protocols and standard operating procedures for Emergency Medical Dispatch and clinical patient care

Operate closely with the educational system to relay appropriate feedback and stimulate necessary changes to accomplish common goals

Incorporate consumers (and other health care providers) input into the evaluation process

Provide positive reinforcement to individuals and the system as well as corrective instruction

Analyze system efficacy and cost effectiveness with respect to patient outcomes

Clinical Supervisors should be considered the Medical Director's representative and be a part of the CQI process

EMS Research

The Medical Director is encouraged to:

Existing practice of high quality; ongoing activities are maintenance level

Existing practice, but little experience or quality requires significant improvement

Non-existing practice; creation, organization, and implementation required

Participate, support, and encourage the asking of questions and the search for answers

Identify local health care and operational issues related to out-of-hospital care that are in need of scientific evaluation and provide leadership to develop research in that area

Identify potential sources of funding for EMS research in the community or at the state and federal level

Establish collaborative relationships with academic institutions and other health care providers involved in scientific research

Incorporate basic principles of conducting research in the objectives for the local Continuing Medical Education curriculum

Assist the development of reliable methods for data collection

Investigate the effectiveness of EMS interventions/treatments and system designs

Medical Director Liaison Activities

The Medical Director should demonstrate leadership through participation in:

Existing practice of high quality; ongoing activities are maintenance level

Existing practice, but little experience or quality requires significant improvement

Non-existing practice; creation, organization, and implementation required

The facilitation of information flow among the community of care givers, from out-of-hospital to emergency department to in-patient care with regard to goals, expectations and priorities of clinical care, and information regarding clinical outcomes

The facilitation of information flow between all EMS personnel

Establishing standards and requirements for concurrent direct (on-line) medical control regarding base station education and physician field experience

Establishing minimal qualifications and training for the delegation of authority for direct (on-line) medical control to surrogates (RNs, etc.)

Resolution of disputes involving medical care occurring within the EMS system

Strategies for integration of out-of-hospital emergency care and the global health care delivery system

Interactions with regional, state, and local EMS authorities regarding standards, requirements, and resource utilization

Coordination of activities such as mutual aid, disaster planning and management, and hazardous materials response

National EMS organizations

Function as educator and liaison to local government

Function as educator and liaison to local medical community

Delegation of authority to other physicians(s) as Assistant Medical Director(s)

Finance

The Medical Director should demonstrate leadership through participation in:

Existing practice of high quality; ongoing activities are maintenance level

Existing practice, but little experience or quality requires significant improvement

Non-existing practice; creation, organization, and implementation required

Budgetary, planning, and management issues

Grant application process for system funding, expansion, and research

Reviewing and recommending EMS equipment

Establish funding priorities regarding issues directly affecting patient care

Public Access

The Medical Director should demonstrate leadership through participation in:

Existing practice of high quality; ongoing activities are maintenance level

Existing practice, but little experience or quality requires significant improvement

Non-existing practice; creation, organization, and implementation required

Collaboration with other health care providers and networks in the community to guarantee public access to EMS for the treatment of perceived medical emergencies

Collaboration with local agencies to assure EMS access to all members of society regardless of socioeconomic status, age, mental disorders, language barriers, etc.

PUBLIC HEALTH

Because of frequent interactions in the community, out-of-hospital providers are able to evaluate many public health issues first hand; their observations and insights should be a source of valuable information to other agencies and the community. The Medical Director should be aware of the community's health care needs and promote full integration of the EMS system as another public health resource.

Public Education

The Medical Director should demonstrate leadership through participation in:

Existing practice of high quality; ongoing activities are maintenance level

Existing practice, but little experience or quality requires significant improvement

Non-existing practice; creation, organization, and implementation required

Assisting in public education regarding appropriate utilization of the EMS system, health promotion, and the prevention of emergencies

Assisting in public education regarding prevention, initial approach, and basic management of common medical emergencies

Collaboration with other community providers and local authorities to assist in community health assessment and surveillance to determine public education needs

Promotion of public recognition of EMS personnel and function

Illness and Injury Prevention

The Medical Director should demonstrate leadership through participation in:

Existing practice of high quality; ongoing activities are maintenance level

Existing practice, but little experience or quality requires significant improvement

Non-existing practice; creation, organization, and implementation required

Promulgation of injury and illness prevention programs

Education out-of-hospital providers in the principles of prevention

Collaboration with other local health care providers and authorities in the assessment of the community's specific needs for prevention activities

Advocate collection and analysis of data identifying factors that contribute to injuries and illness

Promulgation of public education on prevention of injuries and illness

Advocation of legislation that promotes reduction of injury or illness

Legislation and Regulation

The Medical Director should demonstrate active leadership through participation in:

Existing practice of high quality; ongoing activities are maintenance level

Existing practice, but little experience or quality requires significant improvement

Non-existing practice; creation, organization, and implementation required

Analysis and interpretation of legislation affecting local and/or regional EMS practice

Participation in development of legislation related to EMS. Articulation of EMS positions and explain EMS issues to law makers and to solicit support

Participation in local and national EMS organizations

Integration of Health Services

The Medical Director should demonstrate active leadership through participation in:

Existing practice of high quality; ongoing activities are maintenance level

Existing practice, but little experience or quality requires significant improvement

Non-existing practice; creation, organization, and implementation required

Collaboration with other health care providers in the community to integrate EMS interventions as part of the continued health care and follow up to patients accessing the system, whether transported or not.

Collaboration with other health care and social resources in data collection and transmittal of information leading to community's health needs assessment and surveillance.

Developing innovative roles for EMS providers to participate in public health care issues responding to specific needs and resources within the community served.

Information Systems

The Medical Director should demonstrate active leadership through participation in:

Existing practice of high quality; ongoing activities are maintenance level

Existing practice, but little experience or quality requires significant improvement

Non-existing practice; creation, organization, and implementation required

Advocation of uniform data elements and definitions within the EMS system consistent with nationally recognized standards

Working with health care administrators, health care organizations, agencies, and authorities to develop an integrated information system that would allow the exchange of vital information

Obligations of the EMS System

The EMS system has an obligation to provide the Medical Director with the resources and authority commensurate with the responsibilities outlined above, including:

Existing practice of high quality; ongoing activities are maintenance level

Existing practice, but little experience or quality requires significant improvement

Non-existing practice; creation, organization, and implementation required

Compensation for the time required

Necessary material and personnel resources

Liability insurance for duties/actions performed by the Medical Director

(Reprinted with permission of the National Association of Emergency Medical Services Physicians, Lenexa, Kansas.)

Appendix D
Creating an Injury
Prevention Program

Use the following five steps as a guide for developing or expanding an injury prevention effort.

STEP 1: CONDUCT A COMMUNITY ASSESSMENT

Conduct a comprehensive community assessment to identify potential injury prevention interventions. Do this by first reviewing the injury statistics in your state to develop a profile of the injury issue, identify what incidences of injury are most common, and prioritize your targets. This review should provide the demographic characteristics of the populations that are at high risk (i.e., age, ethnicity, income, residence, etc.)

Complete a community resources assessment to determine what is already being accomplished in your state. Because schools, hospitals, and public health and service organizations may all be conducting their own injury prevention campaign, this is another reason to involve a broad range of agency representatives in your planning. Funding agencies look for effective collaborations that produce quantifiable results when deciding which programs to support. Moreover, resources are too precious to create programs that duplicate others or that do not address a high-priority issue or a needy population.

STEP 2: DEFINE THE INJURY PROBLEM

Based on your community assessment, define the injury problem in specific, quantitative (measurable) terms. Find a person with a thorough understanding of injury epidemiology—the who, where, when, what, and how of injuries in your state—to help analyze the data. This analysis will allow you to more narrowly define the most critical injury problems in your state. For example, you should be able to answer the following questions:

- What are the most frequent causes of fatal and nonfatal childhood injuries?
- What populations (age, location, and other characteristics) are at the highest risk for these injuries, and when and where are the injuries occurring?
- What other factors are associated with these causes (host, agent, and environmental factors)?
- What if anything, is being done to prevent these injuries and who is involved?
- Is there an effective intervention available?
- What resources do you have to develop, implement, and evaluate injury prevention initiatives?
- Is there a community/agency *desire* to prevent the injury? Are people more worried about a different issue?

STEP 3: SETTING GOALS AND OBJECTIVES

Now that the injury problem has been identified and an inventory of resources is available you are ready to state the goals and objectives for the prevention plans. To help guide you in writing them a definition of each is provided.

Goals

Make this a broad, general statement about the long-term changes the prevention initiatives are designed to make. For example: "The motor vehicle safety program will decrease preventable injuries on state highways."

Objectives

Make these specific, time-limited, and quantifiable statements about what the prevention initiative will accomplish. There are two types of objectives: process objectives, which state how your program will be implemented and outcome objectives, which state what your program will change, including behaviors, attitudes, and injury incidences.

An example of a process objective would be: "One hundred child safety seats will be distributed to low income families by December 2002." An example of an outcome objective would be: "The bicycle safety program will increase the rate of bicycle helmet use by 15% by the end of 2002." Baseline data are required to determine outcomes. Define how the baseline data were measured. The evaluation of this objective can be done in the same way.

STEP 4: PLAN AND TEST INTERVENTIONS

Interventions are the actions you take to accomplish your goals and objectives. They generally fall into one of the three previously discussed injury prevention categories:

education, enforcement/legislation, or engineering/technology (see Table 1). If possible, choose an intervention that has been tested and proven effective. For guidance, refer to *Injury Prevention: Meeting the Challenge* (see section, Recommended Resources). By using interventions that have been previously tested on populations similar to yours, you might avoid duplicating certain injury rate outcome measures. For example, if smoke detectors have been proven to decrease fire-related burns and deaths, you would only need to document the effective installation and use of the smoke detectors.

When planning interventions, be sure to evaluate the resources available to you and define the priorities for your program. For example: Does your program have an injury prevention objective and allocated resources? Also, review potential partnerships to help determine if other agencies can offer you resources. Other factors to consider are time constraints for launching your initiatives, political factors, and the receptivity of your target population.

As the prevention interventions develop, stay focused on the actions that directly address your objectives. Also, thoroughly evaluate your target population to ensure that your interventions are culturally appropriate, understandable, and acceptable. In fact, conduct focus groups with your target population before implementing a program—it's an excellent way to refine your intervention.

STEP 5: IMPLEMENT AND EVALUATE INTERVENTIONS

Implementation and evaluation are actually a combination of smaller, reoccurring steps. For example, at the time you launch your initiatives, you will at the same time

Table 1   Sample Injury Prevention Interventions

Injury Mechanism	Education	Enforcement/ Legislation	Engineering/ Technology
Motor Vehicle	Implement a media campaign about correct use and positioning of child safety seats; and provide consumer training for correct child safety seat use.	Help to enforce primary restraint laws, improve child safety seat laws, establish child safety seat check points, increase speed limit and DUI enforcement programs, and create "800" safety seat hotlines.	Distribute free child safety seats to low income families, improve signals at problem intersections, and reduce speed limits in neighborhoods with children and around schools.

(continues)

Table 1   *(continued)*

Injury Mechanism	Education	Enforcement/ Legislation	Engineering/ Technology
Pedestrian	Motivate medical professionals to counsel parents about traffic dangers, and provide pedestrian safety programs at elementary schools.	Promote the enactment of pedestrian right-of-way laws.	Improve lighting and crosswalks at problem intersections, and distribute reflector tape products.
Bicycle	Conduct bicycle safety rodeos at schools and community fairs and increase bicycle safety information in health curricula.	Promote bicycle helmet legislation and help enforce current bicycle helmet laws.	Distribute free bicycle helmets to low income families, provide free bicycle repair workshops, and increase bicycle lanes and trails.
Fires/Burns	Educate homeowners and rental property owners about scald burn risks and smoke detectors, and encourage firefighters to conduct school assemblies on fire safety.	Encourage building code officials to enforce building codes for smoke detector use and to require hot water heater settings under 120 degrees.	Promote the use of antiscalding device products.
Home (falls, poison)	Educate parents about gates and stairs; sharp-edged furniture; furniture near windows; proper crib construction; miniblind cords, and locking up poisons, medicines, and alcohol.	Rally against the sale of baby walkers and encourage officials to inspect child care facilities and schools for fall hazards.	Distribute no-choke tubes to determine which objects are safe for small children, encourage use of window guards, and distribute cabinet locking products.

Table 1 *(continued)*

Injury Mechanism	Education	Enforcement/ Legislation	Engineering/ Technology
Firearms/ Violence	Develop a media campaign promoting trigger locks and lock boxes and provide conflict resolution, anger management, and other prevention programs in schools.	Encourage restrictive licensing for handguns and enforcement of existing firearm laws.	Work with local police on community policing initiatives to promote the development of product modifications for handguns.
Child Abuse	Provide parent education programs to young and at-risk parents and develop self-help groups.	Work with local officials to maximize effectiveness of child protective services.	Support home visitor programs for new parents and affordable day care.
Playgrounds	Provide seminars on playground safety for school officials, park and recreation administrators, and child care providers.	Promote mandating the use of U.S. Consumer Product Safety Commission standards for playground equipment and surfaces.	Support community development projects that improve playground equipment and surfaces.
Sports	Provide parents, students, and coaches with educational materials on proper sports equipment and physical conditioning.	Promote mandating the use of proper safety equipment by school and community sports programs.	Promote the use of breakaway bases, mouth guards, and eye protection equipment.
Drowning	Provide information to pool owners about drowning risks and appropriate pool barriers.	Encourage the enforcement of pool barrier codes for community and public pools.	Promote the use of pool barriers, including four-sided isolation fencing.

be evaluating the process and making improvements. Remember, implementation is not a one-time effort. Prevention programs may take place over a number of months and require constant monitoring and improvement.

CONDUCTING AN EVALUATION AND COLLECTING DATA

Program evaluation begins with program design. In essence, by carefully defining your goals and objectives, and carrying out focused prevention initiatives, you are better able to effectively evaluate your prevention. Given limited resources and funding sources, evaluation is now a top priority for community health initiatives. Moreover, evaluation does not signal the end of a program but rather acts as a foundation for building future effective prevention initiatives. In fact, upon completing a community assessment, you will have identified potential data sources and community resources available for tracking the outcomes of your goals and objectives.

PROCESS EVALUATION

Just as there are two categories of objectives, there are two categories of evaluation—process and outcomes evaluation. Process evaluation answers/questions such as: How many people did the program reach and who are they? Was the time schedule for implementation followed? Is the program being carried out within the established budget? These measures will not tell you what behaviors your program changed, or if any injury rates changed, but they will help you identify how the program is being implemented and what changes may be needed to improve the program or its ability to reach the target population.

The National Committee for Injury Control suggests using three methods for collecting data for process evaluation:

- Tabulating and analyzing program records on program activities
- Interviewing or surveying program participants and program staff
- Observing the program in action

Essentially, process evaluation allows you to maintain tight control over program implementation and gauge early quality indicators *(Injury Prevention: Meeting the Challenge)*. For example, measuring how many people attended a class on the proper use of child safety seats, determining the demographics of the attendees with a questionnaire, and measuring what they learned with a posttest are all evaluation tools that would help determine the effectiveness of this intervention.

OUTCOME EVALUATION

Outcome evaluations measure results in changing injury rates, knowledge, attitudes, behaviors, or physical environment of the target population, or the public policy or practice related to the injury. Outcome evaluations tend to be more expensive than process evaluations and usually involve a longer time frame. For example, it may take several years to document changes in injury rates. Also, it may be difficult to control all the other contributing factors, such as high profile media events, new laws, or other programs that may affect large-scale population measures. However, you can use approaches such as surveys and observations to quantify outcomes for injury prevention activities.

Measures of injury morbidity are the most significant indicators, but direct observations of behavior change or the environment modifications are also beneficial. Unfortunately, measures of knowledge and attitudes are ranked lower because they do not always lead to behavior changes. Still, regardless of the outcome measures, it is important to complete baseline measures before launching an injury prevention program. Also, if using an untested intervention, you may need to carry out a more complex evaluation that includes control and experimental groups.

When establishing a budget for injury prevention initiatives, be sure to include funds for evaluation. Some experts recommend that you allocate 15% of a prevention budget to evaluation. You should also identify other resources that can assist with evaluation. The following types of experts may be able to help with your evaluation (National Committee for Injury Prevention and Control 1989):

- Epidemiologists from state health departments, academic and research institutions, and epidemiology consulting firms. Seek the assistance of graduate students, too.
- Statisticians and biostaticians from state health and motor vehicle departments, academic and research institutions, and corporations.
- Nosologists (experts in the classifications of morbidity and mortality data) and medical records technicians from hospitals, state health departments, and the state hospital association.
- Medical record abstractors from academic, hospitals, and clinical settings.
- Individuals with expertise in economics, acute care, rehabilitation, and biomechanics from academic, hospital, and clinical settings, and engineering schools.
- Individuals with knowledge of computers and statistical software from the local health department, academia, hospitals, and corporations.

COLLECTING DATA SOURCES

Finding injury data that can be used to identify risks and plan interventions is a challenge. One issue concerns the fact that data on fatal injuries is much easier to find than information on nonfatal injuries. However, fatal and nonfatal injury data are necessary to develop an accurate view of the broader picture of injuries. Death certificates, trauma registries, and medical examiner reports provide good quality data,

Table 2 Injury Data Resources

Source	Data Type	National and/or State	Available Information
National Vital Statistics	Mortality	Both	Motor vehicle vs. nonmotor vehicle
National Health Interview Survey	Knowledge, attitudes, behaviors	Both	Motor vehicle vs. nonmotor vehicle
National Hospital Discharge Survey	Morbidity	National	When available
National Ambulatory Medical Care Survey	Morbidity	National	None
NHTSA/NCSA Fatal Accident Sampling System	Mortality	Both	Weather, speed, alcohol, etc.
NHTSA/NCSA National Accident Sampling System	Morbidity	National	Road conditions, alcohol use, etc.
Centers for Disease Control, Behavioral Risk Factor Surveillance	Risk factor	Both	Focus on causes
Vital Statistics, State Office of Vital Statistics	Mortality	State, local	Cause of death demographics
Medical Examiner/ Coroner	Mortality	State, local	Varies, often a good source
Uniform Hospital Discharge Data Sets	Morbidity	State	Diagnosis, medical costs, E-codes if available, and disposition
Hospital Emergency Room Data	Morbidity and Mortality	Local	Cause, demographics
Ambulance and EMS Data	Morbidity	State, local	Cause and cofactors, can correlate with hospital data
Trauma Registries	Morbidity and Mortality	Local or regional	Diagnosis, treatment, and outcomes
State Motor Vehicle Data—police, highway patrol, and motor vehicle department reports	MVA, pedestrians, suicide, homicide	State, local	Data collected on motor vehicle, pedestrian, and other

From Emergency Medical Services for Children Resource Center. (1998). *Preventing childhood emergencies: A guide to developing effective injury prevention initiatives* (2nd ed.). Washington, DC: Author.

including cause of injury-related deaths. However, deaths are only a very small portion of the total incidence of injury. Other incidences, including injuries treated in physicians' offices, urgent care centers, or at home, have not been tracked. Estimates indicate that these incidents are twice the number of those seen in the emergency department, or 2,600 nonfatal injuries for every injury-related death. These numbers constitute what is known as the "injury pyramid" (Gallagher et al., 1984).

Another issue confounding injury data collection efforts is the use of E-codes and N-codes, a coding system some hospitals use to describe injuries. Whereas N-codes describe the nature of an injury, E-codes describe the external cause of an injury. For example, an N-code identifies that a patient has a fracture of the left arm (nature of injury), and an E-code identifies that this injury was due to a fall from playground equipment (external cause of injury). Often referred to as the "missing link in injury prevention," E-codes are important factors used to develop injury prevention strategies because they focus on factors leading to the injury (New England Network to Prevent Childhood Injuries, 1989).

If all hospitals were required to consistently record E-codes on hospital discharge and emergency room data sheets, it would help collect "causal" information for planning injury prevention programs. In fact, you may want to consider as one of your injury prevention initiatives an effort to advocate for wider use of E-codes by hospitals in your state. Table 2 is a list of data sources for injury information in your state. For a more complete list, refer to *Injury Prevention: Meeting the Challenge* (National Committee for Injury Prevention and Control, 1989).

BIBLIOGRAPHY

Gallagher, S. S., Finison, K., Guyer, B., & Goodenough, S. H. (1984). The incidence of injuries among 87,000 Massachusetts children and adolescents: Results of the 1980–81 statewide childhood injury prevention surveillance system. *American Journal of Public Health, 14,* 1340–1347.

National Committee for Injury Prevention and Control. (1989). *Injury prevention: Meeting the challenge.* New York: Oxford University Press.

Preventing Childhood Emergencies: A Guide to Developing Effective Injury Prevention Initiatives. Revised Edition. 2000. Producer—EMSC National Resource Center, Washington, D.C.

Glossary

1200 money The term used to describe the federal money given to states to develop EMS systems.

402 funds Federal money flowing into EMS programs through block grants for highway safety programs.

800 megahertz A frequency range used for trunked radio systems.

911 emergency number system A universally accepted number for individuals to call when in need of emergency support.

Academy The focal point of training in the fire service industry.

Accidental Death and Disability: The Neglected Disease of Modern Society A publication of the National Academy of Sciences that detailed the problems of trauma-related injuries in terms of deaths, disability and cost; also known as the White Paper.

Accreditation Approval that a program meets the minimum requirements of the national guidelines.

Administrative law Laws related to the rules and regulations passed by a governmental agency.

Agent Energy.

Algorithm A flowchart that outlines patient care for specific emergencies from patient assessment to management.

Alms houses Facilities that developed to care for individuals who did not have families to provide care such as the poor, orphans, and the insane.

ALS intercept A nontransport vehicle staffed with advanced life support providers who respond to upgrade basic life support teams.

Alternate hypothesis A statement that a significant difference will be seen in the two groups involved in an experiment.

Ambulance trust A method of providing ambulance service in which a board of trustees oversees the operation and management of the service.

American Board of Emergency Medicine (ABEM) Established emergency medicine as the twenty-third recognized medical specialty.

American College of Emergency Physicians (ACEP) Organization representing emergency medicine.

Analysis The assessment of data collected and the transformation of the data into actionable information that can be used to improve the overall system.

Articulation agreement Allows a student who has completed two years at a community college to go on to take two additional years at a four-year college.

Asynchronous learning Availability of resources for learning that can occur in any place and at any time.

Automatic location information (ALI) Provides the system operation with the caller's street address.

Automatic number identification (ANI) Provides the system operator with the caller's phone number.

Baccalaureate education A program that is offered in a college setting in which the student earns a Bachelor's degree in the discipline of EMS.

Balance sheet Reports a business's assets, liabilities, and equity at a particular point in time.

Baldridge Criteria for Performance Excellence Criteria established to use as a tool by organizations to evaluate their overall performance and effectiveness.

Base station The main radio unit in a radio system. A fixed location radio unit.

Basic 911 Provides the system operator with limited information about the caller.

Basic and Advanced Red Cross First Aid Firt aid courses developed by the American Red Cross. Standard training for EMS personnel prior to EMT.

Bias An influence that distorts the results of the test.

Billing for service Charging the patient for the services that are provided.

Biotelemetry Electronic transmission of patient physiological parameters such as an ECG.

Block grant A lump sum of money to be used in broad targeted areas, giving the states more leeway in how to spend it.

Blueprint A document outlining the levels of practice for each prehospital provider.

Call takers Persons who answer 911 line.

Cardiopulmonary resuscitation (CPR) The uses of mouth to mouth ventilations and chest compressions to revive an individual suffering from heart attacks and sudden death.

Career provider An individual whose primary job is in the emergency services.

Catastrophe A situation of extreme proportions with a terribly overwhelming impact.

Categorical funding Funding given by the government to support specific programs or initiatives.

Categorization A process whereby emergency departments in a particular region designate the services they are capable of providing.

Cellular A radio-based mobile telephone system.

Certification Testing of an individual to ensure that they meet the minimum competency level.

Chain of survival A concept developed by the American Heart Association stating that early access, leads to early CPR, and early defibrillation and early advanced care to provide better outcomes.

Charitable giving Monies received by fundraising or donation.

Chase vehicle A motor vehicle that is used to transport personnel (nurses, physicians, paramedics) with advanced training to the scene of an incident to aid the basic level personnel.

Clinical data Data directly related to the assessment, treatment, and clinical outcomes of injuries and illnesses.

Clinical experience Teaching that occurs in a hospital setting and providing direct patient care under supervision of trained professionals.

COBRA See Consolidated Omnibus Budget Reconciliation Act.

Code of Federal Regulations (CFR) Federal regulations derived by federal agencies.

Coding The process of reviewing a patient's medical record and entering it into a registry.

Commercial provider The business of providing ambulance service on a for-profit basis.

Commission on Accreditation of Allied Health Education Programs (CAAHEP) An organization formed to review and recommend accreditation of allied health programs.

Committee on Accreditation of Emergency Medical Services Professions (CoAEMSP) A body of the CAAHEP that serves to review and recommend programs for accreditation of all levels of EMS provider.

Common law Rules and regulations derived from English common law based upon judicial precedent.

Component processes Measures of the processes within the key performance indicators.

Computer-aided dispatch (CAD) The use of computer software to track unit status and dispatch appropriate equipment to an incident.

Consensus standards Rules and regulations developed by professional associations and trade groups related to a particular occupation or service.

Consolidated Omnibus Budget Reconciliation Act (COBRA) Requires hospitals that receive Medicare funding to provide initial assessment and stabilization for any individual presenting to an ED or for a woman in active labor. It also presents guidelines for patient transfers; also known as EMTALA.

Constitutional law Rules and regulations derived from the United States Constitution; examples are civil rights and due process.

Continuing Education Coordinating Board for EMS (CECBEMS) A board established to approve continuing education programs and assign CEU to particular programs.

Continuing education unit (CEU) For courses taken to maintain minimum levels of certification a designated unit is assigned per number of hours of course work.

Continuous quality improvement (CQI) Monitoring the quality of care provided and ensuring that quality is maintained and continually improved based upon outcome evaluation.

Contract An agreement between two parties such as a municipality and a commercial ambulance company.

Cost A financial expression usually in terms of dollars for how efficiently a process is working.

Cost indicator A measurement of the costs related to implementation of a process.

Credit program A program that allows students to earn credits toward a degree or certificate.

Critical care transport The moving of a critical patient (one needing life support measures) from one facility to another.

Critical incident Any event that involves a significant threat to the provider.

Critical incident stress (CIS) An event that poses harm to the provider and results in the inability to function normally in one's job.

Critical incident stress debriefing (CISD) Support program for emergency personnel.

Critical incident stress management (CISM) A systematic approach to prevent and mitigate traumatic stress in emergency personnel.

Critical patient areas Patient populations that require some specific specialized care

Cross-functional team A group composed of suppliers, processors, and customers in a system.

Cumulative stress A buildup that results when general stress is unresolved over time.

Data A record of an event in time

Data elements Specific pieces of data recorded.

Data formats Pieces of information that are precisely defined in regard to the form in which the data is obtained and stored.

Data validation A method of ensuring the accuracy of the data obtained and entered into a system.

Defibrillate The use of electrical shocks to stimulate the heart to pump.

Defusing An informational meeting of work crew members involved in smaller incidents that cause traumatic stress; usually occurs the day of the incident.

Deming Cycle A continuous cycle of planning a change, implementing a change, checking the results, and acting on the results.

Demobilization Brief group informational sessions that occur during the large-scale incidents and disasters as work crews finish their jobs.

Designation The process whereby a hospital is legally approved to provide a specialized service.

Direct medical oversight Real-time physician involvement in a patient encounter with EMS providers; also known as on-line medical oversight.

Disaster Any destructive, dangerous, or life-threatening situation that overwhelms the resources of a community.

Dispatch center A central location for receiving and dispatching 911 calls and coordinating system communications. May be the PSAP or part of the PSAP.

Dispatch life support (DLS) Describes emergency medical dispatching, priority dispatching, and prearrival instructions.

Dispatcher The individual who receives and directs EMS-related calls; also known as a telecommunicator.

Dispensary A facility developed to provide medical care to the poor.

Division of Emergency Medical Services (DEMS) A division of the former Department of Health and Welfare (DHEW) to administer federal EMS programs.

Double blind, randomized control study Each subject has the same chance of being in the control group as the experimental group and neither the experiment or the subject is aware of the interventions being used.

Duplex Two-way transmission of radio messages.

Emergency department A department within a hospital that provides stabilizing care for urgent and emergent conditions. Formally known as the Emergency Room.

Emergency medical dispatch (EMD) The process of sending the right units to the right location with the right resources.

Emergency Medical Services for Children (EMS-C) A program established to focus on the special needs of children in the EMS system.

Emergency Medical Services Systems Act of 1973 Governmental legislation that established the 15 components of an EMS system and provided federal funds for systems meeting these requirements.

Emergency Medical Technician—Basic An individual trained to assess and manage patients at the BLS level. The minimum level of training for ambulance personnel.

Emergency Medical Technician—Intermediate An individual who provides minimal advanced life support for medical and trauma patients.

Emergency Medical Technician—Paramedic An individual who can provide advanced life support using a diagnostic approach. The highest level of prehospital providers.

Emergency Medical Treatment and Active Labor Law (EMTALA) Requires hospitals that receive Medicare funding to provide initial assessment and stabilization for any individual presenting to an ED or for a woman in active labor. It also presents guidelines for patient transfers; also known as COBRA.

Emergency rooms Formal term for an Emergency Department.

EMS Agenda for the Future A consensus document that outlines a future approach for EMS.

EMS council A group representing all of the constituents of a community EMS system.

EMS Education Agenda for the Future: A Systems Approach An extension of the EMS Agenda for the Future, the education agenda provides guidelines for implementation of curriculum, testing, and accreditation.

EMS system The sum of all components involved in delivery of care including the patient accessing the system, management and transport of the patient, and resumption of the patient to daily life.

EMS dispatcher An individual who services to provide prearrival instructions to the caller and dispatch appropriate resources to the scene.

Encryption A security measure used to protect information moved between computer systems by limiting access to the computer or program

Enhanced 911 Provides the PSAP with the caller's phone number and the street address.

Environment The surroundings in which an injury occurs.

Evacuation The process of ridding the body of fluids that disrupted balance and tone.

Event-driven resource deployment A type of delivery system that matches resources to predicted demand based upon data and historical patterns.

Exposure The lack of protection of a community from a hazard.

Fail-safe public utility model The local government establishes a public corporation that owns all the assets of the service. The corporation does the billing and contracts with an ambulance service to provide staffing.

Fast track A branch of the emergency department that treats patients who are nonurgent.

Federal Emergency Management Agency (FEMA) The federal agency that is responsible for disaster management in the United States.

Fee-for-service A transaction in which the patient pays directly for the services that are rendered.

Fellows of the American College of Emergency Physicians (FACEP) Certification of physicians specializing in emergency medicine.

Field internship Teaching that occurs while on the job in the field while under the supervision of a trained professional.

Firewall A security measure used to protect information moved between computer systems by limiting access to the computer or program.

First responder An individual trained to provide initial lifesaving assessment and intervention using minimal equipment.

Fixed-post staffing A type of delivery system in which all response teams operate from a fixed station and the same number of units are available at all times.

Flight nurse A registered nurse who is trained to provide emergency care while in flight.

Flight paramedic A paramedic trained to provide care while in flight.

Formatting standard A data set that is programmed into specific computer programs.

For-profit company A business organized by investors who expect to earn money on their investment.

Frequency A measure of radio waves.

General stress Stressors encountered on a daily basis that are either good, resulting in a positive creative force in one's life or bad, resulting in discomfort and unhappiness in one's life.

Global satellite positioning systems (GPS) A worldwide system utilizing satellites to provide precise geographic location information.

Government services A business authorized by the legislature and operated by the executive branch of the federal, state, and local governments, a yearly operating budget is provided by tax revenues.

Grants Money given to an organization that does not have to be paid back.

Haddon's matrix A concept used to determine factors affecting the extent of injury from which prevention strategies or interventions may be designed.

Hazard A dangerous event or circumstance that may or may not lead to an emergency or disaster.

Hazard analysis The methods used to identify, locate, assess risks, and map risks on a community map.

Heroic medicine The aggressive treatment of disorders through the use of techniques such as evacuation and restorative therapies.

High-performance EMS systems An EMS system that produces clinical quality, response time reliability, customer satisfaction, and economic efficiency simultaneously.

HL7 standards A standard for the collection, integration, and exchange of clinical patient care data among health care data systems.

Hospital based Ambulance service provided by a hospital.

Hospital Survey and Construction Act The first major federal funding put into health care; also known as the Hill-Burton Act.

Host An injured person.

Hybrid paper forms Forms that utilize paper and electronic processes to reduce the need for manually entering data into a computer system.

Incident command system (ICS) An organized method of managing a large-scale incident.

Incident commander The person in charge of all the personnel working at an incident.

Income statement Reports a business's revenues and expenses in a given period.

Indirect medical oversight Physician input that is administrative, involving all facets of emergency medical service, but remote from patient care; also known as off-line medical oversight and system medical oversight.

Individual resources One unit.

Information Data placed within a framework or context to give it meaning.

Injury Any unintentional or intentional damage to the body resulting from acute exposure to energy.

Institutional review board (IRB) A group of individuals whose purpose it is to ensure that an experiment is being done following ethical guidelines.

Intensivist A physician who specializes in the care and stabilization of the critically ill patient.

Intentional injuries Damage caused by the desire to induce harm upon one's self.

Interventional study Events are influenced by the researcher and then analyzed for the effects.

Joint Review Committee on Educational Programs for the EMT-Paramedic An organization developed to review and recommend programs for accreditation. This is now replaced by CoAEMSP.

Key performance indicators A measurement of the processes in an EMS organization such as clinical, operational, or administrative processes.

KKK-A-1822 General Services Administration specifications of ambulances.

Large-scale disaster A situation in which the local resources are overwhelmed and an effective response requires state level resources.

Lead agency The governmental agency at the federal or state level responsible for EMS-related issues and regulation.

Licensure Authorizes an individual to provide care based upon proof that the individual has met the minimum competency level.

Literature review Analyzing and researching documentation of what has already been examined.

Location The placement of a hazardous condition.

Major disaster A situation that has caused damage of sufficient severity and magnitude to warrant assistance from the federal government.

Manageable span of control A commander only receives report and maintains responsibility for between three and seven people.

Mass casualty incident A disaster with over 100 victims.

Med channels Frequencies dedicated for communication of patient information and biotelemetry.

Medevac Use of helicopters to transport trauma victims

Medical command/medical direction Physician involvement in emergency medical service.

Medical communications All communication involved in on-line medical control and notification of receiving facilities.

Medical director A physician who oversees the practice of EMTs and paramedics.

Medical oversight Physical involvement in emergency medical services to ensure quality of care and support.

Medicaid A program in which state and federal funds are used to compensate health care providers for services to program enrollees who otherwise are not able to pay for the services.

Medicare Federally funded health care program for the elderly.

Medium duty ambulance A Type I ambulance mounted on a medium duty truck chassis.

Mission A statement of why an organization exists.

Mitigation Any efforts to identify, classify, and eliminate hazards and reduce the potential that they might produce a disaster.

Mobile health care The ability to take services to the patient instead of the patient coming to the hospital or facility.

Mobile unit A radio unit that is inside a vehicle.

Morbidity Measurement of sickness or disease in a particular population.

Mortality Measurement of deaths in a particular population.

Multiple casualty incident A disaster involving between 11 and 100 victims.

Multiple patient incident A disaster involving between two and ten victims.

National Emergency Medical Services Education and Practice Blueprint A guide for curriculum development and certification that identifies the four levels of providers and the core elements pertinent to all providers.

National EMS Core Content Presents a broad definition of what an EMS provider must know and be able to do.

National EMS Education Standard Defines the terminal objectives for each provider level.

National EMS Radio System A series of frequencies designated by the FCC to be used only for EMS transmissions.

National EMS Scope of Practice Model Defines the levels and skills needed for each provider.

National Highway Safety Act of 1966 Legislation that resulted from a presidential investigation into highway traffic deaths.

National Highway Traffic Safety Administration (NHTSA) A division of the Department of Transportation; this organization was developed to oversee the development of initiatives to make road travel safer.

National Registry of Emergency Medical Technicians A private organization that provides testing and national registration for EMTs.

National Standard Curriculum Standards and guidelines complete with objectives and lesson plans to guide the teaching of Emergency Medical Services that allows commonality across all areas of the United States.

National Standard EMS Data Set A uniform list of information that is to be collected and the format in which the data is recorded for prehospital event, developed by the National Highway and Traffic Safety Administration.

Natural disaster Any disaster produced by the forces of nature: fire, air, earth, and water.

Noncredit program A program that offers training that does not lead to a degree.

Nonemergency access number A number for people to call for general information not related to an emergency.

Not-for-profit company A business that is organized under special provisions within the federal tax code; money comes from donations or loans.

Null hypothesis A statement that no significant difference will result in the two groups involved in an experiment.

Observational study Events that are monitored and analyzed without attempting to manipulate or alter the outcome.

Off-line medical oversight Physician input that is administrative, involving all facets of emergency medical service, but remote from patient care; also known as indirect medical oversight and system medical oversight.

One for Life Program An initiative developed in Virginia to raise funds to support EMS; vehicle registration was raised one dollar and the funds were earmarked for EMS.

On-line medical oversight Real-time physician involvement in a patient encounter with EMS providers; also known as direct medical oversight.

Operational data Data related to the nonclinical activities in support of field operations.

Optical character recognition A form in which the data can be converted into text, numbers, and symbols after being scanned into the computer.

Optical imaging A type of form that can be scanned and stored in the computer system.

Optical mark recognition A form that uses one or more small circles filled in by pen or pencil to return a value for a particular data element.

Organizational assessment An objective and detailed analysis of an organization's overall performance.

Paper forms Forms used in the field for data collection.

Paramedic engine company A fire service vehicle that staffs a paramedic and responds to ALS calls as an upgrade response vehicle.

Pathway management A process in which a managed care organization subscriber calls a central number and speaks with a health care professional and is directed to the proper course of action to take.

Patient care record A report completed by the EMS provider for each patient contact.

Patient dumping The transfer of patients to an alternate facility for economic rather than medical reasons.

Peak hour The period of time in which the most ambulances are scheduled to be on duty at one time.

Peak load staffing Making additional personnel and resources available during times of suspected high use rates.

Performance The combined effects of quality and cost.

Performance and process measures The actions taken and the ability to evaluate those actions to bring about change.

Performance indicator Measure of the aspects within a component process.

Personal data assistant (PDA) A device that integrates voice, data, and GPS functions in a single handheld unit.

Plan-Do-Check -Act (PDCA) Cycle A continuous cycle of planning a change, implementing a change, checking the results, and acting on the results.

Portable A radio unit that an EMT is able to take to a scene.

Posting plans Staging a response vehicle in a location where it is anticipated that demand will be high.

Post-traumatic stress disorder (PTSD) A psychological disorder that results from a life-threatening stressor that is left unresolved over time.

Prearrival medical instructions Information provided by dispatchers to the 911 caller on how to provide immediate care while the ambulance is en route.

Preparedness Resource identification and allocation and the training and drilling of disaster response personnel.

Prevention Stopping the occurrence of injury before it happens.

Primary prevention Strategies to prevent an injury from occurring.

Priority dispatching The process of using a scripted series of questions to interrogate the caller and determine the proper level of EMS system response.

Process A collective means of fulfilling the mission of and organization and serving customers.

Process assurance Ensuring that all teams are performing the same procedures outlined by their system.

Process improvement Attempting to improve overall performance by finding ways to provide higher quality care at lower costs.

Prospective The process of studying something as it happens.

Protocol A preauthorized set of instructions that guide patient care.

Public access The ability of an EMS system to respond appropriately to a caller's needs.

Public education The process of teaching the public about an issue of importance to EMS.

Public information Any news that an EMS organization wants to tell the public in the community about.

Public information officer (PIO) An individual designated by an EMS agency to disseminate public information (news).

Public information, education, and relations (PIER) An acronym to describe activities for disseminating public information developed by the National Highway Traffic Safety Administration.

Public law Laws derived by Congress and state governing bodies.

Public relations The process of shaping public opinion to support EMS initiatives.

Public safety agency A governmental agency that provides all public safety functions such as fire, police, and EMS.

Public safety answering point (PSAP) A center where call takers receive all 911 calls.

Public service announcement (PSA) Free advertising on broadcast media or in print media.

Public utility model A method of providing ambulance service through an established EMS authority that contracts with a commercial provider; the authority owns the equipment and establishes performance standards.

Quality A measure of how well a process is working.

Quality indicator A measurement of the changes expected based on implementation of a specific process.

Rates of reimbursement A set fee that is agreed with being paid for specific services.

Real-time checks The ability of an electronic data system to provide immediate feedback on acceptable response and ranges for specific data.

Reciprocity Acceptance of training and certification by another jurisdiction.

Recovery Any activities designed to put the community back on its feet.

Reliability Repeated observations by different people at different times are in agreement.

Rescue squad A third-service EMS agency.

Response Actions required to save lives, limit destruction, and meet basic human needs in the immediate and short-term effects of a disaster.

Restorative The process of building a body back up to its normal stamina after an illness.

Resuscitator runs Archaic term for the response of a unit with an oxygen-powered resuscitator to fire calls to assist firefighters overcome by smoke.

Retrospective Refers to the process of review and examination of outcomes after occurrence.

Risk The degree of susceptibility of individuals or an entire community to the hazard becoming an emergency or disaster and causing death, injury, or destruction.

Secondary injury prevention Strategies that attempt to minimize further injury or death after the initial trauma or injury event has occurred.

Section A modular structure used in incident command.

Sector An area of responsibility.

Self-study One of the stages in the educational program accreditation process during which the program compares itself to a national standard.

Service providers Any individual or organization that provides EMS.

Shewhart Cycle A continuous cycle of planning a change, implementing a change, checking the results, and acting on the results.

Shock-trauma centers Facilities designated to treat critical patients needing rapid surgical interventions.

Site visit A program director and medical director visit to the institution providing the program to verify compliance with the CoAEMSP guidelines.

Socialized medicine A process whereby the government provides medical coverage for all citizens.

Society for Academic Emergency Medicine (SAEM) Organization representing emergency medicine.

Standard deviation A calculation that allows predictions based upon averages.

Standing order Specific direction given by a physician to support already existing protocols.

Star-of-life ambulance Ambulances designed to meet the General Services Administration specifications.

Start-up money Money needed to get a business off the ground.

Statutory law Rules and regulations derived from a legislative body resulting in federal laws, state codes, and local ordinances.

Strategic information plan Defining the needs of an organization that will enable the organization to achieve its vision and mission.

Strategy The big plan, directed toward achievement of a large goal.

Strike team A combination of same type resources assigned to serve one function.

Subsidy A grant.

Support data Data that comes from processes used to lead, manage, and support the overall organization.

Surveillance Collection of information.

System medical oversight The oversight of an entire EMS system provided by the system medical director.

System status management The process of preparing the system to produce the best possible response to the next EMS call.

Systems communications All communication involved in operating and coordinating an EMS system such as alerting EMS units, dispatching EMS units, and coordination of EMS units.

Tactics The steps or procedures taken in the implementation of the strategy.

Task force A combination of resources that are assigned to deal with one problem in a disaster.

Technological disaster Any disaster produced by mankind or the things that human beings make or use.

Telecommunicator Another term for dispatcher; the individual who receives and directs EMS-related calls.

Telemedicine The ability of a physician to treat a patient in the field without even touching or seeing the patient through the use of technology.

Tertiary injury prevention Medical treatment for injuries upon occurrence.

The golden hour The time a seriously injured patient has to receive definitive care in order to survive his injuries.

Third service A separate public safety service devoted to the delivery of EMS.

Third-party payers An insurance company or medical program pays for a portion of or all of the billed charges.

Three E's of injury prevention Interventions used in injury prevention: engineering, enforcement, and education.

Trauma care system A sub-system of an EMS system designed to provide rapid surgical intervention for moderate to severe trauma victims.

Trauma centers Facilities designated to treat patients seriously injured by trauma.

Trauma registry A uniform means of collecting data on trauma systems and trauma patients.

Traumatic stress An event that poses harm to the provider and results in the inability to function normally in one's job.

Traumatologist A physician who specializes in resuscitation of the trauma victim.

Trepanning Removal of a portion of the skull to relieve pressure on the brain.

Trunked system Radio signals that are transmitted to a local cell and retransmitted to connected cells to allow a wider range.

Type I ambulance A type of ambulance that has a design similar to that of a pick-up truck with the ambulance module in place of the truck bed.

Type II ambulance A type of ambulance that has a design similar to that of a van.

Type III ambulance A type of ambulance that has a design that combines both the modular style of a type I ambulance with the van style of type II; it is the most common configuration in use today.

Ultra high frequency (UHF) A group of radio frequencies above 400 MHz and below microwaves.

Unintentional injuries Damage caused with no intent to do harm.

Universal access number A generic phone number used nationwide to request an EMS response; in the United States it is 911.

Utstein Guidelines An international set of standards and templates for recording of prehospital cardiac arrest and resuscitation.

Validity The instrument is measuring what it is meant to measure.

Value The combined effects of quality and cost.

Value indicator A measurement of the outcomes of specific processes.

Vector Mechanism by which energy is transferred.

Vision A statement of what an organization aspires to be while fulfilling its mission.

Voice recognition The ability of an electronic device to record the spoken word.

Volunteer An individual who gives time and knowledge without compensation.

Vulnerability The potential that a hazard could be attacked, stolen, impacted, or manipulated to become more dangerous and increase the chance of a disaster occurring.

White Paper A publication of the National Academy of Sciences that detailed the problems of trauma-related injuries in terms of deaths, disability, and cost; also known as Accidental Death and Disability: The Neglected Disease of Modern Society.

Wilderness medical training Specialized training for EMTs to meet the needs of those injured in extreme environments.

Years of potential life lost (YPLL) A measurement of the impact injury and illness have on society.

Index